Lasers in Dermatology: Parameters and Choice

Jae Dong Lee • Min Jin Maya Oh

Lasers in Dermatology: Parameters and Choice

With Special Reference to the Asian Population

Springer

Jae Dong Lee
MISODAM Clinic
Daejeon, Korea (Republic of)

Min Jin Maya Oh
ARA Clinic
Incheon, Korea (Republic of)

0th edition: © MDWORLD Medical Publishing Co. 2022

ISBN 978-981-19-7567-7 ISBN 978-981-19-7568-4 (eBook)
https://doi.org/10.1007/978-981-19-7568-4

This Springer imprint is published by the registered company Springer Nature Singapore Pte Ltd.
The registered company address is: 152 Beach Road, #21-01/04 Gateway East, Singapore 189721, Singapore

Preface

I have conducted 11 'Laser Hands-On Courses' from July 16, 2016, to September 1, 2018, which ran for 1 night and 2 days. A total of 70 people came, and most of them were beginners who were new to lasers. They were not interested in the complex principles of a laser, but a parameter that they could apply right away tomorrow. 'Lasers in Dermatology: Parameters and Choice' describes the specific laser parameters for beginners, focusing on each laser instrument. However, since safe and effective laser treatment is not possible simply by memorizing parameters, I have also described an important principle that is essential for parameter control.

Since this book is based on the content of 'Lasers in Dermatology: Choice and Treatment (Korean)', it can be seen as a summary of 'Lasers in Dermatology: Choice and Treatment (Korean)'. For more information, please refer to ‘Lasers in Dermatology: Choice and Treatment (Korean)’.

Since the book needs to describe parameters in detail, I have written down the parameters for specific laser products. However, because each laser product has different parameters, it should not be applied to your own laser, but should be adjusted accordingly taking into account the principles of the laser. There are also some laser instruments in the book that I do not use. For these products, the parameters provided by the laser company and the parameters used by various practitioners were taken into account, as well as principle of lasers. I would like to take this opportunity to express my gratitude to Dr. Min Ho Lee of Besttop urology clinic, Dr. Seung Choi of Ciel clinic, and Dr. Yong Ho Hwang of Wellskin clinic who generously informed me of their parameters and know-how.

The first stage of skin laser treatment is the correct diagnosis of the lesion. However, since this book does not explain the diagnostic criteria or methods of diagnosis, beginners should study the diagnosis of skin diseases additionally. And consultation method is also very important for beginners. Consultation methods vary from practitioner to practitioner, and there are diverse and unique consultation methods. But I didn't include these this book because I thought that it could be an obstacle to your individual creative consultation methods.

Finally, even though it is becoming increasingly difficult for private practices, I hope that my book may be a small beacon for private practice laser physicians. Let's all shout a Korean cheer!

Aza Aza Fighting!

I would like to send my love to my wife Mi Ran and my sons Jeong Jin and Yoo Jin.

Daejeon, Republic of Korea Jae Dong Lee
31 July 2022

Contents

About the Authors

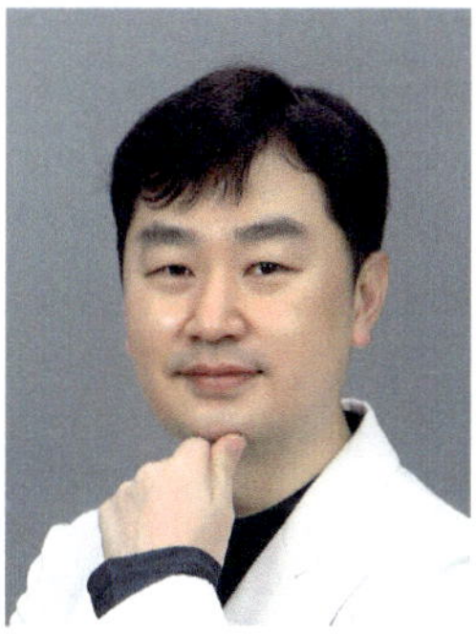

Jae Dong Lee, MD Graduated from Medical College of the Catholic University of Korea. The degree of Master of Medical Science in the Catholic University of Korea. The Chief Academic Officer in Korean Medical Skin Care Society. The Laser Academic Officer in Korean Aesthetic Surgery and Laser Society. The Chairman in Korean Dermatologic Laser Association. Director in MISODAM clinic in Daejeon, Korea (Writing). The principles and choice of laser in dermatology (Korean language). Melasma, diagnosis and treatment of melasma (Korean language). Laser dermatology: Choice and treatment (Korean language). Principles and Choice of Laser Treatment in Dermatology.

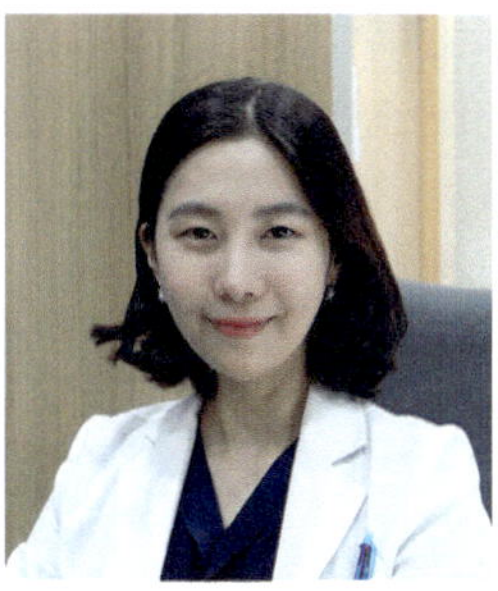

Min Jin Maya Oh, MD Graduated from Medical College of the Catholic University of Korea. The Academic Officer in Korean Academy of Melasma. The Vice-Chairman in Korean Dermatologic Laser Association. Former Asia Pacific Regional Therapeutic Expert for Botox, Allergan. Former Medical reviewer for MFDS (Ministry of Food and Drug Safety). Director in ARA clinic in Incheon, Korea (Writing). Principles and Choice of Laser Treatment in Dermatology.

Part I

Principles of Laser

Six Parameters of Lasers in Dermatology

1

1.1 Light and Matter

The world consists of light and matter (Fig. 1.1). When light and matter meet, they interact with each other and make various physical and chemical changes. For example, if you stand under the clear autumn sky, you can feel your body warming up even in the cool weather. This phenomenon occurs when light is converted into heat in the skin (Light energy → Thermal energy).

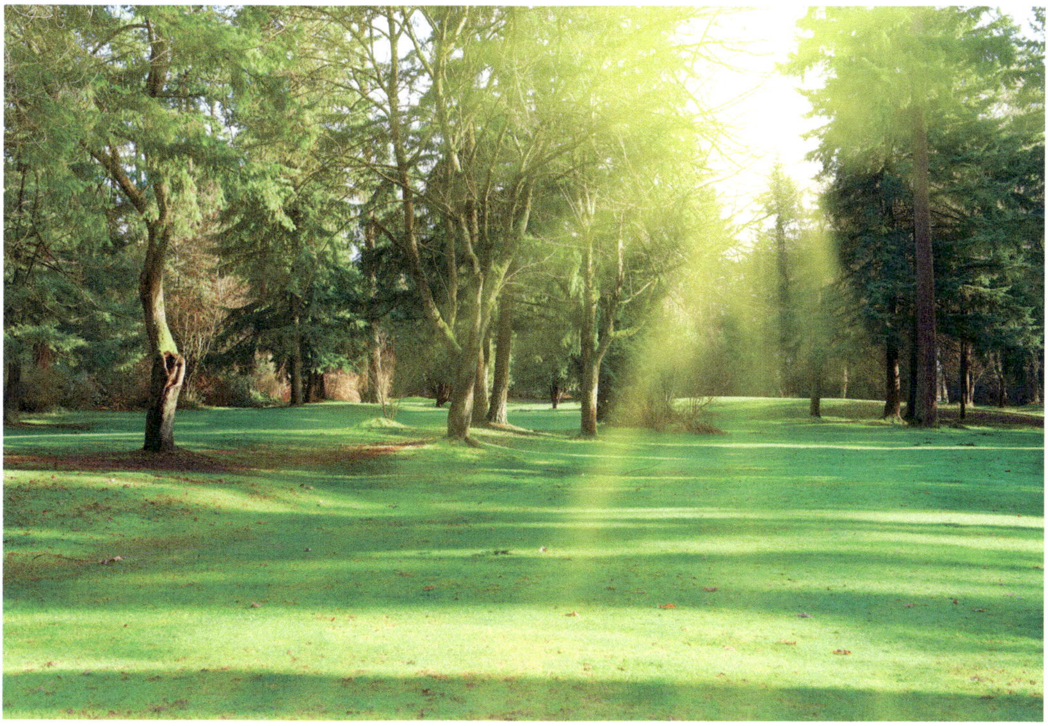

Fig. 1.1 Light and matter

J. D. Lee, M. J. M. Oh, *Lasers in Dermatology: Parameters and Choice*,
https://doi.org/10.1007/978-981-19-7568-4_1

1.2 Electromagnetic Radiation (EMR)

In general, the meaning of light refers to only the visible range (400–760 nm), but strictly speaking, visible light refers to light in the narrow sense, while light in the broad sense refers to electromagnetic radiation (EMR). EMR is all the energy that travels in space in the form of waves by electric and magnetic fields [2]. EMR ranges from visible rays to short wavelengths of γ-rays and X-rays to the long wavelengths of microwaves and radio waves (Fig. 1.2).

Each EMR has its own wavelength and frequency [3]. Lasers used mainly in the dermatological field express EMR with nanometer (nm), which is a unit of wave. The electromagnetic spectrum used in the dermatological field includes ultraviolet (UV), visible, near-infrared (NIR), mid-infrared (MIR), and far-infrared (FIR) (Table 1.1).

Table 1.1 The range and wavelength of electromagnetic radiation [2]

Range	Nanometer
Ultraviolet (UV)	200–400 nm
Visual	400–760 nm
Near-infrared (NIR)	760–1400 nm
Mid-infrared (MIR)	1400–3000 nm
Far-infrared (FIR)	>3000 nm

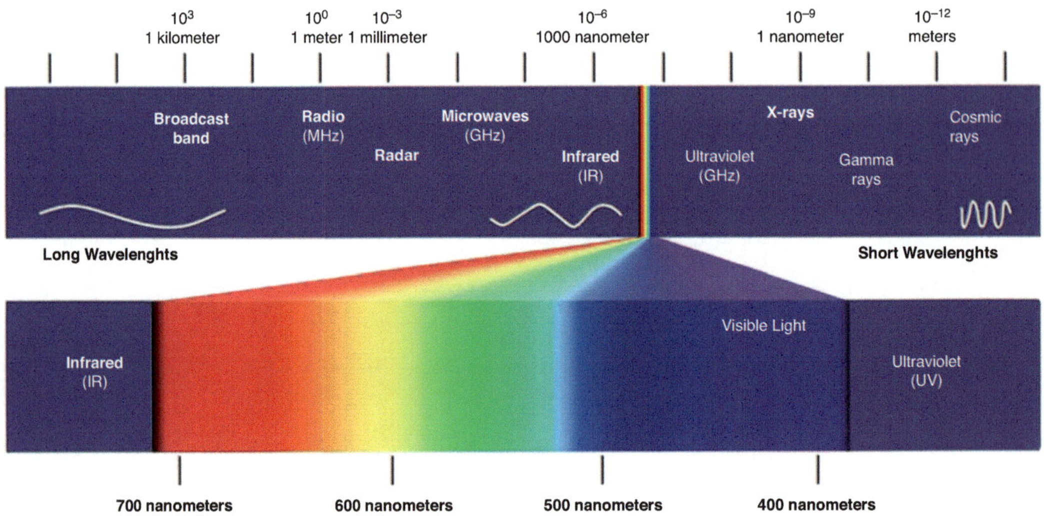

Fig. 1.2 Electromagnetic spectrum. Reproduced from [1]

1.3 Lasing Media

Laser machines consist of three parts: the pumping system, laser medium, and optical cavity with two mirrors. Additional devices are the cooling device and the delivery system. In laser mediums, there are gas types (CO_2 and argon), liquid types (dye), and solid types (ruby, alexandrite, Nd:YAG, and diode) [2]. The wavelength of the laser is determined by the laser medium. For example, CO_2 generates 10,600 nm wavelength, ruby 694 nm wavelength, and alexandrite 755 nm wavelength (Table 1.2).

So, when we talk about the type of laser, when you say ruby laser we know that the wavelength of the laser is 694 nm, and vice versa. Therefore, we must know the wavelength corresponding to the laser medium.

However, some lasers are able to produce multiple wavelengths with one medium. For example, Nd:YAG laser can produce 1064 nm and 1320 nm, and diode laser can produce 808 nm, 810 nm, and 1450 nm. This is why when describing a laser, the wavelength and medium must be described together as in "694 nm ruby laser." In addition, because the laser machine itself varies depending on the pulse duration (PD), PD should also be described as in "694 nm Q-switched ruby laser." However, I say simply "Q694" or "long1064" in conversation or lectures because of its long name.

Table 1.2 Lasing media and wavelength. Modified from [2]

Laser type	Lasing media	Wavelength
Liquid	Dye	585, 595 nm
Gas	CO_2	10,600 nm
	Argon	510 nm
	Excimer	308 nm
Solid	Ruby	694 nm
	Alexandrite	755 nm
	Er:YAG	2940 nm
	Nd:YAG	1064 nm, 1320 nm
	Diode	808, 810 nm, 1450 nm

1.4 Energy Parameters

Laser has various parameters of energy (Table 1.3). Energy is the number of emitted photons during a single pulse. A laser with high energy is a high-quality laser because more photons are emitted during a single pulse enabling higher tissue temperature. Energy is used to represent the power of the laser in pulsed laser in which PD is fixed. On the other hand, power is the number of emitted photons in unit time. The concept of time is included in power, compared with energy. Because power is the number of photons "per hour" in engineering, it refers to the output or "ability (force)" of the machine. Also, since "energy = power × time," meaning energy is the total amount of force applied or the amount of "work" done by the machine. Power is mainly used to represent the output of continuous laser [4].

Thus, energy and power are all used to express the output of laser. But for laser physicians the number of irradiated photons on the skin is important, which is why the concept of unit area is needed. Therefore, the parameters of energy density and power density are used. Energy density is the number of irradiated photons in a single pulse, in unit area of skin. It is often called fluence. Power density is the number of photons which are irradiated on skin, per unit time and unit area.

So which parameter is more important? Fluence or power density? When laser contacts skin, temperature rises. In other words, light energy is converted into thermal energy. The more the number of photons, the higher the temperature will be. Both fluence and power density have the concept of "quantity of photons" in their definition, so the higher the fluence or power, the higher the temperature. However, with the same number of photons, in which condition does the temperature rise more, 10 photons entering the skin in 1 s or 10 photons entering the skin in 10 s? Of course, in the former case, the tempera-

Table 1.3 Energy parameters of optical radiation

Parameter	Units	Formula
Energy	Joule(J)	Energy = power × sec
Power	Watt(W) = J/s	Power = energy/sec
Energy density (fluence)	J/cm^2	Energy density = energy/cm^2
Power density (irradiation)	W/cm^2	Power density = power/cm^2

ture will rise higher. For both the former and the latter, the fluence is 10 J/cm^2. However, the power density is 10 W/cm^2 for the former and 1 W/cm^2 for the latter. In other words, power density is more important to us than fluence.

Other parameters used in lasers are shown in Table 1.4. Also, unit conversion of a second should be understood (Table 1.5). In most laser texts, for example, it is not written as 10^{-3} s, but rather in milliseconds, or simply the abbreviation "ms." The novice laser physician may be confused by the unfamiliar second units. The least you need to know is which units are bigger or smaller. Also, since all units are shorter than 1 s, you might think that there isn't a big difference between each unit, but actually there's more than 1000 times the difference.

Table 1.4 Parameters of optical radiation [2]

Parameter	Units
Pulse duration	Seconds, milliseconds, microseconds, nanoseconds
Frequency	Hertz (Hz) = pulses per second
Wavelength	Nanometers (nm)
Spot size	Millimeters (mm)

Table 1.5 Unit conversion of a second

Units	Second
Millisecond (ms)	10^{-3} s
Microsecond (μs)	10^{-6} s
Nanosecond (ns)	10^{-9} s
Picosecond (ps)	10^{-12} s

1.5 Skin Optics

Four phenomena occur when laser contacts skin. These are reflection, refraction, transmission, scattering, and absorption (Fig. 1.3) [2]. To increase absorption, which is our goal, we must first reduce reflection and refraction and we must understand scattering. Transmission, on the other hand, inevitably occurs depending on the wavelength, in which unabsorbed photons pass through the skin and reach deep tissues such as the subcutaneous fat tissue. First, let's look at scattering among these four phenomena.

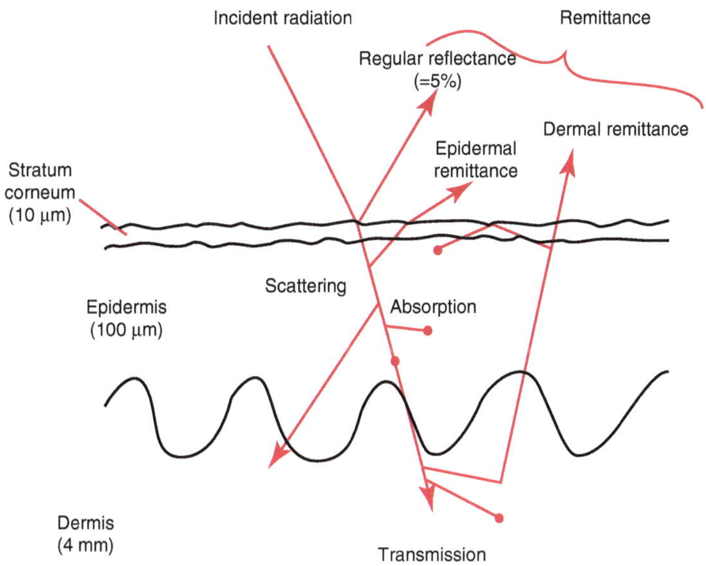

Fig. 1.3 Schematic diagram of optical pathways in skin: Reflection, Transmission, Scattering, Absorption. Modified from [5]

1.6 Scattering and Spot Size

Absorption occurs when the frequency of the photon and the electrons are same (resonance), resulting in conversion of light energy into thermal energy. In contrast, scattering occurs when the frequency of photons and electrons do not match [6].

I like to compare absorption and scattering to billiards. If the cue ball strikes another ball exactly, the cue ball stops and its energy disappears, while the other ball absorbs all the energy and bounces off. This can be compared to absorption. On the other hand, if the cue ball does not strike the other ball exactly, it may bounce off randomly. This may be compared to scattering. (Of course, this is intentional in billiards.)

Scattering is mainly caused by collagen in the dermis [7]. At wavelengths below 300 nm, most light is absorbed by chromophores such as epidermal proteins, DNA, and urocanic acid in the epidermal layer, and scattering does not occur. At wavelengths above 1300 nm, the absorption coefficient for water increases and the laser is absorbed directly in the epidermis and scattering does not occur. Therefore, the wavelength at which scattering occurs is mainly at 300–1300 nm.

When describing scattering, spot size should be considered. The relationship between scattering and spot size is difficult to explain simply, so let's just run to the conclusion. The larger the spot size, the deeper the optical penetration depth (OPD). That is, the spot size and OPD are proportional (Fig. 1.4).

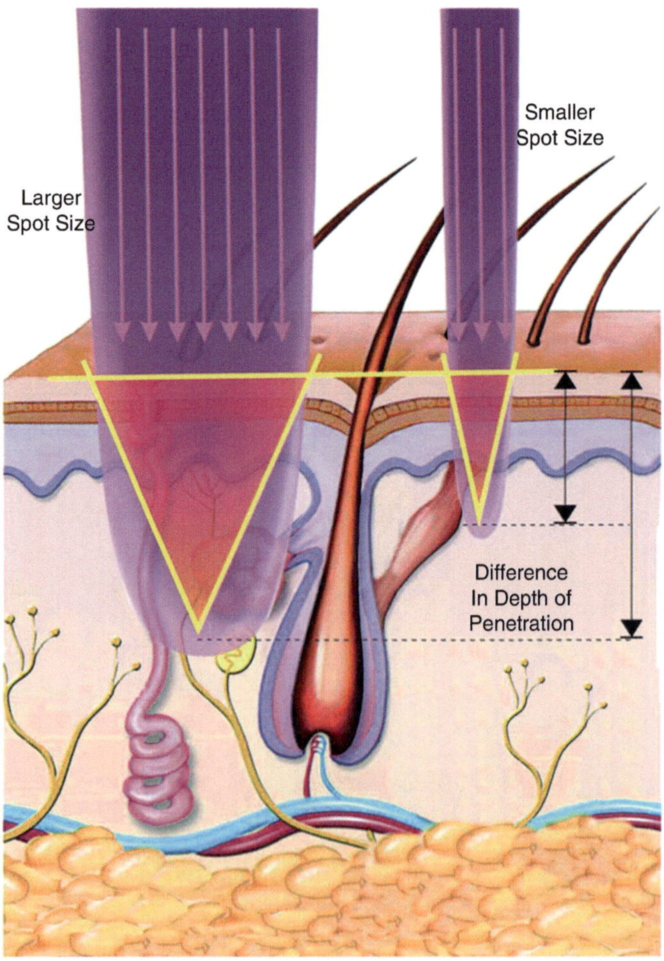

Fig. 1.4 The relationship between spot size and optical penetration depth (OPD). Reproduced from [8]

1.7 Chromophore and Absorption Coefficient

Chromophores are "components of the skin that absorb certain light" [2]. The three major chromophores of the skin are melanin, hemoglobin (Hb), and water. In addition, tattoo ink is also considered as a chromophore.

Simply explained, certain chromophores have a characteristic light absorption rate. This characteristic light absorption rate is the absorption coefficient. For example, melanin, hemoglobin, and water all have different absorption rates for light. In addition, the absorption coefficient not only depends on the chromophore, but also depends on the wavelength [9].

The absorption coefficient depends on the wavelength and the chromophore (Fig. 1.5). For example, when a 694 nm ruby laser irradiates 1000 photons, 90 photons are absorbed in the chromophore melanin and one photons are absorbed in the chromophore hemoglobin. There is a chromophore that absorbs better depending on the wavelength. On the contrary, there is a wavelength that absorbs better depending on the chromophore.

Since the wavelength is determined when purchasing the laser machine, we should purchase a laser for the chromophore we want. For example, for vascular therapy, lasers with a wavelength of 500–600 nm with a high absorption coefficient for hemoglobin is needed. For pigmented lesions and laser hair removal, ruby laser or alexandrite laser with a high absorption coefficient for melanin is needed (Table 1.6).

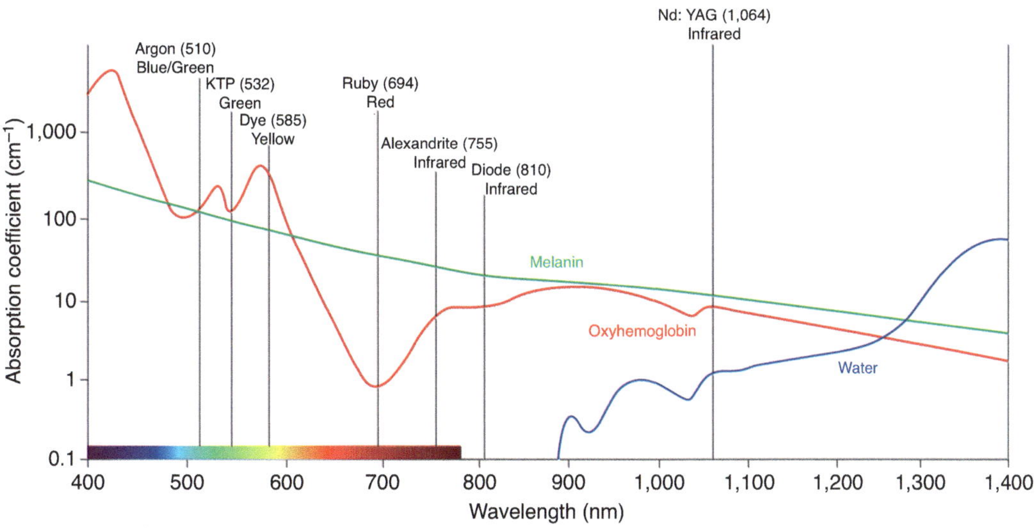

Fig. 1.5 Absorption curves for various wavelengths and chromophores. Reproduced from [2]

Table 1.6 Chromophores and indications by type of laser. NAR: non-ablative rejuvenation. Published with kind permission of © Jeonghyun Yoon MD. 2021. All rights reserved

Wavelength (nm)	Laser	Chromophore	Indications
308 (UV-B)	Excimer	DNA/RNA	Psoriasis, vitiligo
532 (green)	KTP Q-switched Nd:YAG	Hemoglobin Tattoo ink (red) Melanin	Telangiectasia Tattoo removal Benign lentigo
585–600 (yellow)	Pulse dye	Hemoglobin	Port-wine stain Telangiectasia
694 (red)	Q-switched ruby	Tattoo ink (blue, black, green) Melanin	Tattoo removal Benign lentigo
755 (infrared)	Q-switched alexandrite Long-pulsed alexandrite	Tattoo ink (blue, black, green) Melanin	Tattoo removal Benign lentigo Hair removal
810 (infrared)	Diode	Melanin	Hair removal
1064 (infrared)	Q-switched Nd:YAG Long-pulsed Nd:YAG	Tattoo ink (blue, black) Melanin Met-hemoglobin	Tattoo, dermal pigment Hair removal, NAR Telangiectasia
1320 (infrared)	Long-pulsed Nd:YAG	Water	NAR, atrophic scar
1450 (infrared)	Diode	Water	NAR, atrophic scar Acne
1540 (infrared)	Er:glass	Water	NAR, scar
2940 (infrared)	Er:YAG	Water	Ablation, scar
10,600 (infrared)	Carbon dioxide (CO_2)	Water	Ablation, scar

1.8 Laser-Tissue Interactions

What happens after laser is irradiated and absorbed into the skin? Heat is generated. In other words, "light energy" is converted into "thermal energy." When converted to heat, the temperature of the chromophore rises. Then, when the temperature of the chromophore increases, what kind of phenomenon and reaction will occur on the skin?

As the temperature rises in the skin, various phenomena take place. In order from low to high temperature: Denaturation of protein, evaporation of water, carbonization, evaporation, etc., take place. These phenomena result in tissue reactions (effects, interactions) that cause the skin to dry, break, and ablate [10]. As such, physical "phenomena" according to temperature change appear first, and these phenomena affect the skin, resulting in tissue "reactions."

The laser-tissue interactions can be classified into three types: photothermal effects, photomechanical effects, and photochemical effects. The photothermal effect refers to laser-tissue interactions by the phenomena of coagulation, vaporization, carbonization, and melting [11]. For example, coagulation and formation of scabs when treating lentigines with long-pulsed laser or IPL, or vaporization with a CO_2 laser is considered as a photothermal effect. Photomechanical effects exhibit laser-tissue interactions by the phenomena of plasma formation, shock wave, cavitation, and jet formation [11]. For example, bursting of blood vessels resulting in purpura by 585 nm PDL laser and the breakdown of melanosomes and the damage of melanocytes by Q-switched laser and tattoos removal procedures are considered as a photomechanical effect. Photochemical effects include low level laser therapy (LLLT) using light emitting diodes (LEDs) or He-Ne lasers, photodynamic therapy (PDT) using photosensitizers, and excimer lasers for vitiligo.

Previously, we classified laser-tissue interactions into three types, but strictly it can be divided into five types (Table 1.7) [11]. Depending on the laser text, the photodisruptive effect and photomechanical effect are sometimes considered the same while biostimulation is seen as a separate effect, but in other laser texts it is considered as a part of photochemical effect.

Under what conditions will these three effects occur? Different effects occur depending on PD and power density (Fig. 1.6). When PD is in seconds and the power density is low, photochemical effect takes place. When PD is in milliseconds and the power density is about 10–10^3 W/cm^2, photothermal effect takes place. When PD is in nanoseconds and the power density is more than 10^{11} W/cm^2, photomechanical effect takes place. This is called "the rule of one microsecond" because the photomechanical and photothermal effects are divided based on 1 microsecond, usually 10^{-6} s [2].

Table 1.7 Laser-tissue interactions (effects, reactions) and phenomena

	Effects (reactions)	Phenomena
1	(photo)mechanical/photodisruptive effect	Plasma formation, shock wave, cavitation, jet formation
2	(photo)thermal effect	Coagulation, vaporization, carbonization, melting
3	(photo)chemical effect	
4	Plasma-induced ablation effect	Plasma
5	Photoablation effect	Vaporization and liquefication
–	Biostimulation	

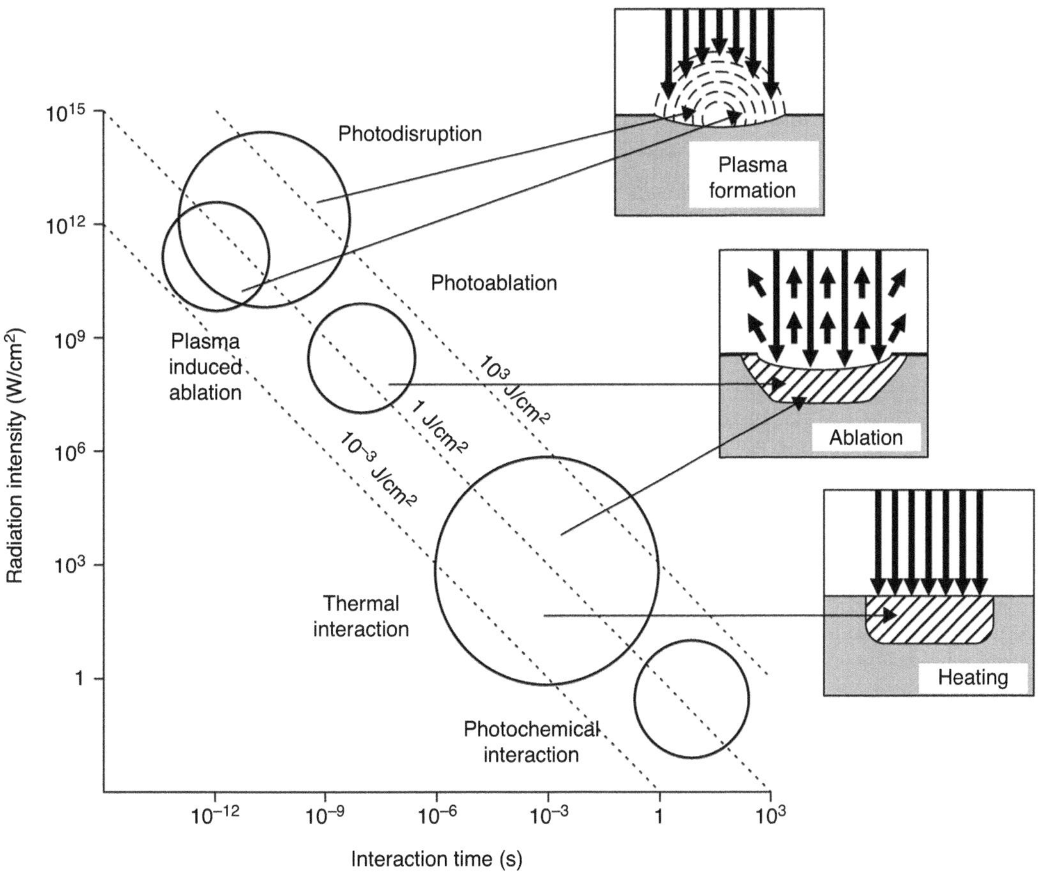

Fig. 1.6 Laser-tissue reactions. Reproduced from [12]

In other words, laser-tissue interaction depends on the correlation between PD and power density. For example, even if PD is short as 10^{-6} s but the power density is as low as 10^{-3} W/cm^2, there will be no effect. In contrast, if PD is as long as 10^3 s but the power density is as high as 10^6 W/cm^2, only side effects such as burn will occur. In both cases, the desired effect cannot be achieved.

It is also important to note that fluence is not important in Fig. 1.6. Diagonally dotted lines show the same 1 J/cm^2 but depending on the PD and the power density, photochemical, photothermal, and photomechanical effects can occur [11]. Therefore, simply increasing fluence does not give the photomechanical effect for a laser that exhibits a photothermal effect.

The five laser-tissue interactions can be thought of as separate reactions (Fig. 1.6), but they are not completely independent and adjacent reactions overlap one another [11]. For example, we assume that there is no temperature change in photochemical effects, but in reality, temperature plays an important role. There are overlapping parts in plasma-induced ablation and photodisruption. Also, temperature elevation is observed when rapidly repeating 10–20 Hz of picosecond laser or femtosecond lasers, which are thought to have no thermal effect due to having a PD of less than 100 ps. For example, water (liquid) must be converted to water vapor (gas) at 100 °C or higher, but water vapor (gas) is also present in indoor air below 100 °C. In addition, since most skin tissues are non-uniform when irradiated with a laser, the phenomenon of overlapping other tissue reactions is more pronounced.

1.9 Selective Photothermolysis

In 1983, Richard R. Anderson and John A. Parrish published the theory of selective photothermolysis in Science [13]. The ultimate goal of skin laser treatment is to precisely apply laser energy to a specific chromophore of the skin (or target tissue) without damaging the surrounding tissues [7]. As seen in absorption coefficients earlier, it was previously thought that this ultimate goal could be achieved by selecting a wavelength with a higher absorption coefficient for the target tissue than the surrounding tissue. But in reality, this does not happen.

In the 1960s, 510 nm argon lasers were used to treat port-wine stains (PWS). Argon lasers were thought to be suitable for vascular therapy because of their high absorption coefficient for hemoglobin, but in fact they affected the surrounding tissues and burned them. Argon lasers have high absorption coefficient for hemoglobin which selectively raises the temperature in blood vessels, but because they irradiate continuous waves, heat spreads and the temperature of surrounding tissues also rise, resulting in burn [15]. On the other hand, a short irradiation with a pulsed wave showed that only the blood vessels were damaged and the damage of surrounding tissues were minimized (Fig. 1.7) [16]. In other words, "heat diffusion" was the problem. To explain this

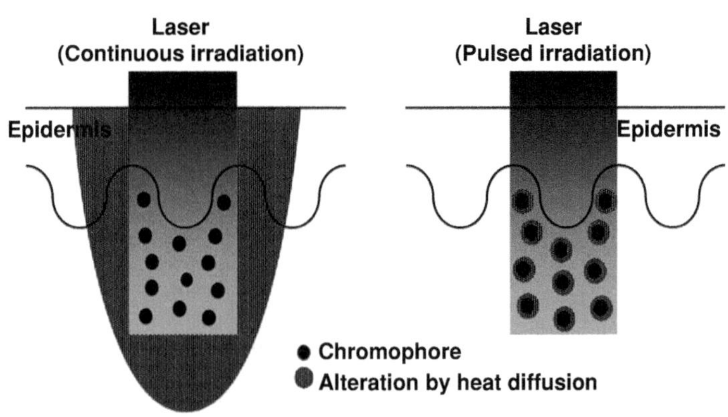

Fig. 1.7 Schematic diagram for laser treatment using continuous wave, and pulsed wave. In this figure, chromophore refers to the blood vessels of port-wine stains. Reproduced from [14]

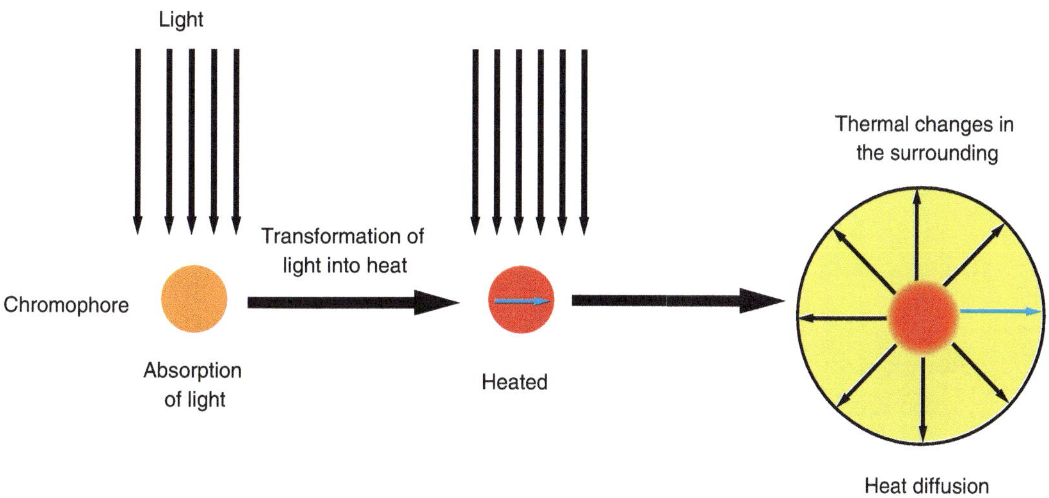

Fig. 1.8 Schematic diagram of change in chromophore after laser is absorbed. Modified from [14]

phenomenon, Richard R. Anderson presented the theory of selective photothermolysis.

During laser irradiation, the light energy absorbed by the target is converted into thermal energy (Fig. 1.8). During laser irradiation, thermal energy raises the temperature of the target tissue, but also diffuses into and out of the target tissue (heat diffusion). However, after irradiation the temperature of the target tissue does not rise any further, it rather cools down while heat diffusion to the surrounding tissue occurs. The target tissue is damaged as the temperature rises to the threshold at which tissue degeneration occurs while the laser is irradiated. However, because part of thermal energy was used to raise the temperature of the target tissue, the thermal energy diffused to the surrounding tissue does not rise up to the threshold for tissue degeneration (Fig. 1.9) [13]. In other words, by adjusting the PD, the extent of damage can be limited to the target tissue. The key of theory of selective photothermolysis is, "When light energy is irradiated for an appropriate time, it is converted into thermal energy in the target tissue and is mainly used to raise the temperature of the target tissue, damaging the target tissue and not damaging the surrounding tissue."

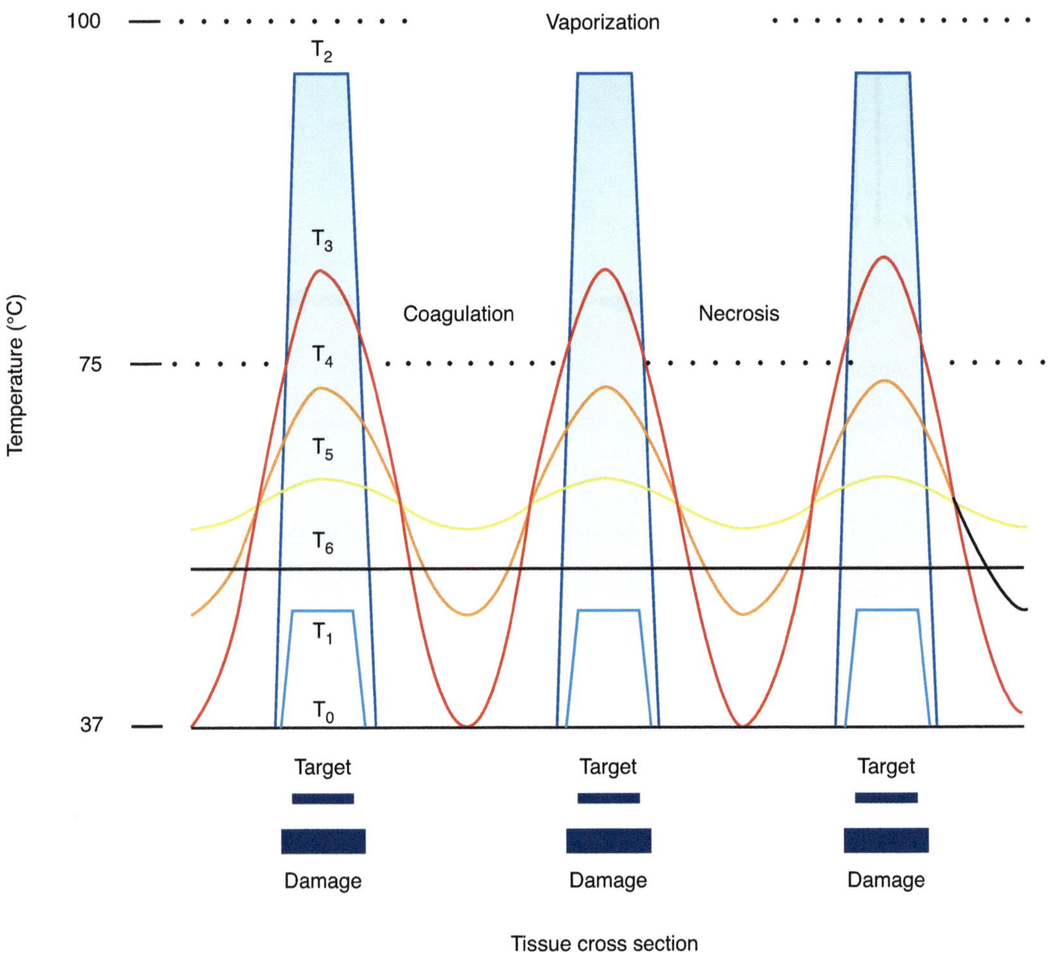

Fig. 1.9 Temperature change during selective photothermolysis. T_0: The temperature of the target tissue before laser irradiation (same as skin temperature). T_1: Temperature during laser irradiation (only the target tissue is heated selectively). T_2: Temperature at the end of laser irradiation (target tissue is irreversibly damaged). T_3, T_4, T_5: Temperature after thermal relaxation time after laser irradiation (target tissue cools while surrounding tissue increases in temperature). T_6: Both the target and surrounding tissues reach the same thermal equilibrium. Reproduced from [13]

1.10 Thermal Relaxation Time (TRT)

$$z_{\text{therm}}(t) = \sqrt{4\kappa t}.$$

$Z_{\text{therm}}(t)$: thermal penetration depth, k: heat conductivity, t: time

Heat diffusion distance (thermal penetration depth) is proportional to time (formula above) [11]. The distance at which heat is diffused will have a distance that damages the target tissue without affecting the surrounding tissue and a distance that affects the surrounding tissue. Similarly, with time, there will be a time that damages the target tissue without affecting the surrounding tissue and time that affects the surrounding tissue. Thermal relaxation time (TRT) refers to the time when only the target tissue is damaged without affecting the surrounding tissue.

If the thermal penetration depth [$Z_{\text{therm}}(t)$] is defined as the diameter (d) of the target tissue and the above formula is arranged based on time, TRT is as follows.

$$\mathrm{TRT} = d^2 / gk$$

d: thickness or diameter of the target, *g*: geometric factor, *k*: thermal diffusivity.

g is a geometric factor known to be 24–27 if the target tissue is a sphere, 16 for a cylinder [13], and 8 for a plane [13, 17]. In other words, temperatures cool slowly in spherical, cylindrical, and planar order. For example, planes like the epidermal layers cool more slowly than spheres like melanosomes or cylinders like blood vessels.

The important thing to note is that TRT is proportional to the square of the tissue diameter (d^2). In other words, the larger the tissue, the larger the TRT and the slower the temperature drop. Conversely, the smaller the tissue, the smaller the TRT and the faster the temperature drop (Table 1.8) [18]. This phenomenon is easily observed in everyday life. For example, the kimchi stew in the pot slowly cools because it is large, but if you spoon the kimchi stew, it will cool down quickly because it is small.

Table 1.8 TRT to remember [2, 4, 6, 10, 18, 19]

TRT to remember	
Melanosome	<1 μs (250–1000 ns)
Tattoo pigment	20 ns–3 ms
Melanocyte	1–30 μs
Basal layer	0.4 ms
Epidermis	2 ms (1–10 ms)
Capillaries	4.5 ms (100 μm: 100 μm corresponds to the size of the smallest visible blood vessel)
Hair follicle	40 ms (10–100 ms)
Water	<1 ms in CO_2 laser, 1 μs in er:YAG

1.11 Pulse Duration (PD) Vs TRT

Until now, we reviewed TRT. But in reality, what we actually adjust is not the TRT, but the pulse duration (PD). What is the relationship between PD and TRT, and how do we adjust it? PD can be divided into three based on TRT [7].

First, PD is longer than the TRT (TRT < PD, middle figure in Fig. 1.10). Temperature of the surrounding tissue rises, resulting in damage to both the target tissue and the surrounding tissue [7]. It is a side effect that we do not want.

Second, PD is shorter than the TRT (TRT > PD, right figure in Fig. 1.10). There is no damage to the surrounding tissue because the temperature of the surrounding tissue does not rise, but there is not enough time to raise the temperature of the target tissue. There will be no side effects, but no effects either [7]. However, photomechanical effects can be used with Q-switched lasers. Because Q-switched lasers have very short PD (nanoseconds), they cannot treat keratinocytes or melanocytes with very long TRTs (TRT 1–30 μs) directly. However, by photomechanical effect, melanosomes (TRT 250–1000 ns) can be exploded by shock waves resulting in indirect destruction and necrosis of keratinocytes or melanocytes.

Third, PD and TRT are the same (TRT = PD, left figure in Fig. 1.10). Only the target tissue is damaged without damaging the surrounding tissues. This is the ideal situation. However, this situation is difficult to create. This is because the formula of TRT itself is based on a general heat equation, not a formula for individual special situations, and the size of the target tissue varies. The TRT that we know is an approximation (Ballpark figures), not an absolute time. Therefore, it would be safe to shorten the PD so

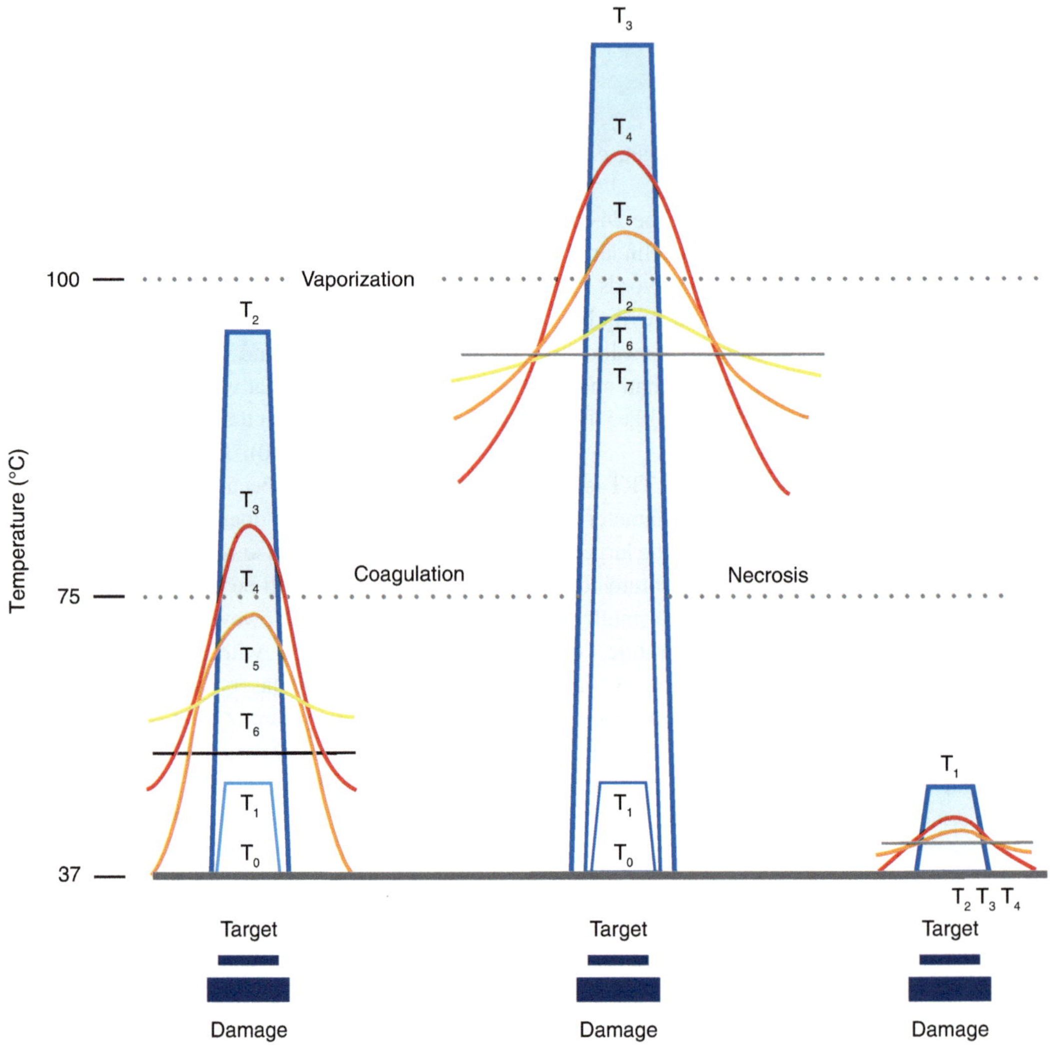

Fig. 1.10 Temperature changes by PD. Left: PD and TRT are the same (TRT = PD). Middle: PD is longer than the TRT (TRT < PD) or the energy is high. Right: PD is shorter than TRT (TRT > PD). Modified from [13]

that it is similar or slightly shorter than TRT. In this case, the photothermal effect is applied.

In summary, the same or shorter PD compared to TRT should be used to selectively treat only the target tissue (TRT ≥ PD).

1.12 Clinical End Point

Observation of skin changes during or after laser irradiation usually determines the appropriate fluence. This is called the clinical end point [20]. In your head, you should imagine the phenomena taking place inside the skin, for each clinical end point [6]. Clinical end points and my thoughts about the possible causes of each clinical end point are described below (Table 1.9).

For example, a 585 nm PDL with 450 μs uses shock waves, a photomechanical effect to rupture vessels for vascular therapy. The clinical end point is purpura (vessel rupture). On the other hand, a 595 nm PDL with millisecond uses photothermal effect for vascular therapy. Darkening may be observed (clot formation) or the blood

Table 1.9 Clinical end points and corresponding causes

Laser	Clinical end point
Lasers for vascular lesions	Purpura—Vessel rupture Darkening, disappearance—Clot formation, vessel coagulation Gray and white discoloration—a sign of necrosis
Lasers for pigmented lesions	Darkening and perilesional erythema—Denaturation of proteins, microvacuole Immediate whitening—Microbubble, Mie scattering Petechial—Vessel rupture
Laser for hair removal	Perifollicular erythema, edema—Peribulbar damage Pop out—Vaporization Gray or white discolorization—a sign of necrosis
Nonablative laser	No clinical end point
Ablative laser	Gray—Coagulation Darkening—Carbonization Disappearance—Vaporization
Fractional photothermolysis	No clinical end point

vessel may disappear (vessel coagulation). Too much energy may result in gray or white discoloration (necrosis).

After the laser procedure, we are only able to see the clinical end point. This is why we need to think about the cause, conversely. We should carefully observe the changes in the skin after the laser procedure, think about why these changes occurred, and determine whether these changes are appropriate and adjust the fluence.

Clinical end points can be defined differently for each lesion. For example, to treat epidermal pigmentation I use coagulation, and consider "delayed perilesional erythema" as an approximate clinical end point. "Delayed" means that erythema does not occur immediately after the procedure. It should only be observed when returning to the initially irradiated lesion after irradiating the entire face from one face to the opposite side. However, patients with freckles (which are also epidermal pigmentations) have bright skin tones and Fitzpatrick skin types I to III, so post-inflammatory hyperpigmentation (PIH) does not occur well. That is why clinical end point for freckles is sometimes "immediate darkening." In addition, different standards may be set for each physician. For example, if you want to get rid of epidermal pigmentations quickly, you can take "immediate whitening" as the clinical end point, risking the risk of PIH.

1.13 Meanings of Parameters

Table 1.10 summarizes the meaning of laser parameters based on what has been explained so far.

Table 1.10 Meanings of parameters

Parameter	Meanings
Wavelength	Kind and depth of chromophore
Pulse duration	Size of chromophore
Spot size	Location of chromophore
Fluence	Clinical end point
Frequency (Hz)	Repeat pulse method
Surface cooling	Epidermal sparing (e.g., vascular lesions, hair removal)

1.14 Strategy

There are three strategies for selectively raising the temperature of only one part spatially (Table 1.11) [21]. First, selective photothermolysis, second, epidermal cooling, and third, fractional photothermolysis. Let's look at these three strategies one by one.

First, selective photothermolysis. The difference in absorption coefficient is used to increase the temperature of only the target tissue while protecting the surrounding tissue.

$$\Delta T = \frac{F_z \mu_a}{\rho c}\left(\frac{\tau_r}{\tau_r + \tau_p}\right)^{g/2}$$

ΔT: temperature increase of a desired target
μ_a: absorption coefficient
F_z: local subsurface fluence
ρ: density
c: specific heat
g: geometric factor (1 for planes, 2 for cylinders, and 3 for spheres)
τ_p: laser pulse duration
τ_r: thermal relaxation time of the target (TRT)

Variables in the above formula include fluence, absorption coefficient, TRT, PD, geometric factors, density, specific heat, etc. It is easy to think that by controlling fluence or PD the lesions may be treated, but this is not true. For example, if a 5 mm lentigo surrounded by normal tissue is irradiated with a 10 mm spot size laser, there will be temperature change in both the lentigo (ΔT in lentigo) and the normal tissue (ΔT in normal tissue) within the 10 mm spot size. There is no difference between fluence and PD within the same spot size. Then what is the difference between the two tissues? First is the absorption coefficient and the second is the TRT. That is, the lentigo can be selectively treated only by using the difference in the melanin absorption coefficient or concentration difference between the lentigo and the normal tissue. In addition, to selectively treat lentigo one by one, PD should be sequentially reduced from long to short using thermal kinetic selectivity (TKS, refer to Sect. 10.4 in Chap. 10).

Table 1.11 Strategies of laser therapy

Spatially selective temperature elevation
1. Selective photothermolysis A. absorption coefficient (wavelengths), concentration of chromophore B. pulse duration (thermal kinetic selectivity)
2. Epidermal cooling
3. Fractional photothermolysis

Second, epidermal cooling. For example, in laser hair removal, both the temperature of epidermal melanin and dermal hair is increased. When epidermal cooling forcibly reduces epidermal temperature, the temperature of dermal hair is selectively increased.

Third, fractional photothermolysis. This method is a method of selectively treating only a partial portion spatially from the first irradiation. Lasers that use fractional photothermolysis are fractional lasers using Er:glass or CO_2 lasers. But is fractional photothermolysis only possible with fractional lasers? Fractional photothermolysis is effective not only with expensive fractional lasers, but also with the pinhole method, where only one shot is shot with a regular CO_2 laser.

What kind of strategy should be applied in each situation? First, the theory of selective photothermolysis mainly applies to horizontal situations. This method is applied when target tissue and competition tissue are located horizontally. For example, this method is used to treat epidermal pigments such as lentigo. Second, epidermal cooling is applied in vertical situations. For example, it is applied when treating dermal lesions such as vascular therapy, hair removal, and nonablative rejuvenation. The third method is applicable to all situations.

Conversely, what is the situation in which these methods cause problems? First, in the theory of selective photothermolysis, problems arise when absorption coefficients are similar or PD is similar. For example, treatment is difficult when the original skin is dark so that the difference in absorption coefficient of the original skin and the lentigo is not large. On the contrary, treatment is difficult when the lentigo is bright so that the difference in absorption coefficient of the original skin and the lentigo is not large. Second, in epidermal cooling, problems can arise if epidermal cooling is poor. Thus, the laser physician should always check the cooling machine. Third, in fractional photothermolysis, problems arise when fractional laser is too dense. In this case, regeneration from the normal tissue to the fractional irradiated tissue is not easy and may cause side effects.

1.15 Conclusions

We can summarize what has been said so far, in the following sentences.

Laser parameters should be selected to selectively increase the temperature of the chromophore (or target tissue) without affecting the surrounding tissues.

1. Laser with a wavelength corresponding to the chromophore should be selected.
2. Pulse duration (PD) equal to or shorter than the TRT according to the size of the chromophore should be selected.
3. Spot size according to the location of the chromophore should be selected.
4. Finally, fluence with desirable clinical end points should be selected.

References

1. Issa MCA, Tamura B. Lasers, lights and other technologies. Springer; 2018.
2. Allemann IB, Goldberg DJ. Basics in dermatological laser applications. Karger Medical and Scientific Publishers; 2011.
3. Goldsmith LA, Katz SI, Gilchrest BA, Paller AS, Leffell DJ, Wolff K, et al. Fitzpatrick's dermatology in general medicine. New York: McGraw-Hill Professional; 2012.
4. Lee W. Principles of IPL and its uses (Korean). Seoul: MDworld; 2008.
5. Anderson RR, Parrish JA. The optics of human skin. J Investig Dermatol. 1981;77(1):13–9.
6. Goldman MP. Cutaneous and cosmetic laser surgery. Philadelphia: Mosby Elsevier; 2006.
7. Stratigos A, Dover JS. Overview of lasers and their properties. Dermatol Ther. 2000;13(1):2–16.
8. Lee M-C, Chang C-S, Huang Y-L, Chang S-L, Chang C-H, Lin Y-F, et al. Treatment of melasma with mixed parameters of 1,064-nm Q-switched Nd: YAG laser toning and an enhanced effect of ultrasonic application of vitamin C: a split-face study. Lasers Med Sci. 2015;30(1):159–63.
9. Carroll L, Humphreys TR. LASER-tissue interactions. Clin Dermatol. 2006;24(1):2–7.
10. Kauvar A, Hruza G. Principles and practices in cutaneous laser surgery. CRC Press; 2005.
11. Niemz MH. Laser-tissue interactions. New York: Springer; 2007.
12. Jelínková H. Lasers for medical applications: diagnostics, therapy and surgery. Elsevier; 2013.
13. Anderson RR, Parrish JA. Selective photothermolysis: precise microsurgery by selective absorption of pulsed radiation. Science. 1983;220(4596):524–7.
14. Watanabe S. Basics of laser application to dermatology. Arch Dermatol Res. 2008;300(1):21–30.
15. Parrish JA, Anderson RR, Harrist T, Paul B, Murphy GF. Selective thermal effects with pulsed irradiation from lasers: from organ to organelle. J Invest Dermatol. 1983;80(Suppl):75s–80s.
16. Franck P, Henderson PW, Rothaus KO. Basics of lasers: history, physics, and clinical applications. Clin Plast Surg. 2016;43(3):505–13.
17. Altshuler GB, Anderson RR, Manstein D, Zenzie HH, Smirnov MZ. Extended theory of selective photothermolysis. Lasers Surg Med. 2001;29(5):416–32.
18. Brazzini B, Hautmann G, Ghersetich I, Hercogova J, Lotti T. Laser tissue interaction in epidermal pigmented lesions. J Eur Acad Dermatol Venereol. 2001;15(5):388–91.
19. Kang WH. Treatment strateties for pigmentation disorders in skin (Korean). Seoul: Hansol Medical; 2013.
20. Wanner M, Sakamoto FH, Avram MM, Chan HH, Alam M, Tannous Z, et al. Immediate skin responses to laser and light treatments: therapeutic endpoints: how to obtain efficacy. J Am Acad Dermatol. 2016;74(5):821–33. quiz 34, 33
21. Keyvan N. Lasers in dermatology and medicine. London: Springer-Verlag; 2012.

Part II

Choice of Laser and Medical Skin Care

2 Choice of Laser

2.1 Aesthetic Procedure Selection

One laser text classifies cosmetic procedures into four types according to the purpose of the procedure and describes them as "4 R's" (Table 2.1) [2]. First, refill. These procedures fill in the gaps. Typical procedures include fillers and fat grafting. Second, relax. These procedures prevent thick wrinkles by relaxing the muscles or reduce the volume of the muscles by contracting them. For example, toxins are used to prevent wrinkles of the glabella, forehead, and crow's feet. They also reduce the volume of the masseter muscles to make the face appear slimmer. Third, resurface. These procedures improve the skin. All the lasers and procedures described in this book fall under this category. Fourth, resuspend or lift. These procedures lift the sagging tissue that has lost its elasticity by pulling it.

Among new private practice doctors, there are those who choose to perform only one of these four procedures, but I think that all four procedures should be performed unless the hospital specializes in one type or one procedure in Gangnam (Seoul's Gangnam district is home to hundreds of cosmetic surgery clinics.). If you look at the horizontal axis instead of the vertical axis in Table 2.1, you can see that it is divided into noninvasive, minimally invasive, and invasive according to the degree of invasiveness of the procedure. Noninvasive procedures have fewer side effects but are not very effective. Also, like the prescription of Stieva-A Cream, it is not very helpful in terms of profit for doctors. The various lasers and procedures described in this book are mainly minimally invasive procedures. Minimally invasive procedures are in high demand because it is effective while the burden of side effects or cost of invasive surgery is low. In addition, patients undergoing skin procedures (resurface) are not only interested in the skin but are also highly interested in other procedures such as toxin, filler, and thread lifting. On the other hand, invasive procedures such as surgery feel burdensome. Therefore, a patient who has received laser procedure may also undergo toxin, filler, or thread lift procedures, thereby creating new demand from the same patient. Invasive procedures are mainly surgical methods, such as fat grafting, double eyelid surgery, and MACS lift. In dermatology, CO_2 laser resurfacing is considered as an invasive procedure. These procedures have a long downtime, often cause serious complications, and, above all, are not in high demand. These are the methods that can only be performed if the clinic is opened in Gangnam or in the heart of the city. Therefore, I think it is better to designate all the minimally invasive "4 R's" as treatment subjects, rather than selecting only one of the "4 R's."

J. D. Lee, M. J. M. Oh, *Lasers in Dermatology: Parameters and Choice*,
https://doi.org/10.1007/978-981-19-7568-4_2

Table 2.1 The 4 R's. Reproduced from [1]

	Refill	Relax	Resurface	Resuspend or lift
Noninvasive			Topical treatment Retinoids	
Minimally invasive	Collagen Cosmoderm/Cosmoplast Restylane/Perlane Juvédem Ultra and Ultra Plus Prevelle Silk	Botox Dysport	Photomodulation IPL Microdermabrasion Light chemical peel Pulsed/diode/Nd:YAG laser Nonablative resurfacing laser IPL + ALA	Radiofrequency Sculptra Aptos threads Ultrasound Intense infrared
Invasive	Sculptra Radiesse Silicone Fat FAMI		Er:YAG laser Medium-depth chemical peel CO_2 laser resurfacing Fractional resurfacing Deep chemical peeling	Blepharoplasty Lifts S-lift Neck liposuction Full rhytidectomy

2.2 Order of Laser Purchase

When you first open a clinic, which laser should you purchase first? If you have enough money, you can buy all the lasers, but to spend as efficiently as possible within the limited funds, you must purchase one by one, starting with the necessary lasers. Then, on what basis will you determine the laser purchase order? It may vary depending on the location of the hospital, but I think it is appropriate to purchase lasers in the order of the most in-demand indications (Table 2.2). I think the order is as follows: laser hair removal, melanocytic nevus removal, acne treatment, pigmentation treatment, scar treatment, and vascular treatment. The most in-demand indication in skin care is laser hair removal, not melanocytic nevus removal. Some people do not have melanocytic nevi on their faces, but all have hair under their armpits. However, since most patients seeking laser hair removal are women and mainly seek a female doctor, male doctors should focus more on removing the next high demand, i.e., melanocytic nevus removal. I think more in-demand for acne treatment than for pigmentation treatment. You can see a lot of acne patients in clinics near middle and high schools. Vascular treatment is described first in many laser texts and is thought to be important because it is described in detail, but the skin of Koreans is different from that of Caucasians, so the demand for vascular treatment in skin care is the least.

Table 2.2 Order of laser purchase. Needle RF: fractional microneedle radiofrequency

Indications	Initial purchase lasers	Later purchase lasers
Hair removal	810 nm diode laser (Female doctors)	Long-pulsed alexandrite laser
Melanocytic nevus removal	CO_2 laser	Er:YAG laser
Acne	LED	1450 nm diode laser
Pigment	Q-switched Nd:YAG laser	Long-pulsed alexandrite laser
Scar	CO_2 fractional laser	Needle RF
Blood vessel	Long-pulsed Nd:YAG laser	Pulsed dye laser

So which laser should we buy for each indication? I think lasers should be purchased separately as "initial purchase laser" and "late purchase laser." In my opinion, the criteria for "initial purchase laser" are first, a laser that is essential for each indication, and second, a laser that is relatively inexpensive. However, "initial purchase laser" has limitations and side effects. So, I recommend purchasing an "initial purchase laser" first, and after you study hard and improve your skills, and if you want to overcome the limitations of the "initial purchase laser," then it is time to purchase the "later purchase laser." For example, the CO_2 laser can be used for most nevi, benign tumors, and epidermal pigmentations, but the risk of side effects is high. If you desire a more precise treatment, then you should purchase the Er:YAG laser. However, if you purchase only the Er:YAG laser without the CO_2 laser, it will be difficult to remove large nevi, and bleeding will not stop, so you will eventually purchase a CO_2 laser.

Finally, which company's laser should you buy? There may be various criteria such as output, beam quality, option, A/S, marketing, design, etc. for individual laser purchase criteria, but I think output is the most important criterion. High output laser can make the pulse duration (PD) shorter. According to the "TRT $\geq$ PD" of selective photothermolysis, a shorter PD can treat a smaller target tissue (refer to Sect. 1.11 in Chap. 1). For example, when treating lentigo with IPL, if the output is low and PD cannot be reduced to 7 ms or less, light lentigo cannot be treated. Then how do we know the output of the laser? You can refer to the specifications of the laser company's website or brochure. If you look at the specifications, pulsed laser has energy displayed as Joule, and continuous laser has power displayed as Watt. For example, the pulsed laser, Q-switched Nd:YAG laser, is marked as 1.2–1.3 J, and the continuous laser, CO_2 laser, is marked as 25–30 W. I think the most important purchase criterion is to compare the laser specifications of several companies and select the laser with the highest output. Sometimes the specifications are not displayed or only the maximum fluence is displayed, not the output. In this case, you can calculate the energy or output or compare the output directly at a conference. A direct way to compare the output is to increase the fluence or output to the highest with the same large spot size and the same shortest PD. The laser with the highest fluence or output is the laser with the highest output.

Generally, high output and good lasers are expensive lasers, so Dr. Young Hoon Han recommends purchasing the most expensive laser when purchasing individual lasers. In addition, he recommends that it is better to purchase one most expensive laser than to purchase several medium-low-cost lasers. For example, if the total laser purchase budget is 100 million won, instead of purchasing all the low-cost CO_2 laser, Q-switched Nd:YAG laser, and CO_2 fractional laser, he recommends purchasing just one 100 million won CO_2 laser. After the profit is equivalent to 100 million, then the most expensive Q-switched Nd:YAG laser should be bought and so forth. (Published with kind permission of © Younghoon Han MD. 2021. All rights reserved).

2.3 Order of Parameter Selection (Optical Thermal Model)

Optical thermal models have been developed to determine appropriate laser parameters [3]. The optical thermal model is divided into three stages in order of laser-induced tissue reactions. First is the optical phase, where photons are absorbed by the target tissue. For the laser to be selectively absorbed by the target tissue, it is necessary to select a wavelength having a higher absorption coefficient for the target tissue than the surrounding tissue. Thus, the optical phase is the phase of selecting the wavelength. In addition, since the optical penetration depth (OPD) is determined according to the wavelength, the depth of the target tissue should also be considered at this stage.

Second is the thermal phase, where photons turn into heat. To minimize damage to the surrounding tissue, the thermal stage should be determined in accordance with the theory of selective photothermolysis so that the target tissue does not transfer heat to the surrounding tissue. Thus, the thermal phase is the phase of selecting the pulse duration.

Third is tissue denaturation process. When heat is applied to target tissue, the optical proper-

Table 2.3 Order of parameter selection

Order of parameter selection
Wavelength → pulse duration → spot size → fluence

ties of the tissue change. For example, after irradiating IPL in lentigines, darkening is examined to determine whether the fluence is appropriate (clinical end point). This stage corresponds to the tissue denaturation process.

Therefore, the order of selecting laser parameters is as follows. First, select the wavelength. Next, determine the pulse duration. Finally, tissue response should be observed to control fluence.

I think that spot size should be added to order of parameter selection. Spot size should be added before fluence. When performing laser treatment, spot size determination is essential, especially when treating the dermis, because fluence varies with spot size (refer to Sect. 4.6 in Chap. 4). Therefore, laser parameters should be determined in order of wavelength, pulse duration, spot size, and fluence (Table 2.3).

2.4 Misconceptions about Peak Power

Peak power refers to the maximum instantaneous output allowed by the original equipment. Peak power is a term mainly used to indicate the maximum characteristics of equipment and is one of the selection criteria when purchasing a laser. Peak power can usually be found in the specification on the back page of the brochure distributed by the company. Power refers to energy per PD. Applying high energy in a short time will increase the temperature of the tissue. So, beginners who know a little bit about power try to increase the fluence or especially reduce the PD to increase the power close to the peak power of the laser when there is no reaction in the target tissue after irradiating the long pulse laser. But there is a problem here. For example, if there is no response when treating capillaries with a 532 nm long-pulsed KTP laser with a spot size of 5 mm, PD 10 ms, and a fluence of 10 J/cm^2, a beginner makes the following error.

First, beginners think that the fluence should be raised to 12 J/cm^2 to see the photomechanical effect by increasing the power. Raising fluence isn't a bad choice, but it's for the wrong purpose. Long-pulsed lasers cannot reduce PD to nanoseconds no matter how much it reduces PD in milliseconds. Photomechanical effects, photothermal effects, and photochemical effects appear depending on the power density, but more important than the power density is PD (refer to Sect. 1.8 in Chap. 1). Only nanosecond or picosecond PDs have photomechanical effects. Therefore, long-pulsed lasers with millisecond PD cannot produce photomechanical effects.

Second, beginners who know the concept of TRT think that the peripheral damage is less when the PD is reduced. This choice is also for the wrong purpose. The order of parameter selection in the photothermal model is wavelength, PD, spot size, and fluence. In the tissue denaturation stage, not only the temperature is important, but also the time required for tissue denaturation according to the Arrhenius formula (refer to the Sect. 7.3 in Chap. 7). The problem is that the "pulse duration" selected in the previous thermal stage and the "time" according to the Arrhenius formula in the tissue denaturation stage may be same or different. In addition, "pulse duration" takes precedence over the "time" according to the Arrhenius formula in the order of the photothermal model. If the two times are the same and there is no response of the target tissue, if the "pulse duration" is reduced by applying the concept of peak power, the laser is absorbed only in a part of the target tissue in the heat stage, so that the sufficient effect is not seen. Also, in the stage of tissue denaturation, the time is shortened in the graph of Arrhenius formula (Fig. 7.4), resulting in no effect. In this case, only the fluence should be raised for tissue denaturation. If the two times are different, first select the "pulse duration" that can be selectively absorbed into the target tissue, and then apply the concept of macropulse (instead of applying the concept of peak power) to determine the "time" of tissue denaturation according to the Arrhenius formula. A multipulse irradiation method should be selected (refer to Sect. 8.4 in Chap. 8).

Third, a beginner who understands the concept up to the Arrhenius formula thinks that PD should be increased to 15 ms to make sure the photothermal effect takes place. But this is also wrong. As explained in the second error, among the "pulse duration" of the thermal stage and "time" of the tissue denaturation stage, the "pulse duration" takes precedence. If the target tissue's TRT is 10 ms, and the PD is increased to 15 ms, it will damage the surrounding tissue. As such, there is no concept of peak power in the photothermal model and Arrhenius formula. Therefore, it is good to forget the concept of peak power when adjusting the laser parameters.

Then, if the target tissue does not respond after irradiating the laser, how should the parameters be adjusted? The reason there is no response to the laser is because some of the parameters such as wavelength, PD, spot size, and fluence that correspond to the desired target tissue are incorrectly selected. For example, in the case of poikiloderma of Civatte, it looks brown, so beginners might choose the Q-switched ruby laser, which is a pigment laser. However, in poikiloderma of Civatte, there are some pigmentations, but the main lesion is blood vessels. DeoxyHb in blood vessels has a high absorption coefficient at 630–700 nm like melanin, and because the blood vessels are thick, light is reflected and the amount of light entering our eyes is reduced by 50%, making it appear brown [4]. Therefore, it does not respond to the use of Q-switched ruby laser, which cannot treat blood vessels due to short PD. In other words, if there is no response to a specific parameter, you should not only adjust the fluence or PD, but check all six laser parameters one by one.

2.5 Fluence Instability

The parameters of the laser instrument panel and the parameters irradiated may be different. As the laser is used, the output of the flash lamp decreases and the actual fluence gradually decreases. To compensate for this, there is also a laser with an added function to adjust the fluence by autocalibration. However, since most lasers do not have this function, you must know the more you use the laser, the lower the actual output.

It is not a big problem when the clinical end point is visible immediately after the procedure, because the decreased output can be immediately recognized. But in case of laser hair removal, where there is no immediate clinical end point caution should be taken.

For example, suppose you initially start laser hair removal for several patients at 8 J/cm^2. As the laser is used, the number on the instrument panel does not change, but the output decreases little by little. After realizing that there is no effect by 8 J/cm^2, the fluence is gradually increased to 10 J/cm^2. After that, if the lifespan of the flash lamp expires and you replace it with a new lamp but still use 10 J/cm^2, the energy is too high and side effects occur. It is difficult to notice this in advance because there is no change immediately after laser hair removal.

Therefore, first, because the output of the laser decreases as it is used, you should raise the fluence if you think the effect is inadequate. Second, after replacing the flash lamp or calibrating the output with laser check, the fluence should be lowered. Third, patients undergoing a procedure without a clinical end point, such as laser hair removal, should be informed of the side effects of the procedure in advance, and instructed to immediately visit the hospital if an abnormality is found after the procedure.

2.6 Effect Versus Safety?

The laser physician must determine three or six parameters. However, in the end, the final decision is in choosing between effect and safety. Choosing effect increases the likelihood of side effects, and choosing safety increases the likelihood of no effect. Which shall we choose? Effect versus Safety?

Some like to compare private practice to martial arts, and like novices and masters of martial arts, they say there are novices and masters in laser physicians. What is the difference between novices and masters in laser physicians? I think if the lasers are the same, there is no difference in effects between novices and masters. Because if the laser is irradiated with high power, it will be effective for both novices and masters. However, there is a difference in the probability of side effects occurring for novices and masters. I think a "master laser physician" is someone who creates similar effects with minimal side effects.

Thus, I believe that to become a "master," safety must be chosen over effect. Of course, safety without effectiveness is also undesirable. Through education and experience, safe and effective parameters must be found.

2.7 Therapeutic Window and Epidermal Bypass Effect

Most procedures have a therapeutic window. Tissue degeneration should also be treated between the damage threshold and the survival threshold [5]. If it is lower than the damage threshold, there is no effect, and if it is higher than the survival threshold, side effects occur (refer to the Sect. 7.3 in Chap. 7).

$$\Delta T = \frac{F_z \mu_a}{\rho c}\left(\frac{\tau_r}{\tau_r + \tau_p}\right)^{g/2}$$

- ΔT: Temperature increase of a desired target
- μ_a: absorption coefficient
- F_z: local subsurface fluence
- ρ: density
- c: specific heat
- g: geometric factor (1 for planes, 2 for cylinders, and 3 for spheres)
- τ_p: laser pulse duration
- τ_r: thermal relaxation time of the target (TRT)

Different lasers have different wavelengths, and each wavelength has its own absorption coefficient. A wavelength with a high absorption coefficient can raise more temperature than a wavelength with a low absorption coefficient. However, according to the above formula [6], the temperature can be the same regardless of whether the absorption coefficient is high or low if the fluence is appropriately adjusted. Then, what is the difference between a laser with a high absorption coefficient and a laser with a low absorption coefficient?

Table 2.4 shows simulated numbers I wrote for better understanding. Assume that the temperature we want is 73 °C and the temperature at which postinflammatory hyperpigmentation (PIH) occurs is 75 °C. 532 nm and 1064 nm have a ten-fold difference in absorption coefficient. Therefore, the temperature of target tissue is the same when 10 J/cm² is irradiated with a 1064 nm laser and 1 J/cm² is irradiated with a 532 nm laser. However, since 532 nm can raise energy by 0.1 J/cm² intervals, the temperature rises by 7 °C. 1 J/cm² is not effective while 1.1 J/cm² is effective but PIH occurs. On the other hand, 1064 nm laser can also raise energy at 0.1 J/cm² intervals, but because the absorption coefficient is one tenth of the 532 nm laser, the temperature increases by 0.7 °C. Therefore, 1064 nm laser is effective at 10.5, 10.6, and 10.7 J/cm², and there is no PIH occurrence.

Lasers with low absorption coefficients can raise temperatures little by little compared to lasers with high absorption coefficients, even if fluence intervals are the same. In other words, a laser with a high absorption coefficient may have a narrow therapeutic window, or none, while a laser with a low absorption coefficient may have a wide therapeutic window. When this is applied to the pigment laser, because the absorption coefficient of melanin decreases as the wavelength increases, shorter wavelength has a narrow therapeutic range, while longer wavelength has a wider therapeutic range.

Table 2.4 Temperature change by fluence. (The numbers are simulated)

532 nm (μ_a = 70 cm^{-1})		1064 nm (μ_a = 7 cm^{-1})	
1.0 J/cm²	70.0 °C	10.0 J/cm²	70.0 °C
1.1 J/cm²	77.0 °C	10.1 J/cm²	70.7 °C
1.2 J/cm²	84.0 °C	10.2 J/cm²	71.4 °C
		10.3 J/cm²	72.1 °C
		10.4 J/cm²	72.8 °C
		10.5 J/cm²	73.5 °C
		10.6 J/cm²	74.2 °C
		10.7 J/cm²	74.9 °C
		10.8 J/cm²	75.6 °C

There is one more thing to consider because Koreans have high levels of epidermal melanin content. There is a wavelength that is better absorbed by epidermal pigmentations, and a wavelength that is better absorbed by dermal pigmentations. Wavelengths below 800 nm are better absorbed by epidermal pigmentations, and wavelengths above 800 nm are better absorbed by dermal pigmentations [4]. Why is this so? Just like scattering occurring in the dermis, short wavelengths meet and absorb melanin pigment in the epidermis and relatively fewer photons enter the dermis. On the other hand, longer wavelengths encounter less melanin in epidermis (epidermal bypass), so that more photons enter the dermis. The boundary of these wavelengths is approximately 800 nm.

So, when the dermis is the target tissue, wavelengths of 800 nm or more are mainly used (e.g., hair removal using 810 nm diode laser, tattoo removal using 1064 nm laser), and wavelengths of 800 nm or less are mainly used when the epidermis is the target tissue (e.g., 694 nm ruby laser, 755 nm alexandrite laser, 532 nm KTP laser to treat epidermal pigmentations).

However, wavelengths above 800 nm are not entirely unabsorbed by the epidermis. Therefore, epidermal cooling is essential during laser hair removal with 810 nm and 1064 nm lasers. Likewise, 1064 nm Q-switched Nd:YAG lasers is not entirely unabsorbed by epidermis. Rather, it is suitable for use in "laser toning" because of its low absorption.

In summary, the following conclusions are reached.

1. Lasers with lower absorption coefficients are safer. In case of melanin, lasers with wavelengths to the right of the absorption curve are safer (longer wavelength).
2. Wavelengths of less than 800 nm are mainly used to treat epidermal pigmentations, while wavelengths of more than 800 nm are mainly used to treat dermal pigmentations (epidermal bypass).

From now on, I will define the two conclusions above as the "epidermal bypass effect" for ease of explanation. Then where can the "epidermal bypass effect" be applied? This is highly applicable in the selection of pigment lasers. When selecting epidermal pigment lasers, a laser with a wavelength of 800 nm or less must be purchased (e.g., 532, 694, and 755 nm). The safest laser is 755 nm alexandrite laser, because lasers with wavelengths to the right of the absorption curve are safer. On the other hand, the laser with the highest side effect is the 532 nm laser. I therefore believe that alexandrite lasers should be chosen over ruby lasers for epidermal pigmentation treatments. The only dermal pigment laser is the 1064 nm Nd:YAG laser. Ruby lasers and alexandrite lasers are also able to treat dermal pigmentations and tattoos, but Nd:YAG laser is more effective because of the epidermal bypass effect.

2.8 Selection of Pigment Lasers for Koreans

In one laser text, it was described that when epidermal pigmentations were treated with CO_2, Q-switched, and long-pulsed lasers, the incidence of PIH was 50%, 10%, and 1% respectively [7, 8]. Long-pulsed laser had the fewest side effects, but they had to be repeated several times. When treating epidermal pigmentations, the order of safety is as follows: Long-pulsed laser > Q-switched laser > Ablative laser.

On the contrary, which laser is most effective? Theoretically, because Q-switched laser breaks cells, it can remove the pigment with just one shot, so the Q-switched laser may be considered most effective. However, the lentigo is composed of melanocytes, and the number of melanosomes is different for each melanocyte. Due to the difference in absorption coefficient, Q-switched lasers can only remove melanocytes with more than a certain number of melanosomes. In other words, melanocytes with less than a certain number of melanosomes cannot be removed. On the other hand, ablative lasers can completely remove the pigment and its surrounding tissues, all at once. So, although PIH occurs, ablative lasers are most effective in terms of effectiveness. Therefore, the order of effectiveness (the oppo-

Table 2.5 Choice of pigment laser

For epidermal pigment	
1. Long-pulsed laser	755 nm > 532 nm
2. Q-switched laser	755 nm > 694 nm > 532 nm
3. Ablative laser	Er:YAG > CO_2
For dermal pigment	
Q-switched laser	1064 nm
Fractional laser	Er:glass, CO_2 pinhole method

site of the order of safety) is as follows: Ablative lasers > Q-switched lasers > Long-pulsed lasers.

Specific wavelengths are as follows (Table 2.5): Due to epidermal bypass effect, to treat epidermal pigmentations, wavelengths below 800 nm should be selected, and the closer to 800 nm, the safer. There are only two long-pulsed lasers below 800 nm, 532 nm long-pulsed KTP lasers and 755 nm long-pulsed alexandrite lasers. 755 nm long-pulsed alexandrite lasers are safer than 532 nm long-pulsed KTP lasers. Also, in the case of Q-switched lasers, the order of safety is as follows: 755 nm Q-switched alexandrite lasers >694 nm Q-switched ruby lasers >532 nm Q-switched Nd:YAG lasers. There are two types of ablative lasers, CO_2 laser and Er:YAG laser. Er:YAG laser has few side effects because the ablation depth is shallower and has less residual thermal damage (RTD) (refer to Sect. 11.7 in Chap. 11). Therefore, Er:YAG laser is safer than CO_2 laser.

There are so many lasers that can be used to treat epidermal pigmentations. Which laser should we buy first? I think it is best to buy the cheapest and the most effective laser first. Next, buy the safest laser. I think lasers in between are ambiguous. Lasers in between do not have a definite effect and they are not without side effects.

Therefore, when buying an epidermal pigment laser, you must first buy the most effective and inexpensive CO_2 laser. After using the CO_2 laser as much as possible, and when you feel the limitations of a CO_2 laser, then buy the safest long-pulsed alexandrite laser. Similarly, if you want to buy a Q-switched laser, first buy a 532 nm Q-switched Nd:YAG laser, then buy a 755 nm Q-switched alexandrite laser.

For dermal pigment lasers, there are Q-switched lasers, fractional lasers, and pinhole therapy. According to epidermal bypass effect, a wavelength of 800 nm or more is needed to treat the dermis, and the only possible Q-switched laser is the 1064 nm Q-switched Nd:YAG laser. Therefore, only Q-switched Nd:YAG lasers are needed to treat dermal pigmentations. Fortunately, the cost of purchase is also lower than other Q-switched lasers. For fractional lasers or pinhole therapy, first purchase a low-cost CO_2 laser and perform pinhole therapy, and if you feel limitations, then consider purchasing a 1550 nm fractional Er:glass laser.

2.9 Strong and Weak Treatment of Lentigines

The histological findings of the lentigines are characterized by proliferation of melanocytes, increased pigmentation around the basal layer, and epidermal growth in which the rete ridges become club shape and is lengthened into the papillary dermis [9]. The mechanism of lentigines is unknown, but histological findings suggest that it is a tumor or hamartoma caused by the proliferation of melanocytes. Therefore, the therapeutic target of laser in lentigines is melanocytes. However, melanocytes do not have enough melanin, the laser chromophore. Melanocytes synthesize melanosomes and deliver them to the supranuclear cap of peripheral keratinocytes through dendrites. Melanosomes are divided into four stages (stage I to IV) according to their maturity level. Melanosomes in the first and second stages are "melanin-free" and have "red melanin only," and melanosomes in third and fourth stages are melanosomes that synthesize eumelanin [10] and are commonly found in dendrites of melanocytes.

Hruza et al. irradiated 694 nm Q-switched ruby lasers on normal skin and lentigines. Transmission electron microscopy revealed that the melanosomes in stages 1 and 2 were intact. Therefore, I believe that irradiation of pigment lasers will not damage melanocytes first, but primarily damages keratinocytes and dendrites of melanocytes, which has the most melanosomes in third and fourth stages. Yamasita et al. observed lentigines disappearing by naked eye after irradiation of lentigines with IPL, but melanocytes remained intact on reflection-mode confocal microscopy (RCM) [11]. Melanocytes also remained after the crust of lentigines exfoliated after Q-switch ruby laser irradiation [12]. Mun et al. performed laser toning with a 1064 nm Q-switched Nd:YAG laser, observed "dendrectomy" phenomenon in which melanocytes did not disappear but only the dendrite disappeared [13]. As such, target and chromophore are different in the treatment of lentigines. In conclusion, the treatment of lentigines remains difficult.

Treatment methods of epidermal pigmentations include long-pulsed lasers such as IPL, Q-switched lasers, and ablative lasers. Recently a new laser, picosecond laser, has been released. I think that theoretically, picosecond laser has similar safety profiles compared to long-pulsed lasers regarding PIH occurrence (refer to Sect. 6.4 in Chap. 6).

Another technique is "one shot toning." 1064 nm Q-switched Nd:YAG laser is performed at 1–2-week intervals at 4–6 J/cm^2, with the "energy level that only damages the target cells without affecting the surrounding cell" (refer to Sect. 5.5 in Chap. 5). Although the epidermal pigmentations do not disappear all at once, repeated treatment 5–10 times can treat the epidermal pigmentations without any side effects. Although not one-shot toning, Nam et al. reported that, for 12 patients with multiple senile lentigines, a 1064 nm Q-switched Nd:YAG laser was applied with 1.62 ± 0.16 J/cm^2 (0.8–2.0 J/cm^2). Immediate moderate erythema was regarded as a clinical end point and was performed 5 to 12 times with an average interval of 28.0 ± 11.4 days [14]. The results showed that 58.3% (7 patients) showed significant improvement, and 25.0% (3 patients) showed moderate improvement. Since one-shot toning is a method of gently breaking cells, there is little chance of PIH unless there is underlying melasma. Therefore, I think one-shot toning is safer than a picosecond laser or a 755 nm long-pulsed alexandrite laser. So, I think the safety of the pigment laser in the treatment of epidermal pigment is as follows:

One shot toning > picosecond laser ≒ long755 > long532 > Q755 > Q694 > Q532 > Er:YAG > CO_2

In conclusion, epidermal pigmentation treatment has a therapeutic spectrum between safety and effect. One end has a laser that is safe but requires multiple treatments and cannot completely treat pigmentations (one shot toning, long755). The other end has a laser that is effective, pigmentations can be treated at once and there is no recurrence. But this laser is highly likely to cause textural imperfection, persistent erythema, and PIH (Er:YAG, CO_2). The pigment laser should be selected after sufficient consultation with the patient about safety and effectiveness. I think it's better to treat sequentially, starting with the safe method, several times.

And I think that there is a "strong treatment" and a "weak treatment" for each pigment laser (Table 2.6). For example, a 755 nm long-pulsed alexandrite laser can remove epidermal pigmentations at once by increasing the fluence, but the possibility of PIH is high, melasma may occur if there is underlying latent melasma. On the other hand, if the fluence is lowered to 7–8 J/cm^2, epidermal melasma can be improved.

"Weak treatment" of 1064 nm Q-switched Nd:YAG laser is one-shot toning, and "strong treatment" is the focusing method (refer to Sect. 5.7 in Chap. 5). However, I do not use the focusing method for epidermal pigmentation treatment because the focusing method generates a lot of PIH in epidermal pigmentations and it is not easy to control.

The "weak treatment" of 532 nm Q-switched Nd:YAG laser is repeat pulse method, a method that repeatedly irradiates low fluence (refer to the Sect. 5.6 in Chap. 5). On the other hand, fluence could be raised so that "immediate whitening" occurs. This is the "strong treatment" of 532 nm Q-switched Nd:YAG laser. However, "strong treatment" that increases fluence with a 532 nm Q-switched Nd:YAG laser often causes PIH.

I think that narrowing blood vessels can lower PIH because (1) recent papers suggest the possibility that blood vessels may be involved in the

Table 2.6 My classification of "strong treatment" and "weak treatment" of pigment laser. Q1064: 1064 nm Q-switched Nd:YAG laser, long755: 755 nm long-pulsed alexandrite laser, Q532: 532 nm Q-switched Nd:YAG laser

	Strong treatment	Weak treatment
Q1064	Focusing method	One shot toning (4–6 J/cm^2)
long755	High fluence (20–25 J/cm^2)	Low fluence (15 J/cm^2)
Q532	Vasoconstriction method	Repeat pulse method
CO_2	Focusing + Q532	Defocusing method

recurrence of the lentigo [12], and (2) inflammatory cells move through dilated blood vessels during inflammation. Therefore, I use anesthesia with dental lidocaine (epinephrine 1:100,000), to make the skin pale before treatment.

"Weak treatment" of CO_2 laser is a defocusing method that induces epidermal coagulation, and "strong treatment" is a method of focusing and removing all epidermis and papillary dermis with rete ridges of lentigines. However, this method may cause skin texture changes or scarring. On the other hand, when sparsely irradiated with a CO_2 laser, it is impossible to remove all the rete ridges because the spot size of the CO_2 laser is small. Another option would be to use the 532 nm Q-switched Nd:YAG laser after the CO_2 laser. However, I haven't used this method yet because I think PIH is very likely in this method.

Based on the above, I treat lentigo as follows. First, the safest one-shot toning is performed on odd number sessions (session 1,3,5...) of the 10 sessions (refer to Sect. 3.6 in Chap. 3). For sessions 2 and 4, the next safest 755 nm long-pulsed alexandrite laser is used. In case of Fitzpatrick skin type IV or V, visible facial PIH, dark knuckles, visible dark skin, soft skin with no visible pores, erythematous lentigo, mottled pigmentation on face (refer to Sect. 19.3 in Chap. 19) low fluence is used. Otherwise, high fluence is used. For epidermal pigmentations that do not have "delayed perilesional erythema" after long-pulsed alexandrite laser, repeat pulse method is used with a Q-switched Nd:YAG laser of 532 nm on the same day. If the lentigo is larger than 1 cm, "strong treatment" is performed for quick treatment. Anesthesia with dental lidocaine (epinephrine 1:100,000) is applied and when the skin becomes pale, it is irradiated once with a fluence (0.6–0.7 J/cm^2) that results in slightly whitening without petechiae (vasoconstriction method). Also, on the same day, small lentigines with a size of 1–2 mm that do not respond to long-pulsed alexandrite laser and 532 nm Q-switched Nd:YAG laser are removed by defocusing with CO_2 laser. The remaining pigmentations after the fifth session is considered as an epidermal pigmentation or PIH that cannot be treated with laser. Epidermal pigment treatment is stopped and only conventional laser toning and one-shot toning of less than 4 J/cm^2 is repeated.

2.10 Skin Types

There are three major variables that affect the results of cosmetic procedures. First, the treatment results are different depending on the treatment tools such as laser devices or peeling agents (laser or chemical dependent). Second, the results of the treatment vary depending on the physician (doctor dependent). If the operator has a lot of knowledge and is skillful, better results will be obtained. Third, the results of the procedure vary depending on the patient (patient dependent). No matter how good the laser machine is, even an experienced physician with a lot of knowledge can have completely different results depending on the patient. Therefore, the physician should know the results may vary depending on the patient and should be able to distinguish the patient's skin types to some extent.

Not everyone has the same skin. Just as the skin color of different ethnicities differ, each person has different skin types, such as wrinkled skin, skin with pores, skin with scars, and sensitive skin. These are called skin types. I believe that the cause of various skin types is due to a combination of genetic causes, environmental causes (such as the latitude and humidity in which you live), and personal causes (such as makeup habits or the habit of rubbing your face with a towel).

Skin types can be classified according to various criteria, and there are various skin type classification methods. For example, the Fitzpatrick skin type, a representative skin type classification method, classified the skin into six skin types according to the tendency of pigmentation to sunlight and the tendency to burn [15]. In addition to that, there are various classification methods, but I classified the procedures according to the skin type based on the Baumann skin type.

2.11 Treatment by Baumann Skin Type

The Bauman skin type classified the skin into 16 skin types based on four criteria such as dryness, irritation, pigmentation, and wrinkles [16]. However, there are five skin types that are problematic in laser treatment, i.e., very oily skin, very dry skin, very sensitive skin, very pigmented skin, very wrinkled skin. Cautions should be taken when treating these five skin types.

Table 2.7 is a table that summarizes the "procedures to avoid" and "helpful procedures" according to the skin type I have experienced while performing laser treatment for 15 years in consideration of Baumann's skin type. Among the five skin types, wrinkled skin was excluded because there were no problems with laser treatment.

First, the oily skin type is mainly related to acne or rosacea, and the skin in which papules and pustules are frequently observed is considered an oily skin type. Previously I had performed fractional laser treatment on acne-prone skin which resulted in aggravated papules, pustules, and acne-like eruptions, so I have set fractional laser as a contraindication for oily skin types. IPL is also used to treat acne, but I have experienced that acne often worsens after IPL with ultrasonic gel application (possibility of ultrasonic gel clogging the pores?) and consider IPL using ultrasound gel as a contraindication. Helpful procedures include drugs such as doxycycline or isotretinoin used for acne, Jessner's peel, which contains salicylic acid (SA), or modified Jessner's peel, and photodynamic therapy (PDT).

Second, in dry skin type, slight erythema, cracks, and dead skin cells are observed due to dry skin, and I consider rough skin as a dry skin type. Patients who have taken isotretinoin within 6 months are also considered dry skin types. Because these skins have a weak skin barrier, excessive dead skin cells and PIH may often occur even with mild peeling. Therefore, it is better to avoid ablative procedures such as various peelings or fractional lasers. Because the skin barrier is considered weak, a moisturizer that can protect the stratum corneum, iontophoresis to strengthen the epidermis, genesis technique to help collagen regeneration in the basal layer and papillary dermis, nonablative rejuvenation (NAR) including needle RF (fractional microneedle radiofrequency) to help the reticular dermis may be helpful for dry skin. I also think that glycolic acid (GA) peeling, which is known to be effective on both the epidermis and dermis, and stimulates fibroblasts, is also helpful. "Injectable glow," which injects hyaluronic acid (HA) directly into the dermal layer, can also be considered.

Third, the sensitive skin type is a skin type in which inflammation occurs easily due to the breakdown of the skin barrier. Patients with this skin type often complain of pain during the procedure, and sometimes complain of discomfort even with weak laser toning. These patients may observe a slight redness even before the procedure, which is easily reddened after the procedure. In addition, I believe that patients with dermographism, in which urticaria occurs after laser or removing sebum with a comedon remover also belong to the sensitive skin type. As with dry skin types, patients with this skin type easily experience side effects from various peeling or ablative lasers. Severe erythema can be seen after applying "soft peel" (1064 nm Q-switched laser after applying carbon powder on face) or skin scrub. Antihistamines are recommended for those with sensitive skin types, and I think the treatments that are helpful for dry skin types will also be helpful for sensitive skin types.

Finally, patients with Fitzpatrick skin type IV or V by questionnaire, visible PIH, melasma, and

Table 2.7 Procedures to avoid and helpful procedures by skin types

Skin type	Diagnosis	Procedures to avoid	Helpful procedures
Oily	Papules, pustules, acne, rosacea.	Fractional laser, IPL (ultrasonic gel)	Acne medications, SA, PDT
Dry	Slight erythema, cracks, dead skin cells, rough skin condition, taking isotretinoin within 6 months	Ablative procedure (various peeling, fractional laser)	Moisturizer, iontophoresis, genesis, needle RF, GA, "injectable glow"
Sensitive	The patient's discomfort (pain), the skin reddens easily. Dermographism, redness	Soft peel, ablative (various peeling, fractional laser)	Antihistamines, GA, PDL, genesis, long1064
Pigmented	Fitzpatrick questionnaire, visible PIH, melasma, dark facial tone	IPL, Q532, CO_2	Long755, toning, GA, tranexamic acid

SA salicylic acid peel, *PDT* photodynamic therapy, *GA* glycolic acid peel, *needle RF* fractional microneedle radiofrequency. *PDL* pulsed-dye laser, *IPL* intense pulsed light

dark facial tone are thought to be pigmented skin types (refer to Sect. 19.3 in Chap. 19). The procedures to be avoided are the 532 nm Q-switched Nd:YAG laser and the CO_2 laser, and IPL should also be treated with caution. Safe treatments are 755 nm long-pulsed alexandrite laser and laser toning. Among peeling, I think that GA peeling without dead skin cells, which does not damage the skin barrier, is helpful, rather than peeling that causes dead skin cells. Tranexamic acid is also recommended, after consultation with the patient.

The above is just my subjective opinion. I hope that you, through your own experience, decide your own skin type identification method or diagnosis method, and decide which are procedures to avoid and helpful procedures.

References

1. Monheit GD. Suspension for the aging face. Dermatol Clin. 2005;23(3):561–73.
2. Tung R, Rubin MG. Procedures in cosmetic dermatology series: chemical peels E-book. Elsevier Health Sciences; 2010.
3. Mordon S, Brisot D, Fournier N. Using a "non uniform pulse sequence" can improve selective coagulation with a Nd:YAG laser (1.06 microm) thanks to Met-hemoglobin absorption: a clinical study on blue leg veins. Lasers Surg Med. 2003;32(2):160–70.
4. Goldman MP. Cutaneous and cosmetic laser surgery. Philadelphia: Mosby Elsevier; 2006.
5. Calderhead RG, Vasily DB. Low level light therapy with light-emitting diodes for the aging face. Clin Plast Surg. 2016;43(3):541–50.
6. Nouri K. Lasers in dermatology and medicine: dermatologic applications. Springer International Publishing; 2018.
7. Allemann IB, Goldberg DJ. Basics in dermatological laser applications. Karger Medical and Scientific Publishers; 2011.
8. Kauvar A, Hruza G. Principles and practices in cutaneous laser surgery. CRC Press; 2005.
9. Kang S, Fitzpatrick TB. Fitzpatrick's dermatology. New York: McGraw-Hill Education; 2019.
10. Textbook compilation committee in Korean Dermatological Association. TEXTBOOK OF DERMATOLOGY, Seventh Edition (Korean). Seoul: McGraw-Hill Education Korea, Ltd; 2020.
11. Yamashita T, Negishi K, Hariya T, Kunizawa N, Ikuta K, Yanai M, et al. Intense pulsed light therapy for superficial pigmented lesions evaluated by reflectance-mode confocal microscopy and optical coherence tomography. J Invest Dermatol. 2006;126(10):2281–6.
12. Yamashita T, Negishi K, Hariya T, Yanai M, Iikura T, Wakamatsu S. In vivo microscopic approaches for facial melanocytic lesions after quality-switched ruby laser therapy: time-sequential imaging of melanin and melanocytes of solar lentigo in Asian skin. Dermatol Surg. 2010;36(7):1138–47.
13. Mun JY, Jeong SY, Kim JH, Han SS, Kim IH. A low fluence Q-switched Nd:YAG laser modifies the 3D structure of melanocyte and ultrastructure of melanosome by subcellular-selective photothermolysis. J Electron Microsc. 2011;60(1):11–8.
14. Nam J-H, Kim H-S, Lee G-Y, Kim W-S. Beneficial effect of low fluence 1,064 nm Q-switched neodymium: Yttrium-Aluminum-Garnet laser in the treatment of senile lentigo. Ann Dermatol. 2017;29(4):427–32.
15. Richter AL, Barrera J, Markus RF, Brissett A. Laser skin treatment in non-Caucasian patients. Facial Plast Surg Clin North Am. 2014;22(3):439–46.
16. Baumann LS, Baumann L. Cosmetic dermatology. McGraw-Hill Professional Publishing; 2009.

Medical Skin Care

3

3.1 Medical Skin Care

Medical skin care refers to a combination of medical treatment performed under a doctor's diagnosis and skin care performed according to an individual's skin characteristics [1]. Medical skin care proceeds in the order of diagnosis, cleansing, moistening, treatment, soothing and moisturizing, sun protection, and makeup (Table 3.1) [2]. An important point in the order of medical skin care is that moistening (moisturizing) is included before and after treatment. To briefly explain the process of medical skin care, the patient visits the hospital and first receives an accurate skin diagnosis, removes foreign substances such as cosmetics on the face, moistening is performed before treatment and soothing and moisturizing is performed after treatment. Finally, cosmetics such as moisturizers or sunscreen is applied and the patient is sent home.

Let's review this step by step.

Diagnosis refers to setting up a skin care plan by accurately diagnosing a patient's disease, identifying the skin type, and the degree of aging [2]. First, history and physical examination are necessary for diagnosis. The patient's history should identify what the patient wants to be treated for (chief complaint), and it is necessary to understand what kind of laser treatment in the past was effective and whether there were any side effects (past history). If there were side effects with a specific laser, cautions should be taken when treating with the same laser. Medical history should also be identified. For example, if the patient is taking isotretinoin, procedures such as peeling or procedures that have peeling effects should be performed with caution because the skin is very dry and skin regeneration is poor. On the other hand, if the patient is taking aspirin, bleeding should be expected during procedures such as melanocytic nevus removal or fractional laser. In addition, skin types such as Fitzpatrick skin type and Baumann skin type should be identified through questionnaire and simple physical examination. Based on the above, three lesions should be identified: First, lesions that should be treated. Second, lesions that can be easily treated without side effect. Third, lesions that have a high risk of side effects and in which caution should be taken.

Table 3.1 Order of medical skin care

Order of medical skin care
Diagnosis → Cleansing → Moistening → Treatment → Soothing & moisturizing → Sun protection → Makeup

Physical examination consists mainly of inspection, but palpation is also important. In the case of psoriasis, hard keratin can be felt by palpation, and in actinic keratosis, the feeling of sandpaper is important for diagnosis. Palpation distinguishes between flat lentigines and raised seborrheic keratosis. Also, in the case of comedones, palpation is as important as inspection

J. D. Lee, M. J. M. Oh, *Lasers in Dermatology: Parameters and Choice*,
https://doi.org/10.1007/978-981-19-7568-4_3

because (1) comedones can be palpated and (2) hidden comedones can be observed only after pulling on the skin [1].

Although there are various examination methods in dermatology, I think that magnifying glass and photography are the most important in medical skin care (Table 3.2). The recommended magnification of a magnifying glass is 7 times, and even a commonly used magnifying glass with a magnification of 3–5 times must be used to thoroughly observe the skin condition [1]. There is an expensive magnifying glass for dermatology (SkinLite II), but I think a cheap magnifying glass purchased online will also do (Fig. 3.1). In addition, a loupe worn on the head is required during laser treatment (Fig. 3.2).

Photography is essential for comparison of results before and after treatment and to avoid disputes. It would be useful to have a photographing equipment such as the recently released box-type skin analysis system (Janus®, PSI corporation, Ltd., Seoul, Korea, Mark-Vu®; PSI PLUS Co., Ltd., Suwon, Korea), but if there is no such equipment, taking a picture directly with a camera will suffice. An important point in photography is reproducibility. It would be ideal to have a separate photo studio, but if this is not possible, the photos should be shot in the same place, with the same lighting and background, in the same posture, and at the same angle. At least five basic photos are required, including a front photo, two side photos, and two 45-degree photos (Fig. 3.3) [1]. In the case of front and side photos, it is possible to take relatively constant photos, but there is no special standard for 45-degree photos, so the location may change each time a photo is taken and with each person taking it. This is why I take the 45-degree photo based on the angle where the patient's nose and cheek meet.

Second, cleansing refers to the process of removing dirty substances, secretions such as sweat, sebum, or exfoliated keratin and corneocytes. There are primary, secondary, and tertiary cleansing methods for skin care. Primary cleansing (point makeup cleansing) is removing makeups of the lip and eye by makeup removers. Secondary cleansing (facial cleansing) is wiping the face with a cleanser suitable for the skin such as lotion, cream, oil, gel, and water. Tertiary cleansing (applying tonic) is a step that uses softening tonic or astringent tonic to neutralize the alkaline components of the soap and cleanser to normalize the skin's pH and supply sufficient

Table 3.2 Dermatology examination method [2]

Dermatology examination method
• Visual examination
– Magnifying glass
• Dermoscopy
• Skin diagnosis device using magnifying lens
• Wood lamp, polarizer
– Photography
• Diascopy
• Skin analysis program
• Biopsy
• Corneometer to measure skin moisture
• Sebumeter to measure oiliness of the skin
• Chromameter and mexameter to evaluate color
• Evaporimeter or tewameter to measure the transepidermal water loss.

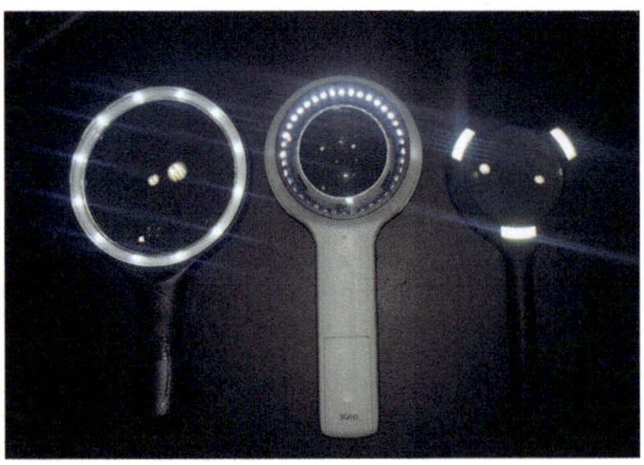

Fig. 3.1 Various magnifying glasses

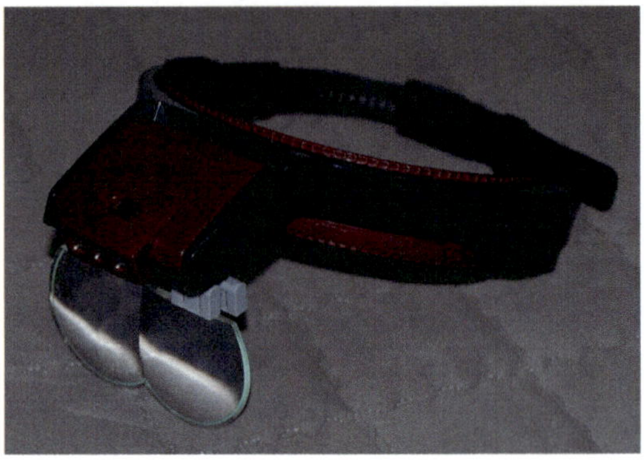

Fig. 3.2 Loupe

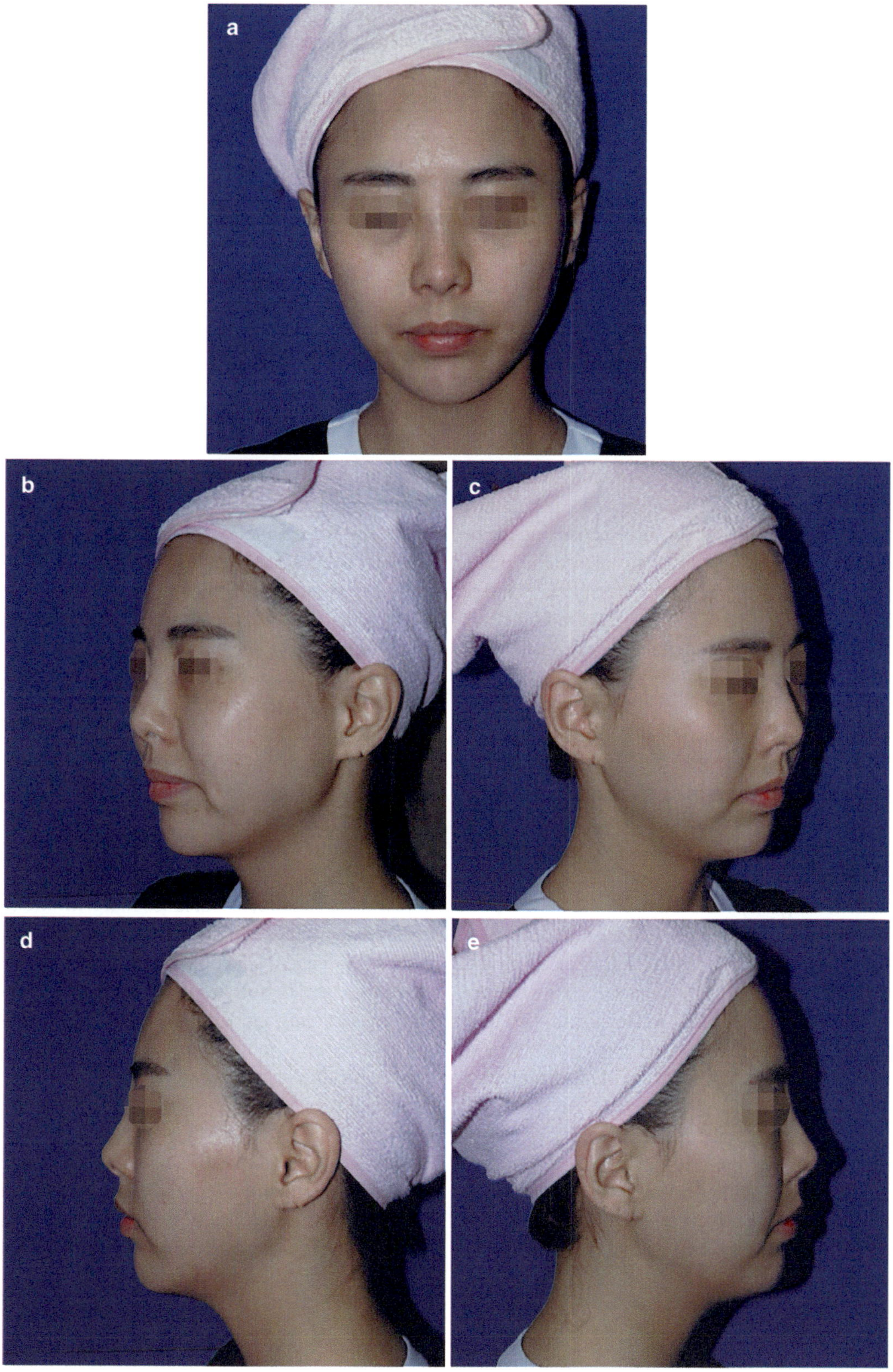

Fig. 3.3 Five basic photos for medical skin care. (**a**) Front photo, (**b**) left 45-degree photo, (**c**) right 45-degree photo, (**d**) left side photo, (**e**) right side photo

moisture to the skin [2]. The skin scrub method is also a cleansing method that uses beauty device.

Sometimes, deep cleansing is performed after tertiary cleansing. Depending on the method, deep cleansing includes physical deep cleansing, biological deep cleansing, chemical deep cleansing, and complex deep cleansing. Physical deep cleansing has scrub types and gommage types, biological deep cleansing uses enzyme for deep cleansing, and chemical deep cleansing uses AHA (alpha-hydroxy acid) or BHA (beta-hydroxy acid) [1].

Now let's take a brief look at tonics. There are softening tonics and astringent tonics [1]. First, softening tonic refers to skin, lotion, and toner. "Skin" and "lotion," which patients often talk about, are softening tonics. Softening tonic provides moisture to the skin, making it soft and moist, and helps the next stage of cosmetics to be absorbed well. It also helps to restore the skin's pH to normal. The pH of normal skin is 5.5–6.5. However, when the skin is damaged, the pH changes to neutral or alkaline, allowing bacteria to penetrate, and the softening tonic restores the pH to normal. Therefore, it is essential to apply softening tonic after all procedures. Second, astringent tonic, called an astringent, has a soothing effect by cooling the skin, temporarily constricting pores, and removing sebum. I use alum containing astringent tonic when I apply soothing pack after a procedure.

Cleansing steps are complicated and take a long time, such as primary cleansing, secondary cleansing, tertiary cleansing, and deep cleansing. Because the purpose of cleansing is to remove foreign substances and wastes from the skin before the procedure, I let my patients self-cleanse and then only perform skin scrub with a cosmetic device.

Third, moistening (moisturizing) is the process of restoring the lost moisture of the stratum corneum. Moistening increases skin temperature and expands skin blood vessels to promote microcirculation. In addition, as the moisture of the skin increases, the skin becomes soft and the effect of cosmetic procedures performed afterward can be enhanced. The moistening method generally uses a facial steamer or a steam towel [2]. A facial steamer is a machine that uses boiling water to spray steam on the face, but it takes a lot of time, so I mainly use the steam towel. The towel soaked in water is stored in the heating cabinet, and when the patient enters the skin care room it is used to cover the patient's face. Steam towels also have the effect of wiping away sebum and waste from the face.

After the above, if necessary, topical anesthesia can be applied or injection may be performed for local anesthesia or nerve block. Anesthetic eye drops (alkyne 0.5% eye drops) may be used before eye shield (corneal protector) is placed under the eyelids. Lidocaine spray can also be used for mucosal anesthesia, but it is usually not necessary for cosmetic procedures. Anesthesia time can be reduced when using topical anesthesia by using occlusive therapy, which increases the percutaneous absorption by 10–100 times [1]. When treating the entire face, topical anesthesia should be applied to the entire face and it should be sealed with a plastic wrap for 20–40 minutes.

Fourth, treatment refers to the process of treating diseases or damage to the skin using laser, ablation, ultrasound device, iontophoresis, and functional products for whitening or anti-aging. That is, it refers to the main treatment we want to implement. Treatment includes surgical treatment (laser treatment, ablation, surgical treatment of acne, electrosurgery, liposuction, vascular sclerosis, soft tissue correction, ambulatory phlebectomy, etc.), medical skin care (ultrasound device, iontophoresis, microablation, oxygen treatment, etc.), and aesthetic skin care (exfoliation using cosmetics, etc.) [2].

Fifth, soothing and moisturizing refers to the process of soothing and moisturizing the irritated skin after treatment. Face packs or low-power lasers are frequently used. The functions of face pack include moisturizing due to occlusive effect, increase of blood circulation, increase of active ingredient penetration due to absorption effect, cleansing to remove contamination of the skin surface, acne treatment, comfort and stability. There are tissue off type, wash off type, and peel off type face packs [1]. Since I mainly use laser, I use a peel off type cool modeling face pack. First, gauze moistened with alum is applied on the skin (Fig. 3.4) and then cool modeling face pack is applied. After 15–20 min, the face pack is removed and a low-power laser, LED (light emitting diode) is performed,

Sixth, sun protection and makeup refer to the process of protecting the skin from UV rays and applying cosmetics to areas that need to be covered and emphasized. First, the face pack is removed and the softening tonic described above is applied. After moisturizer cream applied, sunscreen and make-up may be applied. However, I usually only apply BB cream according to the patient's request and finish medical skin care (Fig. 3.5).

3.2 Homecare

Patients visit the clinic at most once a week, and skin care is about 1–2 h. In addition, laser treatment takes only 10–20 min at most. The rest of the time is entirely dependent on the patient. In other words, no matter how good the laser treatment, patient's exposure to sunshine for an hour can result in new pigmentation and aggravation of melasma.

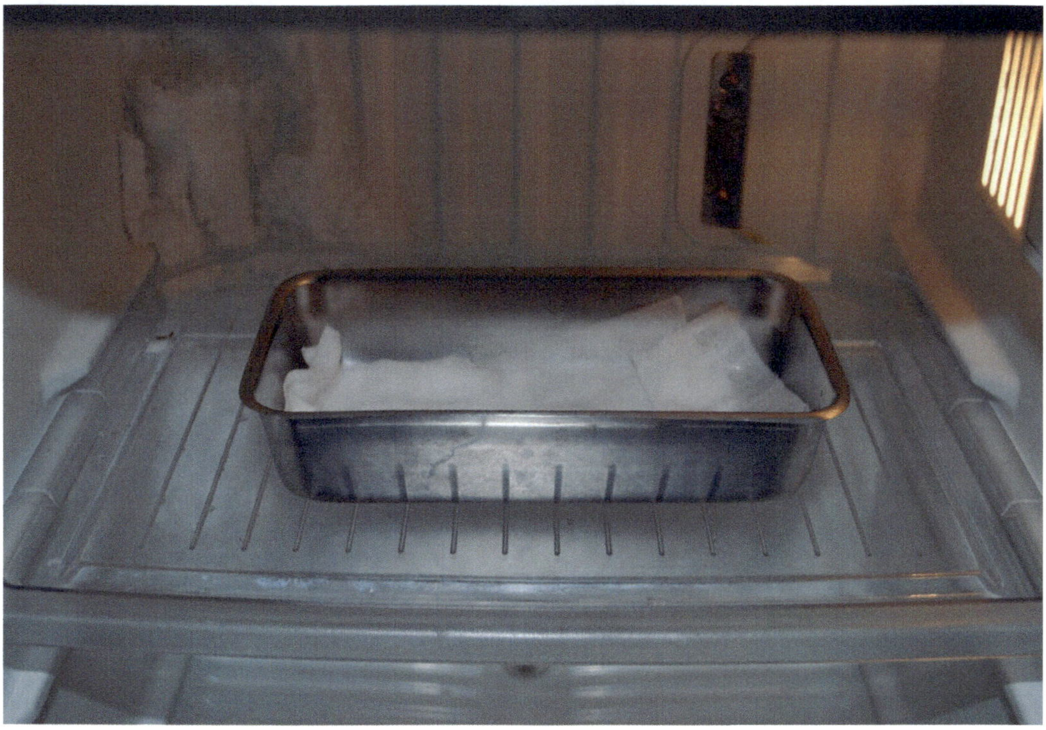

Fig. 3.4 Alum. 4 × 4 inch gauze is spread multi-layer and placed on a tray. Solution diluted with 3% alum is poured into a tray and stored in the refrigerator

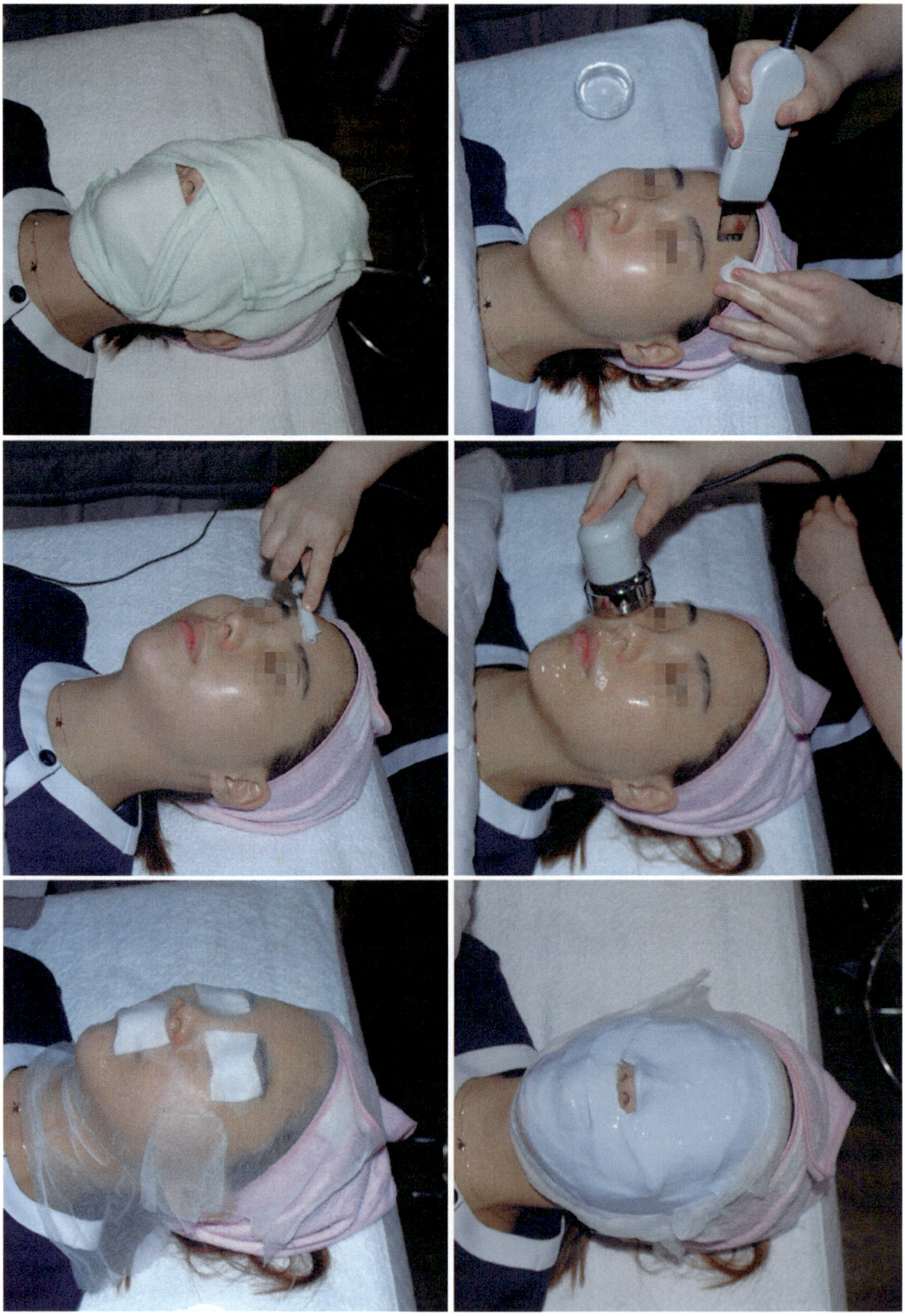

Fig. 3.5 Medical skin care. From above, moistening, skin scrub, iontophoresis, sonophoresis, gauze moistened with alum, peel off type modeling face pack, LED, moisture cream, BB cream, finishing touch

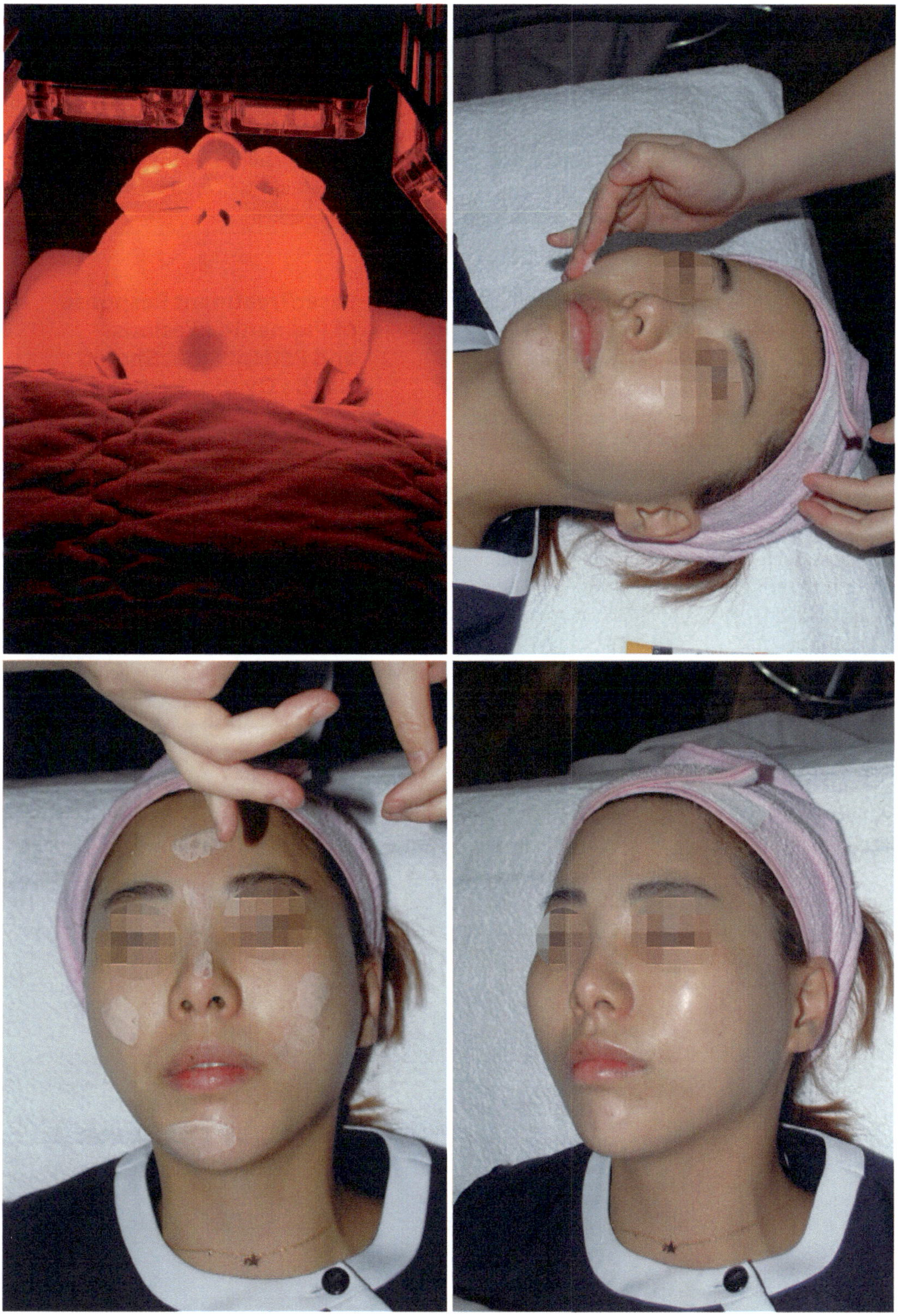

Fig. 3.5 (continued)

I emphasize three things for homecare.

First, you must wear sunscreen. The most important thing in using sunscreen is the amount you apply. Because sunscreen is easily erased after friction, sweating, and especially swimming, the dermatology text, "Text book of Dermatology, 7th Ed. (Korean)," recommends applying sunscreen 20 ~ 30 minutes before outdoor activity and reapplying every two to three hours [3]. In reality, however, it is not easy to apply every two to three hours, so I recommend applying it in the morning and applying it before going out, i.e., applying at least twice a day. I also recommend wearing a hat or a sunshade.

Second, moisturizers should be applied. The basic function of the skin is the "skin barrier" that protects the skin. In particular, it plays a role in confining moisture in our bodies. But due to aging, lipid contents drop resulting in reduction of moisturizing power, and ultimately breaking down the "skin barrier." Therefore, intercellular lipids should be supplemented with the moisturizer.

Finally, skin should not be irritated. Kenichirou Kasai, the author of the book, "Skin Spot Treatment Clinics," describes the causes of melasma as the breakdown of barriers caused by chronic hyper-irritation [4]. Just irritating the skin can cause melasma and darken the skin. Therefore, when washing the face, rubbing with a lot of friction should be avoided. A lot of soap bubbles should be made to gently "pump" them to the face, so that the hands do not touch the face. Trying to remove all makeup should be discouraged and one should believe "It doesn't matter if there's makeup left." Cosmetics irritating the skin should be avoided and when applying makeup and irritation should be minimized by "softly tapping" on the skin rather than rubbing. Finally, skin irritation should be reduced by reducing the number and type of cosmetics applied to the face. Rather, it may be better not to put on any makeup.

3.3 Laser Treatment Response of Pigmented Lesions and Patients that Should Not Be Overlooked

For pigmentation treatment, the principle and parameters of laser are important, but accurate diagnosis and differential diagnosis of various pigmented lesions are also important. It is also important to know the response to laser treatment for each pigmented lesion. In other words, there are pigmented lesions that are effective with laser, but there are also pigmented lesions that are not very responsive to laser. If you do not specialize in pigmentation treatment, there is no need to treat pigmented lesions that are difficult to treat. Rather, side effects such as hyperpigmentation, hypopigmentation, and scarring may occur, which may cause patient complaint. Therefore, private practice physicians should not attempt to cure all pigments.

I actively treat "pigmented lesions that respond well to laser/IPL treatments" while rarely treat "pigmented lesions that sometimes respond to laser treatments" (Table 3.3). For example, I

Table 3.3 Classification of melanocytic nevi and tumors according to the response to laser treatment [5]

Pigmented lesions that respond well to laser/IPL treatments	Pigmented lesions that sometimes respond to laser treatments	High-risk lesions that should not be treated with lasers
1. Simple lentigo and freckles 2. Labial lentigo (i.e., associated with Peutz-Jeghers) 3. Nevus of Ota, Ito, residual Mongolian spot, simple blue nevi 4. Acquired bilateral nevus of Ota-like macule (ABNOM, Hori's nevus) 5. Palmoplantar congenital nevi	1. Café-au-lait macules (CALM, called nevus spilus in Japan) 2. Nevus spilus (CALM-like lesion speckled, often with junctional nevi) 3. Congenital nevus 4. Becker's nevus 5. Melasma	1. Dysplastic nevi 2. Lentigo maligna

explain to my patients that Café-au-lait macules treatments are "1/3 effective, 1/3 not effective, and 1/3 effective but may relapse" and let the patient decide. In nevus spilus only the melanocytic nevi inside the brown nevus are removed, and in Becker's nevus, only laser hair removal is performed. Congenital melanocytic nevus is treated repeatedly with pinhole method only for small congenital melanocytic nevus (less than 1.5 cm) or small medium-sized congenital melanocytic nevus.

There are also skin lesions that are very responsive to treatment and should not be overlooked. I think that patients with the following four lesions are "patients that should not be overlooked" (Table 3.4). First, "freckles" are effective with any laser treatment and has few side effects. This is because freckles have a genetic origin [6] and patients with freckles usually have bright skin tones and Fitzpatrick skin types I, II, and III are not prone to PIH. Second, "PIH induced by acne" disappears naturally with good acne treatment. In particular, there are case reports of dramatic improvement in PIH as well as acne by taking low-dose isotretinoin [7]. Third, despite the fact that "ABNOM (Acquired bilateral nevus of Ota-like macule)" treatment frequently causes PIH and melasma, and that the treatment period is long, eventually ABNOM will disappear if treatment is continued. If the ABNOM patient can be convinced to go through the treatment, ABNOM will be cured and the doctor will become a "great doctor." Fourth, although it is not a pigmented lesion, I believe that patients with rosacea should not be overlooked. Recurrence is common, but it can be easily treated only by medication such as doxycycline or the genesis technique.

In addition to pigmented lesions, the laser reactions to blood vessels, hair removal, nevi, and tumors are described in Table 3.5. However, since Table 3.5 is a table created based on my personal experience, this is just for your information.

Table 3.4 Patients that should not be overlooked

Patients that should not be overlooked
1. Freckles
2. PIH induced by acne
3. ABNOM
4. Rosacea

Table 3.5 Classification of various lesions by response to laser treatment

	Lesions that respond very well to laser treatments	Lesions that respond moderately to laser treatments	Lesions that do not respond very well to laser treatments and frequently recur
Blood vessel	Senile hemangioma Port-wine stain (by only PDL)	Rosacea Spider nevus Venous lake Pyogenic granuloma Acne	Erythema
Pigmentation	Ephelis Melanonychia	Lentigo smaller than 1 cm ABNOM Nevus of Ota Acne PIH	Lentigo larger than 1 cm Melasma CALM Nevus spilus Becker's nevus
Tattoo	Black tattoo Amateur tattoo	Red tattoo Green tattoo (by ruby)	Yellow tattoo Semi-permanent tattoo
Hair removal	Thick hair (armpits, calves)	Thin hair (mustache)	

(continued)

Table 3.5 (continued)

	Lesions that respond very well to laser treatments	Lesions that respond moderately to laser treatments	Lesions that do not respond very well to laser treatments and frequently recur
Nonablative		Elasticity	Pores, wrinkle
Nevus, tumor	Acquired nevus Seborrheic keratosis Milia Soft fibroma	Congenital nevus (small) Sebaceous gland hyperplasia Seborrheic keratosis larger than 1 cm	Congenital nevus (medium, large) Epidermal nevus Syringoma Porokeratosis Dermatofibroma Xanthoma palpebrarum
Scar		Atrophic acne scar Keloids Hypertrophic scar	Burn scar, Post-operative scar Striae distensae Chicken pox scar

3.4 One-Time Treatment Vs Package Treatment

Most patients want to get rid of 100% pigmentations on their face with a single laser treatment session, but this is impossible, and there is a high risk of side effects. I recommend that laser procedure should be performed in multiple sessions rather than in a single procedure. You have to do what is called "ticketing." The advantage of "ticketing" is, first, a stepwise treatment is possible as pretreatment. For example, first, the epidermal pigmentations are treated, and later, the blood vessels in the dermis may be treated. Also, low fluences may be shot first and skin reactions are observed later to decide whether to raise the fluence or stop the treatment. Second, post-treatment can be included in the course of treatment. If PIH occurs during the course of treatment, there is time to treat PIH itself.

3.5 Package Therapy and Combination Therapy

Package therapy is not simply receiving various lasers or procedures but must be performed in order with a purpose (sequential procedure). For example, in the case of melasma treatment, I think it is safer to perform laser toning first to lower the activity of melanocytes than to use long-pulsed alexandrite laser first. In addition, package therapy also enables increasing of the energy of the long-pulsed alexandrite laser little by little so that PIH does not occur and securing time to treat PIH in advance if PIH occurs.

Combination therapy, in which several procedures are performed simultaneously on the same day, has several advantages. First, each treatment can be effective even if it is treated weakly, and it can be safe because it is performed weakly. Second, it is possible to see a synergy effect.

In case of package therapy, by what principle should the procedure sequence be determined? Also, in case of combination therapy, by what principle should the procedure sequence be determined?

First, let's consider the procedure sequence of package therapy. In order to determine the procedure sequence, it is necessary to fully understand the structure and function of the skin as well as the principle and side effects of each laser or procedure. Here, I will describe only a few principles that I consider. First, in the case of a procedure in which the epidermis is damaged, it takes at least a month for normal epithelialization to proceed. Therefore, in the case of ablation or ablative laser, the treatment should be performed with an interval of at least 1 month. However, in the case of epidermal pigmentation treatment such as shallow ablation or IPL, which produces crusts in places, I think treatment interval of 2 weeks is adequate, given that the skin barrier is strong. Second, dermal pigmentations such as nevus of Ota, ABNOM, and tattoos take 1–3 months to be removed after laser. Therefore, the procedure should be performed every 1–3 months. A faster procedure, e.g., every 1–2 weeks, does not result in faster removal. Third, melanocytic nevus removal or strong CO_2 fractional laser treatment for scar treatment should be performed with at least 2–3 months interval. Although epithelialization has already been completed, the dermis has not been completely regenerated. Thus, I postpone the procedure even if 2–3 months have passed, especially if erythema remains. Fourth, the upper part of the skin is treated first and the lower part is treated later. For example, if epidermal pigmentations and dermal blood vessels need to be treated together, removing the epidermal pigmentation first and then treating the blood vessels in the dermis will be more effective and will have fewer side effects.

In combination therapy, as opposed to package therapy, I think that deeper procedures or lasers should be performed first and then shallower procedures or lasers should be performed later. For example, in tattoo removal, CO_2 pinhole therapy followed by 1064 nm Q-switched Nd:YAG laser is effective, but considering the side effects, it is a dangerous method. In other words, since we have to give priority to safety first, we must perform procedures in order of "deeper procedure → shallower procedure."

3.6 My Procedure Sequence

For those who are new to laser, I will describe my sequence of brightening procedure and scar procedure as an example. Since each hospital has different lasers and different patient groups, my procedure sequence is not the correct answer, and I also change the procedure little by little over time, so please refer to it only as a reference (Table 3.6).

First, I repeat laser toning and epidermal pigmentation treatment (long-pulsed alexandrite laser, repeat pulse method, CO_2 defocusing method) targeting epidermal pigmentations. Generally epidermal pigmentation improves after 2 times of treatment (after session 4). Then instead of epidermal pigmentation treatments, other treatments may be performed depending on the patient. If erythema treatment is required, PDL or needle RF is used, and if pores, scar, wrinkle, and elasticity treatment are required, CO_2 fractional laser or needle RF is added to the even number of sessions instead of epidermal pigmentation treatment. After the fourth session, it is necessary to distinguish whether the remaining pigment is PIH or dermal pigmentations. For PIH, laser toning, one-shot toning, or long-pulsed alexandrite laser with low fluence may be performed. For dermal pigmentations, the energy is increased by using the focusing method (refer to Sect. 5.7 in Chap. 5) for treatment. If melasma does not respond to treatment after the fourth session, the fluence of one-shot toning should be raised.

If you purchased only the basic lasers, CO_2 laser, LED, and Q-switched Nd:YAG laser, and would develop a package therapy for the first time, I recommend the procedure sequence shown in

Table 3.6 My brightening treatment protocol

Session	Procedure
1	Scrub+laser toning+one shot toning+genesis technique+GA50 + brightening skin care+face pack
2	Topical anesthesia+long-pulsed alexandrite laser+CO_2 + repeat pulse method+face pack+LED
3	Scrub+laser toning+one shot toning+genesis technique+GA50 + brightening skin care+face pack
4	Topical anesthesia+CO_2 laser+repeat pulse method+focusing method+skin pack+LED
Erythema	Scrub+(PDL or needle RF) + GA50 + LED
Pores, scar, wrinkle, elasticity	Topical anesthesia+CO_2 + (CO_2 fractional laser or needle RF) + PDRN+LED

A total of 10 treatments are performed at intervals of 1–2 weeks, and if a lot of epidermal pigmentations have disappeared after 1–4 treatments, additional erythema, pores, scar, wrinkle, and elasticity treatments are added depending on the patient. If PIH occurs after the fourth episode, PIH treatment is performed, and if dermal pigmentation is suspected, the focusing method is used

Table 3.7 Brightening treatment protocol recommended for beginners

Session	Procedure
1	Scrub+laser toning+one shot toning+MJP(modified Jessner's peel) + brightening skin care+face pack
2	Topical anesthesia +CO_2 + repeat pulse method(Q532) + face pack+LED
3	Scrub+laser toning+ one shot toning+MJP + brightening skin care+face pack
4	Topical anestheisa+CO_2 + repeat pulse method+face pack+LED or scrub+laser toning+one shot toning+(MJP X) + brightening skin care+face pack
5	Scrub+laser toning+one shot toning+MJP + brightening skin care+face pack
6	Scrub+laser toning+one shot toning+(MJP X) + brightening skin care+face pack
A total of 10 treatments are performed at intervals of 1–2 weeks, and after session 4, repeat session 5 and 6.	

Table 3.8 My scar treatment protocol

Session	Procedure
1	Topical anesthesia+subcision+CO_2 pinhole+CO_2 fractional laser (FAST method) + PDRN+face pack+LED
2	Scrub+laser toning+one shot toning+genesis technique+GA50 + brightening skin care+face pack
Session 1 and 2 are performed, 1 week apart. They are then repeated after 1–2 months, for a total of 10 treatments, and the results are judged after 6 months	

Table 3.7. Laser toning is the backbone and MJP (modified Jessner's peel), a mild peeling is performed every 2 weeks. In session 2, melanocytic nevus and lentigo should be removed by CO_2 laser and small epidermal pigmentations should be removed by the defocusing method. Relatively large epidermal pigmentations are carefully removed using the repeat pulse method by the 532 nm Q-switched Nd:YAG. If there is remaining pigmentations during session 4, pigmentation treatment should be performed again (same as session 2) On the other hand, if there are no remaining pigmentations, laser toning is performed without MJP. For remaining pigmentations after session 4, laser toning and one-shot toning are used for PIH, and focusing method for dermal pigmentations.

For scar treatment, several procedures are combined and performed on the same day and brightening and regeneration procedures are performed the following week (Table 3.8). After 1–2 months, scar treatment, brightening, and regeneration procedures are repeated again. A total of 10 treatments are performed. Since collagen regeneration lasts up to 6 months after the procedure, the results are judged after 6 months.

I perform subcision to rolling scars, and then CO_2 pinhole therapy to icepick and boxcar scars (refer to Sect. 17.4 in Chap. 17). In addition, the FAST method is used to treat rolling scars and boxcar scars, by using a CO_2 fractional laser with increased density and energy, so that only areas with scars are treated, usually with a 5 × 5 mm area (refer to Sect. 12.8 in Chap. 12).

References

1. Jeong JY. Clinical skin care (Korean). Seoul: MDworld; 2010.
2. Textbook compilation committee in Korean Dermatological Association. Text book of dermatology 6th edition (Korean). Seoul: Daehanuihak; 2014.
3. Textbook compilation committee in Korean Dermatological Association. TEXTBOOK OF DERMATOLOGY, seventh edition (Korean). Seoul: McGraw-Hill Education Korea, Ltd; 2020.
4. Kasai K. Skin spots treatment clinics (Korean edition). Seoul: Shinheung med science; 2007.
5. Suzuki H, Anderson RR. Treatment of melanocytic nevi. Dermatol Ther. 2005;18(3):217–26.
6. Allemann IB, Goldberg DJ. Basics in dermatological laser applications. Karger Medical and Scientific Publishers; 2011.
7. Winhoven SM, Ahmed I, Owen CM, Lear JT. Postinflammatory hyperpigmentation in an Asian patient: a dramatic response to oral isotretinoin (13-cis-retinoic acid). Br J Dermatol. 2005;152(2):368–9.

Part III

Lasers and Parameters

4 Q-Switched Ruby Laser, Absorption Coefficient, and Spot Size Effect

4.1 Introduction of Q-Switched Ruby Laser

Wavelength of Q-switched ruby laser is 694 nm, which has the highest absorption coefficient for melanin compared to hemoglobin (Table 4.1). The pulse duration (PD) of the Q-switched ruby laser is 40 ns and TRT of melanosome is 250–100 ns [1, 2], and because TRT > PD in selective photothermolysis, Q-switched ruby laser is suitable for treating melanosomes. However, in Q-switched ruby lasers, our actual target is not melanosomes, which are subcellular organelles, but rather cells such as keratinocytes or melanocytes that have melanosomes. Since TRT (15–30 μs [3]) of cells is too large compared to PD (<50 ns) of Q-switched laser, Q-switched laser cannot directly destroy the cells, but a photoacoustic effect (a type of photomechanical effect) that causes shock waves or cavitation can be used to blast melanosomes to damage the nucleus or cell membrane of cells, thereby indirectly destroying keratinocytes or melanocytes to cause necrosis (refer to Sect. 1.11 in Chap. 1).

Table 4.1 Specifications of Q-switched ruby lasers (TattooStar R, Asclepion Laser Technologies GmbH, Jena, Germany)

Laser type	Q-switched ruby laser
Wavelength	694 nm
Spot size	2.5, 4, 5, optional 6 mm
Pulse duration	Approx. 40 ns
Energy density	Max. 23 J/cm^2 (1.2 J)
Pulse rate	0.5–2 Hz

Because wavelength of Q-switched ruby laser has a low absorption coefficient for hemoglobin, the risk of vascular damage is low. But post-inflammatory hyperpigmentation (PIH), our main concern, does not result from vascular damage alone (refer to Sect. 19.6 in Chap. 19). Shock wave is more important for PIH than blood vessel damage. The shorter the wavelength, the higher the absorption coefficient of melanin and larger the shock wave. Therefore, Q-switched ruby laser has a lower PIH rate than 532 nm, but a higher PIH rate than 755 nm or 1064 nm (The longer the wavelength, the safer. Refer to Sect. 2.7 in Chap. 2). Also, because of the strong shock wave, hypopigmentation, which is rarely observed in 1064 nm Q-switched Nd:YAG laser, is often observed with Q-switched ruby laser treatment. The optical penetration depth (OPD) is 750 μm [1], which is effective for the treatment of the epidermal layer and the upper dermis [the thickness of the epidermis is 100 μm, and the thickness of the skin is 1000 to 2000 μm (1–2 mm) [4]]. Therefore, although the therapeutic effect on epidermal pigmentations and ABNOM located in the upper dermis is high, it is difficult to completely remove tattoo particles or nevus of Ota which are located deeply.

J. D. Lee, M. J. M. Oh, *Lasers in Dermatology: Parameters and Choice*,
https://doi.org/10.1007/978-981-19-7568-4_4

4.2 Three-Level and Four-Level Lasers

To produce stimulated emission, theoretically, a laser medium only needs to be in an excited state and a ground state (resting state). But mediums with metastable state—which is a stable state between ground state and excited state—are used in real lasers [5].

Thus, the laser which has ground, excited, and metastable state is called a three-level laser, and the laser that has two metastable state is called a four-level laser. The typical three and four-level lasers are ruby laser and Nd:YAG laser, respectively (Figs. 4.1 and 4.2) [7].

In a three-level laser, the lower laser level is in the ground state so there are many electrons in the low energy level. Therefore, high energy is needed for population inversion and a flash lamp with high output is used. Thus three-level lasers are usually pulsed wave lasers. Because three-level laser needs high output, this makes them expensive but, the laser can produce very high energy (pulse energy 20 J). On the other hand, four-level lasers need low energy for population inversion so that low output flash lamp can be used. Therefore, most continuous wave lasers use four-level lasers [7].

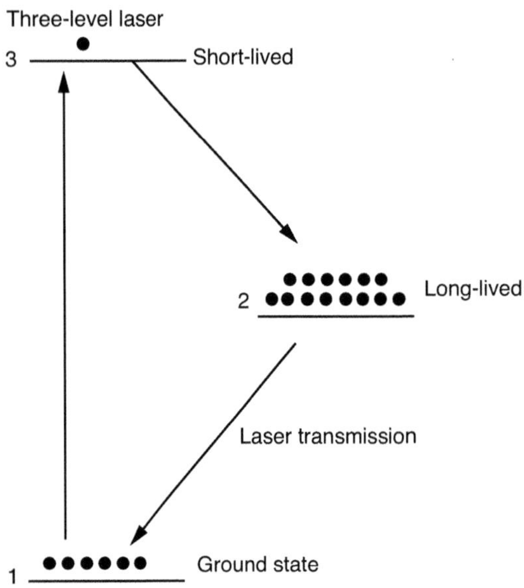

Fig. 4.1 Three-level laser. Reproduced from [6]

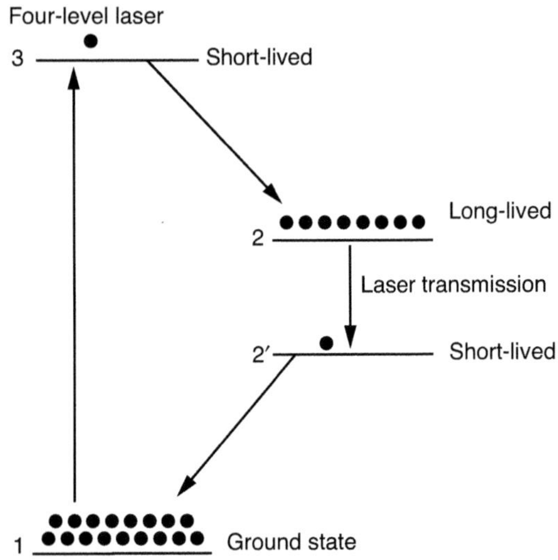

Fig. 4.2 Four-level lasers. Reproduced from [6]

Since Q-switched ruby laser is a three-level laser, it requires a high-output flash lamp, so the purchase cost is high, and the maintenance cost is high because the flash lamp needs to be replaced frequently and there is much machine damage. In addition, the speed is slow (up to 2 Hz), the spot size is small, and the output is also unstable.

4.3 Indications

Since the target chromophore is melanin, Q-switched ruby laser is used for epidermal and dermal pigmentations (Table 4.2), and tattoo removal located deep in the dermis. Although Q-switched ruby laser can be used to treat melanocytic nevus, it cannot be removed all at once because photons cannot penetrate deep into thick nevus with dark pigment (mass effect). Therefore, Q-switched lasers are not used alone for the treatment of melanocytic nevus but is used as an adjunct after ablative lasers such as CO_2 lasers. In the case of tattoo treatment, the treatment effect differs depending on the color of the tattoo. Because the complementary color of green is red, green tattoo is well absorbed by Q-switched ruby laser with a red wavelength and is effective, while a red tattoo cannot be absorbed, and has almost no

Table 4.2 Melanocytic nevi and tumors [8]

Epidermal melanocytic lesions	Dermal melanocytic lesions	Melanocytic nevus
1. Freckle (Ephelides) 2. Lentigo 3. Café-au-lait macule (CALM) 4. Nevus spilus (speckled lentiginous nevus) 5. Becker's nevus	1. Mongolian spot 2. Nevus of Ota 3. Nevus of Ito 4. Acquired bilateral nevus of Ota-like macules (ABNOM)	5. Acquired melanocytic nevus 6. Congenital melanocytic nevus 7. Special forms

Table 4.3 Tattoo colors and corresponding Q-switched lasers. Reproduced from [2]

Tattoo colors	Pulse duration (ns)	Wavelength (nm)	Q-switched lasers
Red	5–10	532	Frequency-doubled Nd:YAG
Black, blue, green	25–40	694	Ruby
Black, blue, green	50–100	755	Alexandrite
Black, blue	5–10	1064	Nd:YAG

effect [2]. Also, Q-switched ruby laser is effective for black tattoo treatment like other Q-switched lasers (Table 4.3) [1].

In addition, Q-switched ruby laser can be used to treat melasma and PIH, but because the spot size is not large, the speed (frequency, Hz) is slow, and the lamp lifespan is short and expensive, this is not recommended. Thus, Q-switched ruby laser is not suitable for performing conventional laser toning.

4.4 Absorption Coefficient

All Q-switched lasers have a fixed pulse duration and do not require epidermal cooling, so if you purchase a specific laser (if you chose a wavelength), you only need to adjust a spot size, fluence, and speed (Hz) among the six parameters of the skin laser. Since Q-switched ruby laser is not fast (Hz), the parameters we need to adjust are fluence and spot size. Next, we will learn about absorption coefficient and appropriate spot size related to fluence.

It may be thought that absorption coefficient of a specific chromophore has a constant value, but this is not true. Even with the same chromophore, absorption coefficient depends on the "concentration of the chromophore" [9]. Also, our hypothesized chromophore is a single target, but the actual chromophore is a target group. For example, when treating pigmentations, a single target is a melanosome, but melanosome concentrations are different for each melanocyte containing melanosomes. Also, the concentration of melanocytes is also different in each lentigines containing melanocytes. Therefore, even though the same melanosomes are targets, light lentigines have a low absorption coefficient while dark lentigines have a high absorption coefficient. Since the temperature must be located within the therapeutic window (refer to Sect. 2.7 in Chap. 2), when the absorption coefficient is high, fluence must be lowered to prevent side effects caused by high temperature, and when the absorption coefficient is low, fluence must be increased to see the effect (formula below [10]). That's why we know empirically that we should irradiate "dark lesions weak and light lesions strong."

$$\Delta T = \frac{F_z \mu_a}{\rho c}\left(\frac{\tau_r}{\tau_r + \tau_p}\right)^{g/2}$$

- ΔT: temperature increase of a desired target
- μ_a: absorption coefficient
- F_z: local subsurface fluence
- ρ: density
- c: specific heat
- g: geometric factor (1 for planes, 2 for cylinders, and 3 for spheres)
- τ_p: laser pulse duration
- τ_r: thermal relaxation time of the target (TRT)

From these, we can draw two conclusions:

1. Different lesions have different concentrations, so energy must be controlled differently. In other words, we should irradiate "dark lesions weak and light lesions strong."
2. There is no absolute parameter.

4.5 Defocusing Method

Since fluence must be adjusted according to the concentration of the lesion, fluence must be varied for each lesion. However, treating one lesion, and then adjusting the fluence of the instrument panel, and then treating the next lesion is too cumbersome and takes a lot of time, so there are often physicians who use defocusing method. Q-switched ruby laser, like the CO_2 laser, has the same number of photons as the handpiece is lifted higher from the skin, but the spot size increases, so the fluence, which is the number of photons/area (unit J/cm^2), decreases. Therefore, light lesions can be treated by focusing, and dark lesions can be treated by defocusing and lowering fluence. The important point in defocusing method is the concept that tissue change of the lesion should be the same regardless of focusing or defocusing, so the clinical end point should be the same.

Large spot sizes and fast speed (Hz) are unavailable for Q-switched ruby lasers. Thus, many physicians use defocusing method to enable fast procedure. When melasma and epidermal pigmentations are present at the same time, the handpiece can be raised high when irradiating melasma and lowered when irradiating epidermal pigmentations, using the defocusing method to perform the procedure quickly. In addition, Q-switched Nd:YAG laser can control fluence at 0.1 J/cm^2 intervals, but the Q-switched ruby laser can control fluence at 0.5 J/cm^2 intervals, so precise fluence control is difficult. To compensate for this, defocusing method is used in the Q-switched ruby laser.

However, the defocusing method requires experience because the distance must be precisely adjusted by judging the concentration of the lesion instantaneously. This method that relies on experience is very inaccurate and the results vary depending on the physician. Therefore, I do not actively recommend the defocusing method.

4.6 Spot Size Effect

Let's learn about the spot size effect. Let's assume that there is a large spot size of 1 cm^2 and a small spot size of 0.5 cm^2, 10 and 5 photons were shot respectively, and there is 2 unabsorbed photons outside the beam. Eight photons will be absorbed by the large spot size and 3 by the small spot size (Fig. 4.3). Fluence is the number of photons per unit area, so the fluence of the laser is 10 J/cm^2 in both spot sizes, but inside the skin, the fluence is different (8 J/cm^2 and 6 J/ m^2, respectively). In other words, the larger the spot size, the higher the actual energy in the skin. The reason for this is because photons that are deviated from the laser direction, and thus not absorbed are constant. Thus, the larger the spot size, the higher the proportion of the relatively absorbed portion. In other words, the unabsorbed portion is a "constant," and the fluence is an energy density, which is a "ratio."

In summary, the energy in the skin is relatively low at small spot sizes and relatively high at large

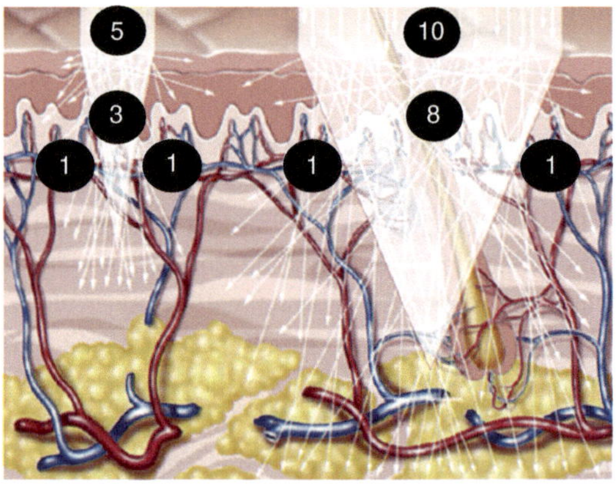

Fig. 4.3 Number of photons according to spot size. If the spot size is 1 cm^2 and 0.5 cm^2 and the fluence is both 10 J/cm^2, the number of photons is assumed to be 10 and 5, respectively. Modified from [11]

spot sizes. Then, what should we do when converting the spot size in the same fluence? Reducing the spot size at the same fluence will result in lower energy absorption resulting in no side effects, but less efficacy. If the spot size is increased, the actual energy becomes higher than the original energy, so there is a high possibility of side effects. Therefore, when increasing spot size, fluence should be reduced.

So, what should we do to get equal energy in the skin at different spot sizes? Figure 4.4 shows the number of photons converted to fluence from Fig. 4.3. Previously, at 10 J/cm^2 of the handpiece, the fluence in the skin was 8 J/cm^2 for the large spot size and 6 J/cm^2 for the small spot size. To create the equivalent energy in the skin with small spot sizes, the fluence of handpiece should be increased. To create the same energy at 8 J/cm^2 in the skin with a small spot size, the energy should be raised above the original handpiece's energy of 10 J/cm^2, for example, it should be raised to 12 J/cm^2. It is important to note that scattering occurs mainly in dermis. Scattering does not occur in epidermis. The energy of the large spot size in the epidermis is therefore 10 J/cm^2 but the energy of small spot size is 12 J/cm^2. In other words, small spot sizes have a relatively high epidermal energy compared to large spot sizes and are more likely to cause side effects on the epidermis. Therefore, to create the same

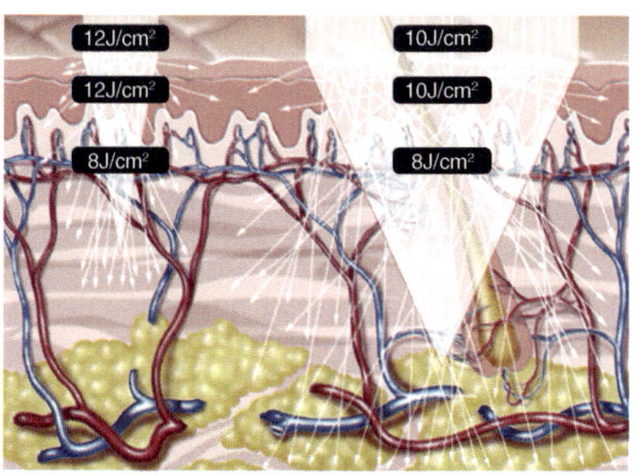

Fig. 4.4 The number of photons is converted to fluence from Fig. 4.3. The value of the "small spot size" is the assumed value of the fluence needed for the epidermis and the handpiece when adjusting the fluence of the dermis to 8 J/cm^2. Modified from [11]

effect in the dermis, increasing the spot size is a method to protect the epidermis.

The spot size effect can be summarized as follows.

1. The larger the spot size, the deeper the penetration depth of laser.
2. When increasing spot size at the same fluence, the fluence should be reduced.
3. When treating the dermis, large spot sizes should be used to protect the epidermis.

4.7 Determination of Spot Size

How should we determine spot size? Let's think about epidermal treatment and dermal treatment, respectively. First, deeply located chromophores can be treated with larger spot size. However, when treating the epidermis, there is no scattering, and spot size is not relevant because the depth of the chromophore is shallow. But if spot size is large, laser procedure can be performed quickly. On the other hand, if spot size is large, for example, when patient has dark facial tone in the treatment of lentigo, "relative" hypopigmentation may occur due to reaction in both lentigo and normal tissue (refer to Sect. 20.3.2 in Chap. 20). A typical example is the bar-shaped "tiger print" that occurs after IPL. Tiger print recovers faster than other hypopigmentation and is not permanent, but color contrast appears artificially and later, rod-shaped PIH may occur. To reduce this, smaller spot size should be used for epidermis treatment in patients with dark facial tones.

Second, a large spot size is advantageous when treating the dermis (spot size effect). However, if the spot size is increased, there is a limit to the output, so high fluence cannot be created. Then what is the appropriate spot size to treat the dermis? There are various opinions regarding this. Ross et al. stated that spot size should be at least four times greater than optical penetration depth (OPD) [12]. The OPD of 694 nm is 750 μm, so according to this logic, the spot size should be 3 mm or more. Dr. Minho Lee suggested that, regardless of wavelength, half of the spot size corresponds to the target depth for a spot size of 10 mm or less, so that a target at this depth can be safely treated. In other words, the "half rule" was suggested: the spot size should be set to 2 times the target depth (Published with kind permission of © Minho Lee MD. 2019. All rights reserved). Since the thickness of the skin is 2 mm on average, according to the half rule, when treating the entire epidermis and dermis, the spot size should be 4 mm or more.

When I use the Q-switched ruby laser, I mainly use the 4 mm spot size. This is because, when treating the epidermis, relative hypopigmentation of 3–4 mm or less is not very noticeable, and to treat the dermis, the spot size must be 3–4 mm or more. A wider spot size is better when treating the dermis, but because the Q-switched ruby laser has the inconvenience of replacing the handpiece when changing the spot size, I use the 4 mm spot size without changing it unless necessary.

4.8 Parameters

The indications for Q-switched ruby lasers are epidermal pigmentation, dermal pigmentation, and tattoo treatment. Let's look at the parameters for each indication (Table 4.4).

First, the fluence of epidermal pigments, freckles, and lentigines should be set for coagulation. The clinical end point should be darkening and slight peripheral erythema. Usually 3 J/cm^2 is adequate. Of course, dark lesions should be irradiated weakly or defocused, while light lesions should be irradiated strongly and focused (refer to Sect. 4.4 and 4.5 in Chap. 4). The appropriate treatment interval is 4 weeks or more so that the epidermis is regenerated (keratinization cycle, epidermal turnover). However, I do not treat the entire face, but only the pigmented area, so I sometimes set the treatment interval to every 2 weeks. Freckles usually disappear after one or at most two treatments. However, freckles often recur when exposed to sunlight, and patients usually come for treatment once a year. So, I inform my patients that when they receive strong sunlight after laser treatment, freckles may continue to recur, but if treatment is repeated from time to time, it will disappear easily. Also, I reassure my patients that freckles gradually decrease with age, so management with laser until then is needed.

Second, ABNOM, which is a dermal lesion, can cause PIH and worsen melasma. I consider the clinical end point as darkening or graying to slightly destroy the cells with shock wave and cavitation. Considering the skin regeneration of the dermis, I recommend 3–4 J/cm^2 3–4 treatments or more at 3-month intervals. However, Kenichirous Kasai, author of "Skin Spot Treatment Clinics," uses 5–8 J/cm^2 with immediate whitening and recommends 1–2 treatments at

Table 4.4 Parameters of Q-switched ruby laser (TattooStar R, Asclepion Laser Technologies GmbH, Jena, Germany)

Indications	Spot Size (mm)	Fluence (J/cm^2)	Remarks
Freckles	4	3	They will come back again
Lentigines	4	3	1–2 treatments
Café-au-lait macule (CALM)	4	3–4	Not successful in every case
ABNOM	4	3–4	Clinical end point: Darkening or graying
Nevus of Ota	4–6	4–6	
Amateur Tattoo	4–6	3	5–6 treatments
Professional Tattoo, very black	4–6	2	5–10 treatments, sometimes up to 20 treatments
Professional Tattoo, dark	4–6	3	5–10 treatments, sometimes up to 20 treatments
Professional Tattoo, green	4–6	3	5–10 treatments, sometimes up to 20 treatments. Change of color may occur
Permanent make-up	4–6	3	Change of color may occur
Dirt Tattoo	4–6	2	Be careful! Dirt particles can blow up

6-month intervals, considering the time for PIH to disappear even if it occurs [13]. Since ABNOM is sometimes accompanied by melasma, and PIH frequently occurs during the procedure, I set the treatment period for more than a year and reassure the patient that although the face may get darker and worse during treatment, it will surely disappear if treatment continues.

Third, it is better to treat nevus of Ota and tattoos with a wide spot size because they are located deep in the dermis layer (spot size 5–6 mm). In the case of retattooing, although the visible color is not dark, the laser reaction can be strong due to the high concentration of the chromophore. Thus, before the procedure, patient history of retattooing should be asked in advance, and the energy should be increased little by little from low energy for shock waves and cavitation to occur resulting in "immediate whitening with delayed petechiae." The treatment should be performed slowly (1 Hz) observing the reaction. Colored tattoos or semi-permanent tattoos may have paradoxical darkening after laser irradiation, which in turn darkens and may not disappear easily. But recently, paradoxical darkening is considered as part of the treatment process [14]. Therefore, it is necessary to fully explain to the patient in advance the fact that colored or semi-permanent tattoos may turn black during treatment and the number of treatments and treatment period may increase. Traumatic tattoos caused by gunpowder are not common in Korea, but if a substance such as gunpowder is in the skin as a tattoo, it can explode when irradiated with a laser, so the cause of the traumatic tattoo should be asked before the procedure. Since Q-switched ruby laser has a red wavelength (694 nm), it is effective for a complementary green tattoo, but not for a red tattoo of the same color. Nevus of Ota nevus usually disappears after 6 treatments at 3-month intervals in consideration of the regeneration of the dermal layer, and it usually takes 1–2 years. The interval between tattoo treatments is 2–3 months. Amateur tattoos usually require 5 treatments, and professional tattoos usually require 10–15 treatments, but up to 20 treatments may be needed.

Since Q-switched laser is not very painful, topical anesthesia is seldom needed. But for a more comfortable procedure, and in the case of a procedure that confirms a clear clinical end point, I apply 20 minutes of occlusion therapy with topical anesthesia before laser treatment is performed.

References

1. Goldman MP. Cutaneous and cosmetic laser surgery. Philadelphia: Mosby Elsevier; 2006.
2. Allemann IB, Goldberg DJ. Basics in dermatological laser applications. Karger Medical and Scientific Publishers; 2011.
3. Kang WH. Treatment strateties for pigmentation disorders in skin (Korean). Seoul: Hansol Medical; 2013.
4. Textbook compilation committee in Korean Dermatological Association. TEXTBOOK OF DERMATOLOGY, seventh edition (Korean). Seoul: McGraw-Hill Education Korea, Ltd; 2020.
5. Kauvar A, Hruza G. Principles and practices in cutaneous laser surgery. CRC Press; 2005.
6. Berlien H-P. Applied laser medicine. Springer Science & Business Media; 2003.
7. Raulin C, Karsai S. Laser and IPL technology in dermatology and aesthetic medicine. Heidelberg: New York; 2011.
8. Jeong JY. Clinical skin care (Korean). Seoul: MDworld; 2010.
9. Goldman MP. Lasers and energy devices for the skin. [S.I.]: Taylor & Francis; 2013.
10. Keyvan N. Lasers in dermatology and medicine. London: Springer-Verlag; 2012.
11. Gold MH. Lasers and light sources for the removal of unwanted hair. Clin Dermatol. 2007;25(5):443–53.
12. Ross EV, Ladin Z, Kreindel M, Dierickx C. Theoretical considerations in laser hair removal. Dermatol Clin. 1999;17(2):333–55. viii
13. Kasai K. Skin spots treatment clinics (Korean edition). Seoul: Shinheung med science; 2007.
14. Serup J, Bäumler W. Diagnosis and therapy of tattoo complications: with atlas of illustrative cases. Karger Medical and Scientific Publishers; 2017.

5 Q-Switched Nd:YAG Laser and Subcellular Selective Photothermolysis

5.1 Overview of Q-Switched Nd:YAG Lasers

Q-switched Nd:YAG laser basically produces a wavelength of 1064 nm, but it can also make a wavelength of 532 nm, which is a frequency-doubled wavelength of 1064 nm, using KTP crystal [1] (Table 5.1, Fig. 5.1). Being able to use two wavelengths in one laser is a huge advantage. However, I observed that the beam quality of the 532 nm wavelength produced by the Q-switched Nd:YAG laser is not uniform, and the output is higher than the fluence displayed on the instrument panel at a small spot size. This is why I use a 5 mm spot size when using a 532 nm wavelength. Pastelle laser (WONTECH Co. Ltd. Daejeon, Korea) provides an additional replaceable dye handpiece that can convert 532 nm wavelength to 595 nm or 660 nm wavelength.

Table 5.1 Specifications for Q-switched Nd:YAG laser (Pastelle, WONTECH Co. Ltd. Daejeon, Korea)

System type	Nd:YAG
Wavelength	1064 nm, 532 nm Option: 595 nm, 660 nm
Max. energy	532 nm: 500 mJ 1064 nm: 1300 mJ PTP mode: 1600 mJ Genesis mode: 3500 mJ
Pulse duration	4 to 48 ns (Q-switched mode) 80 to 480 μs (Genesis mode)
Repetition rate	Up to 10 Hz
Spot size	2 to 10 mm (1 mm step)

The method of Q-switch is as follows: Both of the mirrors in the optical cavity of Q-switched lasers are 100% reflective, so that the photons move back and forth between the mirrors increasing exponentially (Fig. 5.2). When a certain number of photons are collected, one mirror uses pockels cell to open and close (switching) only for a very short time, emitting photons [2]. Thus, very high outputs are possible and Q-switched laser makes very short pulse duration (PD) in nanoseconds. At this time, the method to create a quasi-continuous wave by keeping one mirror open like a CO_2 laser without using a pockels cell is genesis mode (or non-Q mode). Genesis mode usually has a pulse duration of 300 μs, which is the same as the pulse duration of genesis technique. At first glance, it can be thought that the same effect as the genesis technique of a long-pulsed Nd:YAG laser can be performed by a Q-switched Nd:YAG laser. However, I believe that the Q-switched Nd:YAG laser's genesis mode has a very low output, so it is difficult to see the effect of genesis technique. And although it may be effective if it is irradiated for a long time, but I do not think it is economical because the lifespan of the flash lamp would be quickly exhausted. So, instead of using the genesis mode in the Q-switched Nd:YAG laser, I use genesis technique by long-pulsed Nd:YAG laser.

PTP™ (photoacoustic twin pulse) mode refers to a method in which two subpulses are irradiated with a time difference of about 100–150 μs

J. D. Lee, M. J. M. Oh, *Lasers in Dermatology: Parameters and Choice*,
https://doi.org/10.1007/978-981-19-7568-4_5

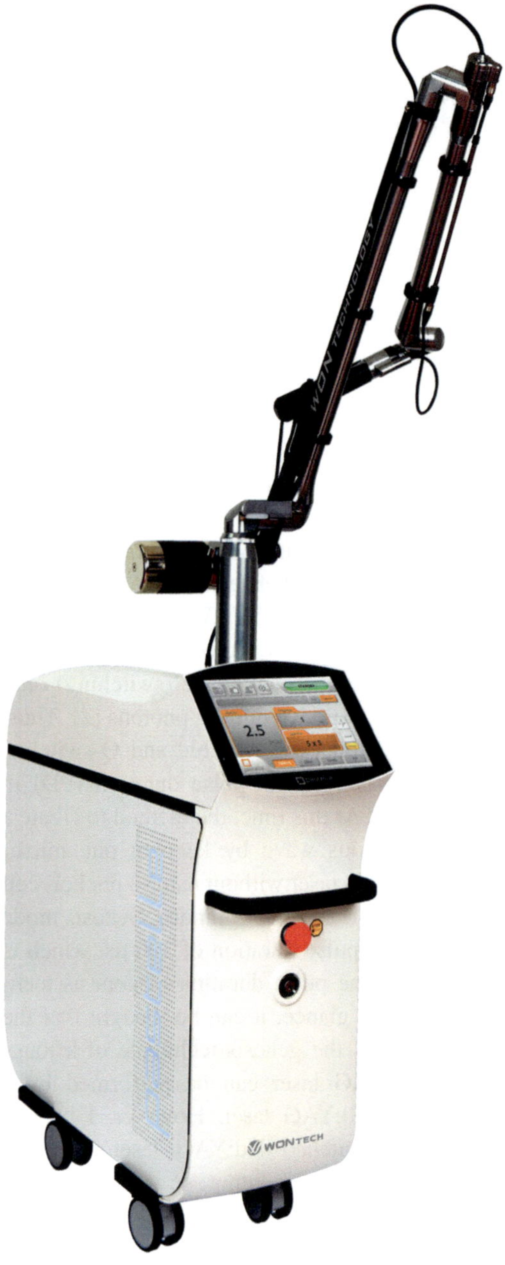

Fig. 5.1 Most Q-switched Nd:YAG lasers can use both 1064 nm and 532 nm wavelengths. (Pastelle, WONTECH Co. Ltd. Daejeon, Korea)

during one pulse [4]. Recently, a Q-switched Nd:YAG laser that irradiates 4–6 subpulses during one irradiation has also been released. There is a lot of controversy about the mechanism and effect of the PTP™ mode, but I think the main effect is simply increasing the frequency. For example, if 10 Hz is irradiated via the PTP™ mode, 20 Hz is actually irradiated. Of course, by repeatedly irradiating like macropulse, the Q-switched laser can also have a similar effect as genesis technique by slowly raising the tissue temperature by the photothermal effect. The fluence in PTP™ mode is displayed by adding the fluences of the two subpulses. For example, in PTP™ mode, 2.5 J/cm^2 means that a subpulse of 1.25 J/cm^2 is irradiated, and after 100 μs, a subpulse of 1.25 J/cm^2 is irradiated again. Therefore, half of the fluence value of the PTP™ mode is the same as the fluence value of the basic mode. The spot size of Pastelle laser (WONTECH Co. Ltd. Daejeon, Korea) can be adjusted from 2 to 10 mm by 1 mm increments. The handpiece of Pastelle laser acts as a zoom handpiece with a spot size of 6 mm or less, where the spot size decreases as the handpiece is removed from the skin. From spot size of 7 mm or more, it is suitable for laser toning because it is collimated through optical control. And as the laser is used, actual fluence becomes lower than the fluence on the instrument panel (refer to Sect. 2.5 in Chap. 2), but Pastelle laser has an autocalibration function so the operator can correct the fluence.

Q-switched Nd:YAG laser is a four-level laser, and as opposed to Q-switched ruby laser, a flash lamp with low output can be used, so the purchase cost is low, the life of the flash lamp is long, and it has also stable output and little mechanical damage (refer to Sect. 4.2 in Chap. 4). And above all, the frequency is as fast as 10 Hz, so it is suitable for laser toning.

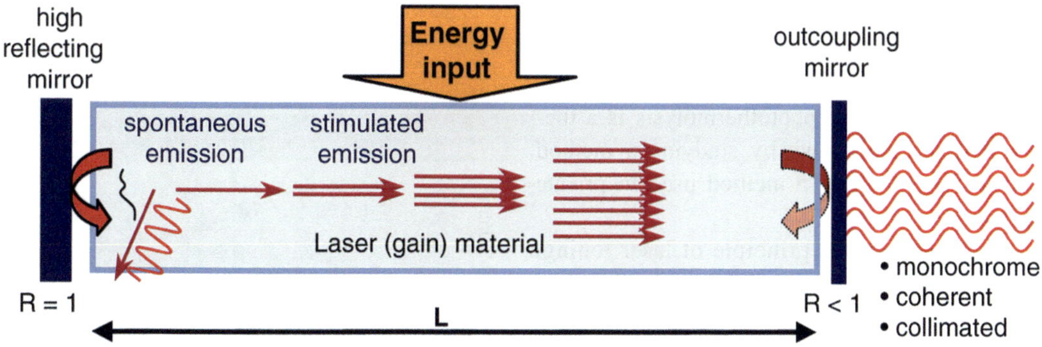

Fig. 5.2 In an optical cavity, photons are amplified in both mirrors. In continuous laser, one mirror is not a 100% reflective mirror, so some photons escape the optical cavity. But Q-switched laser has a 100% reflective mirror, so photons increase exponentially in the optical cavity. Reproduced from [3]

5.2 Indications

Q-switched Nd:YAG laser is a basic laser that every clinic must have, and it is an essential laser for pigmentation treatment. The most frequently performed procedure with Q-switched Nd:YAG laser is "laser toning," which is used not only for the purpose of treating melasma, but also for improving facial tone and preventing and treating PIH.

Since the chromophore of Q-switched Nd:YAG laser is melanin, it can be used for epidermal pigmentations, dermal pigmentations, and tattoo removal similar to Q-switched ruby lasers (refer to Sect. 4.3 in Chap. 4). For epidermal pigmentations, a wavelength of 532 nm, which is mainly absorbed by the epidermis, is used, and for dermal pigmentations, a wavelength of 1064 nm, which is mainly absorbed a lot by the dermis, is used. However, 1064 nm wavelength is not entirely unabsorbed by epidermis. Rather, it is suitable for use in "laser toning" because of its low absorption (refer to Sect. 2.7 in Chap. 2). In tattoo treatment, red tattoos are treated by 532 nm, which is a complementary color to green. Black and blue tattoos are treated by 1064 nm.

Although wavelength of 532 nm is used for epidermal pigmentation treatment, the absorption coefficient for melanin is very high, so the risk of side effects such as PIH is high. So, I treat epidermal pigmentations using repeat pulse method, which repeatedly irradiates the 532 nm wavelength of Q-switched Nd:YAG laser with low energy (refer to Sect. 5.6 in Chap. 5).

5.3 Subcellular Selective Photothermolysis

Subcellular selective photothermolysis is a theory that became known by studying a method called "laser toning," a method used in private practice.

To investigate the principle of laser toning, Kim et al. irradiated 1064 nm Q-switched Nd:YAG lasers on zebrafish and observed the change through microscope and biopsy [5]. They observed changes in melanosomes by irradiating fluence from 0.3 J/cm^2 to 0.9 J/cm^2 with 7 mm spot size and pulse duration 5–7 ns. Melanosomes are partially destroyed even at 0.3 J/cm^2, but fluences of at least 0.4 J/cm^2 are required to observe complete destruction of melanosomes (Fig. 5.3).

Figure 5.4 shows staining results; blue means normal nuclei, and red means apoptotic cells, i.e., the cells that will soon die. Below 0.4 J/cm^2, the nucleus and the cells are both normal, but above 0.5 J/cm^2, apoptotic cells are observed despite normal nucleus.

Taken together, these results show that at 0.4 J/cm^2, only the melanosomes are broken and the cells are not damaged. In other words, there is an "energy level that can break only the melanosomes without damaging the cells." For example, laser toning in melasma does not affect melanocytes or keratinocytes and does not cause side effects, and it is effective in treating melasma by eliminating only the melanosomes contained in melanocytes and keratinocytes.

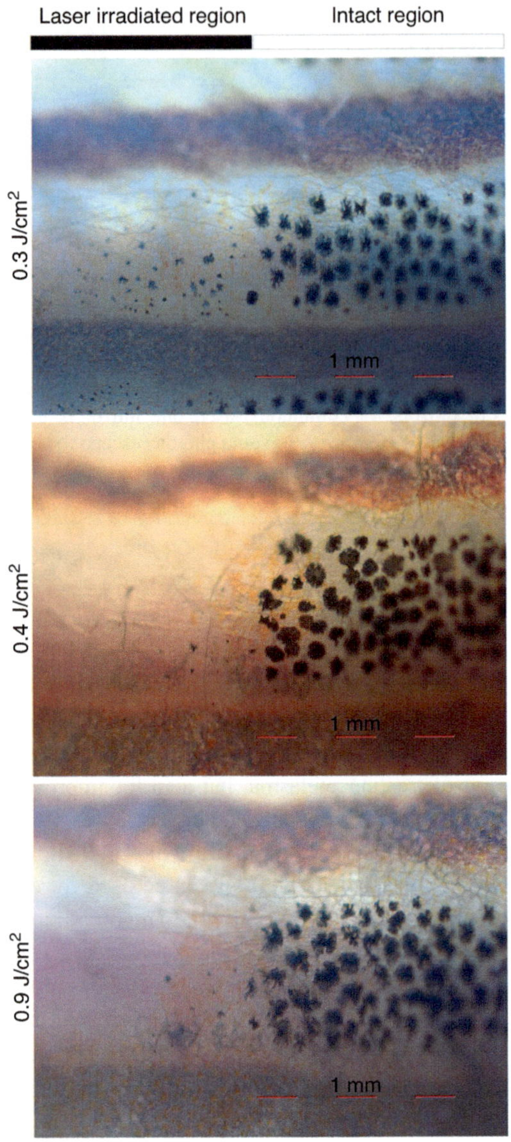

Fig. 5.3 Changes in melanosomes in zebrafish 5 days after 1064 nm Q-switched Nd:YAG laser. The left part of each figure is the irradiated portion. Reproduced from [5]

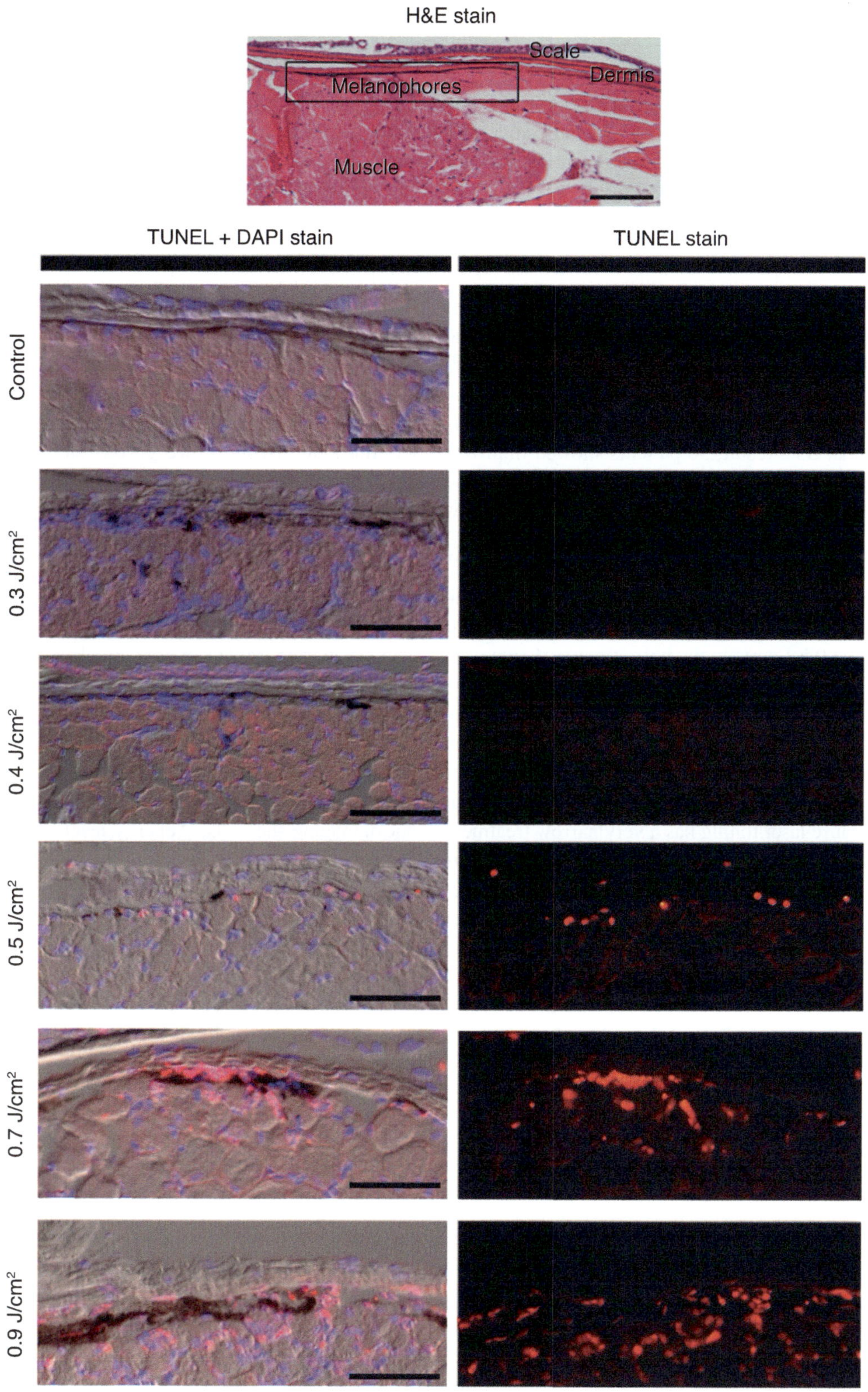

Fig. 5.4 TUNEL and DAPI staining of zebrafish 1 day after 1064 nm Q-switched Nd:YAG laser. Reproduced from [5]

5.4 Golden Parameter of Laser Toning

Is there a golden parameter for laser toning? One laser text suggests 3.0 J/cm^2 in PTP mode and 1.5 J/cm^2 in conventional mode as golden parameters [6]. But I think this energy is still high.

Choi et al. performed laser toning and genesis technique with 1064 nm Q-switched Nd:YAG laser and 1064 nm long-pulsed Nd:YAG laser on 30 patients with aggravated melasma after previous therapy such as laser toning, IPL, fractional lasers, and chemical peels [7]. The parameters were spot size of 6 mm, 10 Hz, 2.1–2.5 J/cm^2 on PTP mode, and the end point was slight erythema. As a result, 30 patients showed improvement without any side effects, even though the patients had aggravated melasma after previous therapy such as laser toning.

As seen in the above paper by Kim et al., melanosomes are partially destroyed at less than 0.3 J/cm^2 in zebrafish, and side effects occur above 0.5 J/cm^2, so the best effect is shown only at 0.4 J/cm^2 [5]. That is, laser toning has a narrow therapeutic window. When laser toning is performed, it may be ineffective, melasma may worsen, or side effects that are difficult to treat such as mottled hypopigmentation may occur. Because laser toning has a very narrow treatment range, even with effective energy, side effects may occur. So, it is safer to use less than the adequate energy because it is better to be less effective, than to have side effects. This is why I think that 1064 nm Q-switched Nd:YAG laser with a spot size of 9–10 mm, 10 Hz and a fluence of 2.0–2.5 J/cm^2 in PTP mode and 1 ~ 1.25 J/cm^2 in conventional mode, is the golden parameter of melasma treatment.

5.5 One Shot Toning

Let's think about the method of irradiating multiple passes, one of the parameters of laser toning. "Laser toning" which is frequently performed in private practice, irradiates more than 1000 shots at 10 Hz. Why irradiate so much at 10 Hz? In the above paper by Kim et al., only one shot (one pulse) was irradiated [8]. Also, if there is an "energy level that can break only the melanosomes without damaging the cells," isn't one shot enough? So, I perform the so-called "one shot toning" where melasma are shot one by one. What is the essence of theory of subcellular selective photothermolysis? There is an "energy level that can break only the melanosomes without damaging the cells." In other words, there is a concept of a therapeutic window. The concept is that it is ineffective at low energy and has side effects at high energy, and that there is an adequate energy that is effective without side effects. If we go one step further down from this concept, wouldn't there be an "energy level that only damages cells without affecting the surrounding cells"? Thus, for treatments of lentigines or post-inflammatory hyperpigmentation (PIH) without inflammation, I use higher energy for one shot toning. There will also be an "energy level that break down not only the cells but also the surrounding blood vessels." That is why petechia occurs during treatment of tattoo and ABNOM.

Then, what is the standard energy for "energy level that can break only the melanosomes without damaging the cells," "energy level that only damages cells without affecting the surrounding cells," and "energy level that break down not only the cells but also the surrounding blood vessels." After reviewing fluences for pigmented lesions in various papers, I concluded that:

In 1064 nm Q-switched Nd:YAG laser a fluence of 4 J/cm^2 and 6 J/cm^2 with a 4 mm spot size should be the standard energy for one shot toning.

Thus, I recommend that with one shot toning, laser must be used below 4 J/cm^2 for melasma, which is an "energy level that can break only the melanosomes without damaging the cells." And for treatments of lentigines or PIHs without inflammation, energy level between 4 J/cm^2 and 6 J/cm^2 should be used, which is an "energy level that only damages

Table 5.2 Parameters of one shot toning

1064 nm Q-switched Nd:YAG laser, 4 mm spot, 1 Hz, one shot	
Indications	Fluence (J/cm^2)
Melasma	3–3.5
Lentigo, ABNOM	4.5–5
Nevus of Ota	≥6
PIH with erythema (inflammation)	3–3.5
PIH without erythema (inflammation)	4.5–5

cells without affecting the surrounding cells." And for treatments of tattoos or melanocytic nevi, energy levels should be above 6 J/cm^2, which is an "energy level that break down not only the cells but also the surrounding blood vessels" (Table 5.2).

5.6 Repeat Pulse Method

Repeat pulse method refers to a method of repeatedly irradiating laser with low energy. If the laser is repeatedly irradiated to the epidermal pigmentation, the temperature rises little by little at first, but when the temperature is above coagulation, melanin and melanin-containing melanocytes and keratinocytes will coagulate. As the tissue becomes darker during coagulation, the absorption coefficient rises. Therefore, the temperature may rise rapidly if repeated irradiation is performed afterwards. If the temperature rises rapidly, there is a high risk of side effects because vaporization or shock waves occur rather than coagulation. Therefore, the laser should not be repeatedly irradiated "after coagulation occurs" for epidermal pigmentation treatment without side effects in the repeat pulse method.

In repeat pulse method, temperatures may vary depending on frequency, pulse count, and fluence (Fig. 5.5). Because there are three variables, various parameters can exist. I chose to fix two variables, frequency and pulse count, and decided to adjust fluence only. I mainly use the repeat pulse method to treat epidermal pigmentations. The parameters are as follows: In 532 nm Q-switched Nd:YAG laser, 5 mm spot size with a frequency of 4 Hz and a pulse count of 4 shots. Fluence starts at 0.3 J/cm^2. The clinical end point is "moderate darkening and delayed perilesional erythema." Fluence is increased by 0.1 J/cm^2 if there is no change. Specifically, 4 shots are irradiated at 0.3 J/cm^2 and, if there is no change, 4 shots are irradiated again at 0.4 J/cm^2 after at least 10 s interval to rule out heat accumulation effect. Usually fluence does not exceed 0.4 J/cm^2, but in case of very light lentigines, the fluence may be higher. Conversely, if 0.3 J/cm^2 is used and immediate whitening is produced, it can be lowered to 0.2 J/cm^2.

How can we fine tune the repeat pulse method? I fine tune in order of fluence, pulse count, and frequency. For example, if the reaction is too strong at 0.3 J/cm^2, 4 Hz, 4 shots and it is too weak at 0.2 J/cm^2, I try 3 shots at 0.3 J/cm^2. If this is still too strong, frequency is lowered to 3 Hz and only 3 shots are irradiated.

Caution should be exercised in the repeat pulse method of epidermal pigmentation treatments because in the tissue degeneration process of the pigmented lesion, the absorption coefficient rises rapidly at a temperature higher than the coagulation. Pulse stacking after darkening state may result in a high risk of side effects due to rapid temperature rise. Therefore, after darkening additional irradiation must be avoided. This is why the repeat pulse method for pigmentation treatment is very difficult and should be used with caution.

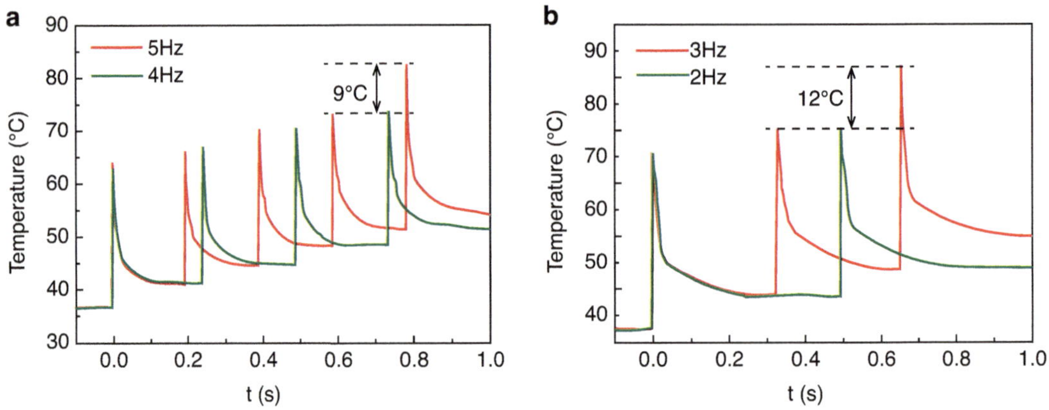

Fig. 5.5 Temperature change when Q-switched Nd:YAG laser is repeatedly irradiated to a capillary tube containing blood with a pulse duration of 300 μs, (**a**) 30 J/cm^2, (**b**) 40 J/cm^2. It can be seen that the temperature change varies according to frequency, pulse count, and fluence. Reproduced from [9]

5.7 Focusing Method

Since wavelength and pulse duration of Q-switched laser are fixed, among three parameters (wavelength, pulse duration, fluence), we can get the desired result by adjusting only fluence. Fluence can be determined based on clinical end points. Then, what is the clinical end point of Q-switched laser in pigmentation treatment? Since Q-switched laser mainly uses shock wave and cavitation, which are phenomena of photomechanical effect, the clinical end point can be clearly seen with our eyes (whitening). However, I think that clear and uniform whitening phenomenon means too much energy. It is known that cavities are observed in histological examination even without visible whitening. So, I take "immediate, uneven, slight whitening" as the clinical end point. However, it is very cumbersome to adjust these fluence differences one by one on the instrument panel.

Dr. Po Lee suggested a method of finely controlling fluence with a Q-switched Nd:YAG laser. The procedure is performed using the zoom handpiece of Q-switched Nd:YAG laser, and the handpiece is lifted from the skin little by little to stop the irradiation when the clinical end point is visible in the eyes. As the spot size decreases when the zoom handpiece is raised, the actual fluence increases gradually. It is similar to the defocusing method of CO_2, but because the spot size gradually decreases when the zoom handpiece is used, it can be named as a "focusing method." (Dr. Po Lee named it "focusing toning." Published with kind permission of © Po Lee MD. 2021. All rights reserved).

First, I attach the zoom handpiece of 1,064 nm Q-switched Nd:YAG laser to the skin with a spot size of 6 mm, 3 J/cm^2, 2 Hz. Then, I irradiate the laser with lifting the handpiece from the skin little by little and stop the laser if "immediate, uneven, slight whitening" occurs. The reason I use 1064 nm instead of 532 nm is that 1064 nm, which has a longer wavelength than 532 nm, is safer because of the epidermal bypass effect, and because 1064 nm has a lower absorption coefficient for blood vessels, the effect on blood vessels is less than 532 nm. The zoom handpiece of Pastelle laser (WONTECH Co. Ltd. Daejeon, Korea) is designed so that in a spot size of 7 mm or more, collimation occurs and zoom is not possible. The spot size that actually touches the skin increases when the spot size is made as large as possible, so I use a spot size of 6 mm. For laser equipment capable of a larger spot size, I recommend the use of maximum spot size. For frequency I use a slightly slow 2 Hz so that I can stop immediately when the clinical end point is visible. The fluence can be raised up to 4.6 J/cm^2 with a spot size of 6 mm, but above 4 J/cm^2 may be too strong for darker pigmentations and for melasma, 3 J/cm^2 is used because side effects may occur. However, in the case of a light lentigo or light tattoo, fluence may be raised up to 4 J/cm^2.

The biggest advantage of Q-switched Nd:YAG laser focusing method is that it can precisely adjust the fluence up to the desired reaction. However, the disadvantage is first, because it uses the shock wave and cavitation of Q-switched laser, the risk of PIH is higher than the repeat pulse method that induces coagulation. (In order of high to low risk: vaporization of photothermal effect > photoacoustic effect > coagulation of photothermal effect) Second, because there is an absorption coefficient for blood, petechia occurs. Third, when the spot size is reduced by half, the fluence increases by 4 times the square of the radius, so even if the handpiece is lifted even a little, plasma is generated and the skin may be ablated. In the case of the epidermis, PIH can occur, especially pigment incontinence, which lasts for a long time. In the case of dermal pigments and tattoos, scarring may occur. Therefore, it is necessary to finely control the distance between the skin and the handpiece. Fourth, in order to quickly treat various pigments on the skin, the distance between the skin and the handpiece could be fixed, but in this case because the concentration is different for each pigmentation, it may not be effective for some pigmentations. On the other hand, in the case of dark pigments, the reaction may be too strong, and side effects may occur. The principle is to adjust the distance between the skin and the handpiece for each pigmentation and repeat this for each pigmentation by attaching the handpiece close to the skin and then lifting it, but this takes a long time.

Because of these shortcomings of the focusing method, I only use this method for dermal pigmentation and tattoo treatment, while carefully adjusting the distance between the skin and the handpiece. For epidermal pigmentations, I set the clinical end point as perilesional erythema, and by lowering the handpiece, use low energy.

5.8 Parameters

Since all Q-switched lasers have a fixed pulse duration and do not require epidermal cooling, if you have purchased a specific laser (if you have chosen a wavelength) you only need to adjust spot size, fluence, and speed (Hz) among the six parameters (Table 5.3).

The indications for Q-switched Nd:YAG laser are epidermal pigmentation, dermal pigmentation, tattoo treatment, and melasma treatment (Fig. 5.6).

Table 5.3 Parameters of Q-switched Nd:YAG laser (Pastelle, WONTECH Co. Ltd. Daejeon, Korea)

Lesion	Mode	Fluence (J/cm^2)	Frequency (Hz)	Spot (mm)	Sessions	Interval (weeks)
One shot toning	1064 nm	≥3	2–3	4	5	2
Lentigo, freckles	532 nm (repeat pulse method)	0.2–0.4	4	5	1–2	2–4
ABNOM	1064 nm	4.0–6.0	2	4–6	≥ 10–20	1–2, 4–8
Ota, Ito	1064 nm	≥ 6.0	2	4–6	3–7	8–12
Tattoo	1064 nm	≥ 4.0	2	4–6	3–7	8–12
Tattoo red	532 nm	1.5	2	4	3–7	8–12
Tattoo green	660 nm (dye handpiece)	≥ 1.5	2	3	≥ 3	6–8
Focusing method	1064 nm	3.0–4.0	2	6		
Laser toning	1064 nm (PTP™ mode)	2.0–2.5	10	9–10	5	2

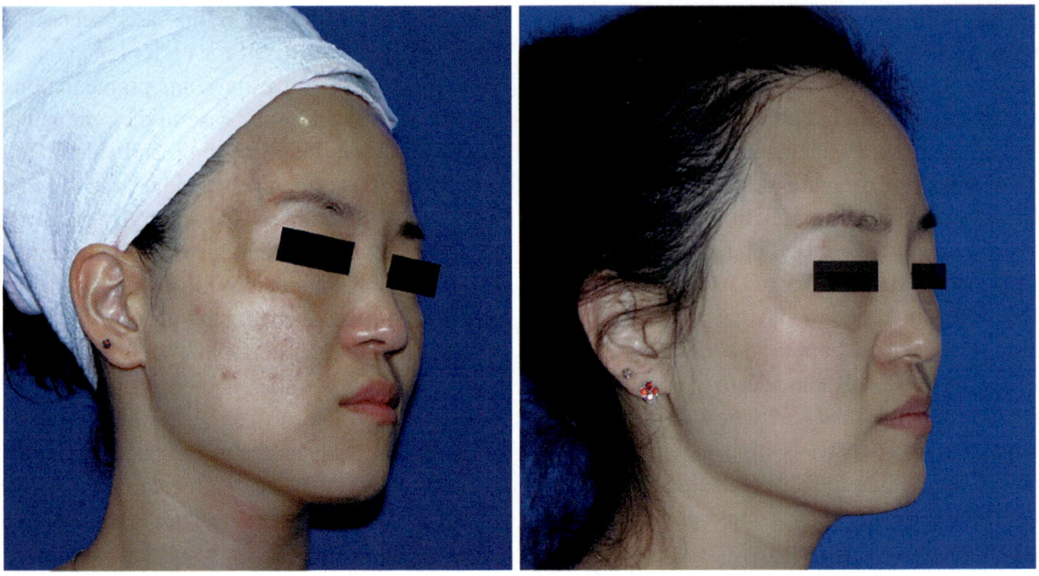

Fig. 5.6 Photographs before and after 10 sessions of laser toning of Q-switched Nd:YAG laser in the treatment of melasma. Laser used: Pastelle, WONTECH Co. Ltd. Daejeon, Korea

First, for epidermal pigments such as lentigo and freckles, one-shot toning or repeat pulse method can be used. In my clinic, out of the 10 laser sessions, I use 1064 nm Q-switched Nd:YAG laser for odd number of sessions, i.e., sessions 1, 3, 5, 7, and 9. On the same day, first, conventional laser toning (PTP™ mode, 2.5 J/cm^2, spot size 9 mm or 2.0 J/cm^2, spot size 10 mm, 1000 shots at 10 Hz) is performed followed by one shot toning (refer to Sect. 3.6 at Chap. 3) One shot toning uses an energy level of 4 J/cm^2 or higher that can break cells, and for the purpose of photoacoustic effect by shock wave the clinical end point is set as "immediate slight erythema." For faster epidermal pigmentation removal, the repeat pulse method using the 532 nm wavelength of Q-switched Nd:YAG laser is used during sessions 2 and 4. Repeat pulse method often causes PIH even when used with caution. Also, if the repeat pulse method is used again in the area where PIH has occurred, PIH will become more severe. This is why I rarely use the repeat pulse method after session 4.

Second, dermal pigmentations, ABNOM, nevus of Ota, and tattoo treatment may be treated by using one-shot toning of 1064 nm Q-switched Nd:YAG laser. It can be treated by controlling the fluence while checking the clinical end point at the 4 mm spot size, but due to the hassle of continuously checking the instrument panel and the pigmentations alternately and the difficulty in fine-tuning, I mainly use the focusing method.

Because PIH is common in ABNOM treatment and because ABNOM is often accompanied by melasma, the clinical end point should be "delayed petechia" and the handpiece should be lowered to decrease energy. But in nevus of Ota and tattoo treatment, the clinical end point should be "immediate whitening with delayed petechia" and the handpiece should be raised to increase energy. There are various treatment methods for ABNOM, but I prefer breaking melanocytes with low power repeatedly so that PIH or melasma do not occur [10]. The first 10 treatments are performed every 1–2 weeks, and the next 10 treatments are performed at 1–2 month intervals. I tell my patients that it takes 1–2 years for complete resolution. For nevus of Ota, considering the regeneration of the dermis layer, 3–7 treatments at intervals of 2–3 months are recommended. Q-switched Nd:YAG laser's 532 nm wavelength is green, so it is effective for a complementary red tattoo, but not for a green tattoo of the same color. Pastelle laser (WONTECH Co. Ltd. Daejeon, Korea) is able to use the wavelength of 660 nm with a dye handpiece. 660 nm is effective for green tattoos that are complementary to red, similar to ruby lasers. The interval between tattoo treatments is 2–3 months. Amateur tattoos usually require 5 treatments, and professional tattoos usually require 10–15 treatments, but more than 20 treatments may be needed.

Third, I use 1064 nm Q-switched Nd:YAG laser to treat melasma, and both conventional laser toning and one-shot toning are performed on the same day. The purpose of conventional laser toning is to temporarily suppress the melanogenesis of the entire face (refer to Sect. 18.7 in Chap. 18). In addition, considering subcellular selective photothermolysis, there is no clinical end point like perilesional erythema because it only breaks melanosomes with shock waves and does not break keratinocytes or melanocytes. Rather, if perilesional erythema occurs, it should be considered as a warning end point. So, for patients who complain of redness or pain during conventional laser toning, the energy is lowered to 2.0 J/cm^2 in PTP™ mode and if there is still complaint, the energy is further lowered to 1.0 J/cm^2. The purpose of one-shot toning is to precisely inhibit melanin synthesis only in melasma lesions. Fluence should be such that erythema does not occur, and it is usually performed at 3.0–4.0 J/cm^2. However, since there is no clinical end point, the exact fluence cannot be confirmed. This is why I set the clinical end point to "delayed perilesional erythema" only for patients taking tranexamic acid.

References

1. Kauvar A, Hruza G. Principles and practices in cutaneous laser surgery. CRC Press; 2005.
2. Jelínková H. Lasers for medical applications: diagnostics, therapy and surgery. Elsevier; 2013.
3. Raulin C, Karsai S. Laser and IPL technology in dermatology and aesthetic medicine. Heidelberg: New York; 2011.
4. Jang HW, Chun SH, Park HC, Ryu HJ, Kim IH. Comparative study of dual-pulsed 1064 nm Q-switched Nd:YAG laser and single-pulsed 1064 nm Q-switched Nd:YAG laser by using zebrafish model and prospective split-face analysis of facial melasma. J Cosmet Laser Ther. 2017;19(2):114–23.
5. Kim JH, Kim H, Park HC, Kim IH. Subcellular selective photothermolysis of melanosomes in adult zebrafish skin following 1064-nm Q-switched Nd:YAG laser irradiation. J Invest Dermatol. 2010;130(9):2333–5.
6. Park SH, Yeo WC, Koh WS, Park JW, Noh NK, Yoon CS. Laser dermatology plastic surgery 2nd ed (Korean). Seoul: Koonja; 2014.
7. Choi CP, Yim SM, Seo SH, Ahn HH, Kye YC, Choi JE. Retreatment using a dual mode of low-fluence Q-switched and long-pulse Nd:YAG laser in patients with melasma aggravation after previous therapy. J Cosmet Laser Ther. 2015;17(3):129–34.
8. Kim JH, Jeong SY, Shin JB, Hc P, Kim IH. Subcellular selective photothermolysis in zebrafish: an electron microscopic evidence after Q-switched Nd:YAG laser ablation. Korean. J Dermatol. 2008;46(20):187.
9. Jia H, Chen B, Li D. Dynamic optical absorption characteristics of blood after slow and fast heating. Lasers Med Sci. 2017;32(3):513–25.
10. Cho SB, Park SJ, Kim MJ, Bu TS. Treatment of acquired bilateral nevus of Ota-like macules (Hori's nevus) using 1064-nm Q-switched Nd:YAG laser with low fluence. Int J Dermatol. 2009;48(12):1308–12.

6 Picosecond Alexandrite Laser and Stress Relaxation Time

6.1 Overview of Picosecond Alexandrite Lasers

The wavelength of picosecond alexandrite laser is 755 nm, which is effective for epidermal pigmentation treatment due to the epidermal bypass effect and is the safest wavelength (refer to Sect. 2.7 in Chap. 2, Table 6.1). Of course, 755 nm wavelength can penetrate deep into the dermis and can be used for dermal pigmentation and tattoo treatment. The pulse duration is less than 700 ps, which is about 10 times shorter than the nanosecond Q-switched laser, so that the peak tensile stress is 100 times greater (refer to Sect. 6.4 in Chap. 6). Therefore, picosecond laser breaks melanosomes or tattoo particles better than Q-switched lasers (Fig. 6.1).

Table 6.1 Specifications for picosecond alexandrite laser (Picowon, WONTECH Co. Ltd. Daejeon, Korea)

Wavelength	755 nm
Laser type	Picosecond alexandrite laser
Pulse energy	230 mJ
Pulse width	<700 ps
Peak power	0.33GW (700 ps)
Pulse rate	1 to 5 Hz
Spot size	2, 3, 3.5, 4, 5, 5.5, 6, 8 mm
Handpiece	Zoom H/P, Fractional H/P

Originally, a picosecond laser showing the effect of plasma-induced ablation or photodisruption should have a pulse duration of several tens of picoseconds. But since the currently released laser has a pulse duration of several hundred picoseconds, it is not a picosecond laser in the true sense. This is why some papers name the currently released picosecond lasers as "pseudo picosecond laser" or "subnanosecond laser" [1].

Recently, lasers that attach fractional handpieces to Q-switched lasers or long-pulsed lasers are emerging. I think that using a fractional handpiece at a wavelength where scattering occurs, without targeting water is not consistent with fractional photothermolysis (refer to Sect. 10.1 in Chap. 10). This is why I do not use the picosecond laser fractional handpiece for the purpose of pigmentation treatment. In addition, when treating scars with picosecond laser, photodisruption effect is induced by using MLA (micro-lens arrays) or DOE (diffractive optical elements) handpiece. However, at 755 nm wavelength, the chromophore is melanin in the epidermis, and scar treatment must occur in the dermis, so I think that the 755 nm picosecond laser will have only a minimal effect on scar treatment.

J. D. Lee, M. J. M. Oh, *Lasers in Dermatology: Parameters and Choice*,
https://doi.org/10.1007/978-981-19-7568-4_6

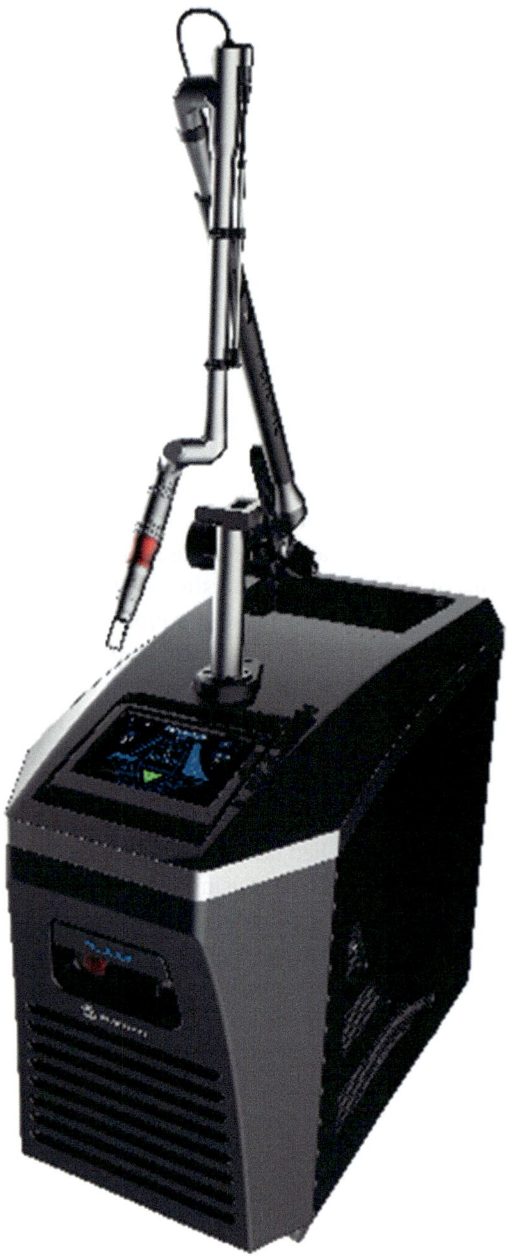

Fig. 6.1 Because picosecond laser has 10 times shorter pulse duration than Q-switched laser, it breaks melanosomes or tattoo particles 100 times better (Picowon, WONTECH Co. Ltd. Daejeon, Korea)

6.2 Indications

The indications for picosecond alexandrite laser are treatment of epidermal and dermal pigmentations and tattoo removal, similar to Q-switched alexandrite laser or Q-switched ruby laser (refer to Sect. 4.3 in Chap. 4, Table 6.2). In particular, picosecond laser is known to be superior to Q-switched laser in tattoo removal.

There are four advantages of picosecond laser over Q-switched laser in tattoo removal (Table 6.3): First, fewer number of treatment sessions is needed. Second, less time is required for complete removal. Third, better clearance of colors, especially blue, green, and yellow. And fourth, after removing the tattoo with a Q-switched laser, the blurry remaining tattoo (ghost of tattoo) can be removed with picosecond laser [2].

When removing tattoos, picosecond laser has not only advantages but also disadvantages as well [2]. First, blister formation is common. If the tattoo is located superficially or the tattoo is on the lower extremities, blisters occur in more than 50% of the first treatment. The mechanism by which blisters occur is still unknown. However, with proper treatment, it subsides quickly without complications within 4–5 days. There are some proposed methods to prevent blisters: (1) a method of using picosecond laser and CO_2 fractional laser together, (2) method of re-irradiating with a fractional handpiece immediately after picosecond laser irradiation, (3) method of covering a silicone gel sheet before treatment. Second, there are tattoos that cannot be removed despite using a picosecond laser. In terms of stress relaxation time (SRT), it can be seen that even picosecond laser cannot remove all tattoos (refer to Sect. 6.4 in Chap. 6).

Table 6.2 Indications of picosecond alexandrite laser

Epidermal melanocytic lesions	Dermal melanocytic lesions	Tattoo
1. Freckle (Ephelides) 2. Lentigo 3. Café-au-lait macule(CALM) 4. Nevus spilus (Speckled lentiginous nevus) 5. Becker's nevus	1. Mongolian spot 2. Nevus of Ota 3. Nevus of Ito 4. Acquired bilateral nevus of Ota-like macules (ABNOM)	1. Black 2. Blue 3. Green 4. Yellow

Table 6.3 Advantages of picosecond laser over Q-switched laser in tattoo removal. Reproduced from [2]

Benefits
1. Fewer number of treatment sessions 2. Less time required for complete removal 3. Better clearance of colors, especially blue, green, and yellow 4. Removing ghost of tattoo remaining after multiple sessions with nanosecond

6.3 Plasma-Induced Ablation, Photodisruption, and Photoacoustic Effect

Figure 6.2 shows the areas of plasma-induced ablation and photodisruption that occur by pulse duration and fluence. The curve shows the threshold at which the plasma occurs. The area under the curve is an area where a photoacoustic effect occurs in which plasma is not generated [4].

Let's look closely. Area 1 is the area of Q-switched laser that we use. That is, in this area, plasma is not generated and phenomena such as shock wave generation, cavitation, and jet formation occur. Area 2 is the area where plasma is made by using a zoom handpiece with a Q-switched laser. Currently released picosecond laser (pseudo picosecond laser, subnanosecond laser) falls in area 3. This is because plasma does not occur during pigmentation or tattoo treatment with a picosecond laser. Nowadays, picosecond lasers are used to treat scars and wrinkles with zoom handpieces. This area is area 4. There is no laser for areas 5 and 6 yet.

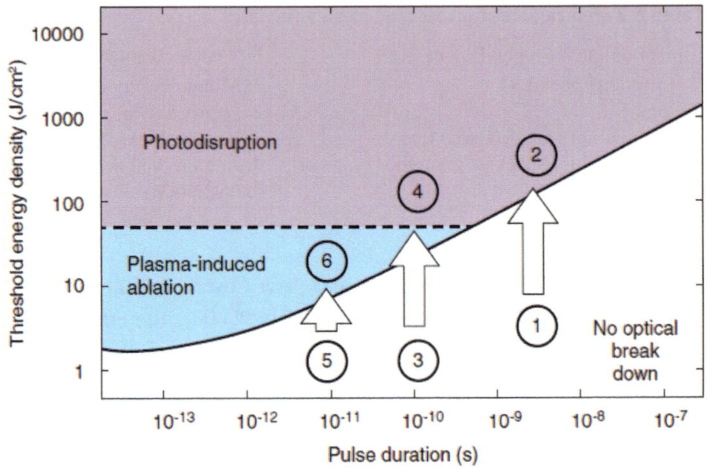

Fig. 6.2 Distinction of plasma-induced ablation and photodisruption according to applied pulse duration and energy density. Modified from [3]

6.4 Stress Relaxation Time

Q-switched lasers and currently released picosecond lasers are in the region of photoacoustic effect which does not produce plasma. Then what is the difference between Q-switched and picosecond lasers?

The keyword in selective photothermolysis is thermal relaxation time (TRT). In other words, the idea is that "if light energy is irradiated for an appropriate amount of time, the light energy received by the target tissue is used only to raise the temperature of the target tissue and does not transmit heat to surrounding tissues." In other words, heat is confined in the target tissue (thermal confinement). Similarly, stress confinement can be thought of stress confined in the target tissue [5]. In other words, "if light energy is irradiated for an appropriate amount of time, the light energy received by the target tissue is used only to give stress and damage the target tissue and does not transmit stress to surrounding tissues."

Figure 6.3 shows the zone of thermal confinement and stress confinement and the corresponding laser. The zone corresponding to the theory of selective photothermolysis is the thermal confinement zone. On the other hand, there is a stress confinement zone which is affected by shock waves, and the corresponding lasers are 1064 nm Q-switched Nd:YAG lasers and picosecond lasers. To put it simply 1064 nm Q-switched Nd:YAG lasers and picosecond lasers are lasers that break target tissue. These zones are not clearly divided [7]. For example, Q-switched Nd:YAG lasers have both mechanical and thermal effects. But the main effect is mechanical.

Similar to thermal relaxation time (TRT), stress relaxation time (SRT) or stress confinement time can be considered in the stress confinement zone. The formula of SRT is as follows [8]:

$$\tau_S = \frac{\Delta}{c_S}$$

- τ_S: stress confinement time,
- c_S: sonic velocity inside the tattoo, $c_S \fallingdotseq 4X10^5$cm/s,
- Δ: characteristic length in the tattoo material.

SRT is a concept to mainly use in tattoo treatment so that Δ depicts the size of tattoo particles. Let's look at SRT in tattoo treatment. The size of tattoo particles varies from text to text, but it is known that the size usually is from 0.5 to 5 μm and as small as 25 nm (1 μm = 1000 nm). Calculated SRT are from 125 ps to 1.25 ns and as small as 10 ps (1 ns = 1000 ps). Therefore, it is difficult to treat tattoos of all size with a 1064 nm Q-switched laser or currently released picosecond laser with a 450–750 ps pulse duration.

Let's consider the therapeutic effect of Q-switched laser and picosecond laser in relation to SRT of melanosomes, which is the goal of pigmentation treatment. The sizes of the melanin

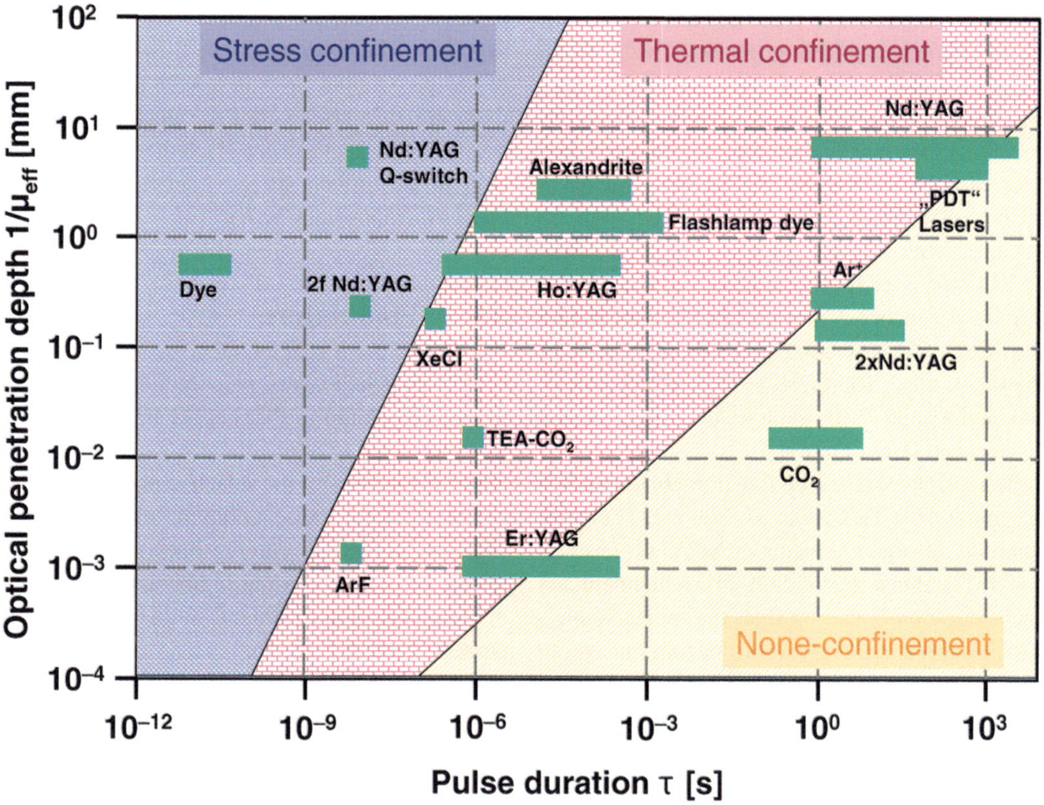

Fig. 6.3 Zone of thermal confinement and stress confinement and the corresponding laser according to pulse duration and optical penetration depth (OPD). Reproduced from [6]

granules and melanosomes are 15 nm and 0.5 μm, respectively, and SRT is 10 ps and 300 ps, respectively [9]. In terms of stress confinement, both lasers cannot treat melanin granules nor melanosomes. In summary, both Q-switched Nd:YAG laser and picosecond laser are lasers in the stress confinement zone, but because the pulse duration is longer than the SRT of some of the tattoo particles and melanosomes, perfect stress confinement is not achieved. Then what is the difference between these two lasers?

The difference between the two lasers can be explained by peak tensile stress. Peak tensile stress is expressed by the following formula [2]:

$$\sigma = -3\gamma\mu F\left(\frac{\tau_a}{\tau}\right)^2$$

- σ: the peak tensile stress, obtained at the center of the tattoo target,
- F: the laser irradiance (fluence).
- τ_a and τ: the acoustic transit time and laser pulse duration, respectively,
- μ: the absorption coefficient of the target material at the laser wavelength,
- γ: a constant that depends only on the properties of the target.

The peak tensile stress formula shows that even though the absorption coefficient and fluence are important, the pulse duration has a very significant effect. For example, in a picosecond laser with 600 ps pulse duration, the pulse duration is 10 times than that of a Q-switched laser having 6 ns pulse duration and the tensile stress is 100 times than that of a Q-switched laser. In other words, the picosecond laser is able to break 100 times better than the Q-Switched laser. However, for the same reason that side effects occur when the pulse duration is longer than TRT in the selective photothermolysis, side effects may occur because the pulse duration is longer than SRT. However, since the picosecond laser has a short pulse duration, the same effect can be achieved with a lower fluence compared to the Q-switched laser (power density = fluence/pulse duration). Fluence is the concept of quantity, and the fluence of picosecond laser means the zone of the shock wave. Therefore, the side effect zone of the picosecond laser is less than that of the Q-switched laser (Table 6.4).

Let's look closely. The size of melanosomes is 0.5 μm and the TRT is 0.5 μs (500 ns). The pulse duration of the Q-switched Nd:YAG laser is 5–10 ns, and in terms of thermal confinement, the pulse duration is shorter than the melanosome's TRT resulting in melanosome coagulation and no side effects. However, because Q-switched Nd:YAG lasers are in the stress confinement zone, the coagulation effect is not large and the main effect is destroying the melanosome with a shock wave. Since the pulse duration of the Q-switched Nd:YAG laser is longer than the SRT (300 ps), the possibility of side effects is high while the effect of destroying melanosomes is low. Picosecond lasers also belong to the stress confinement zone, so when treating melasma, melanosomes are broken by shock wave, similar to the Q-switched laser. Since the pulse duration of the picosecond laser is longer than the SRT, there are side effects, but the pulse duration is shorter than that of the Q-switched Nd:YAG laser, so side effects are less likely to occur and it breaks melanosomes better.

Table 6.4 The comparison of Q-switched Nd:YAG laser versus subnanosecond laser targeting melanosome

	Q-switched Nd:YAG laser	Picosecond laser (Subnanosecond laser)
Pulse duration	5–10 ns	450–750 ps
TRT of melanosome (500 ns)	TRT > PD	TRT ≫ PD
Tissue reaction	Stress confinement	Stress confinement
SRT of melanosome (300 ps)	SRT ≪ PD	SRT ≤ PD
Peak tensile stress	Lesser	Greater
Spatial extent of the shock wave	Large	Small

6.5 Parameters

Like Q-switched lasers, picosecond lasers have a fixed pulse duration that cannot be adjusted, so you only need to adjust fluence among the three major parameters of the selective photothermolysis: wavelength, pulse duration, and fluence. In addition, epidermal cooling does not affect the results of both epidermal pigmentation and dermal pigmentation treatment, so this can be disregarded (Table 6.5, Fig. 6.4).

In the case of dermal pigmentation treatment, the larger the spot size, the deeper the penetration, so it is better to increase the spot size as much as possible. However, if a high fluence is required due to the limitation of the output, the spot size should be reduced and the fluence should be increased. For example, with a spot size of 3.5 mm, the fluence can be raised to a maximum of 2.4 J/cm^2, so to use a fluence of 2.5 J/cm^2, the spot size must be reduced to 3 mm.

Fluence should be set to the appropriate clinical end point, so that the irradiation for "dark

Table 6.5 Parameters of picosecond alexandrite laser (Picowon, WONTECH Co. Ltd. Daejeon, Korea)

Lesions	Spot size (mm)	Fluence (J/cm^2)	Frequency (Hz)
Café-Au-Lait	4	1.6	>2
Freckles	3.5	>1.9	>2
ABNOM	3.5–4	1.9–2.4	>2
Ota, Ito, Blue nevus	3–4	2.0–2.5	>2
Tattoo (eyebrow)	3.5	>2.0	>2
Tattoo (eyeliner)	3.5	>1.8	>2
Tattoo (body)	3	>2.4	>2
Laser toning	8	0.4	10
	7	0.6	10

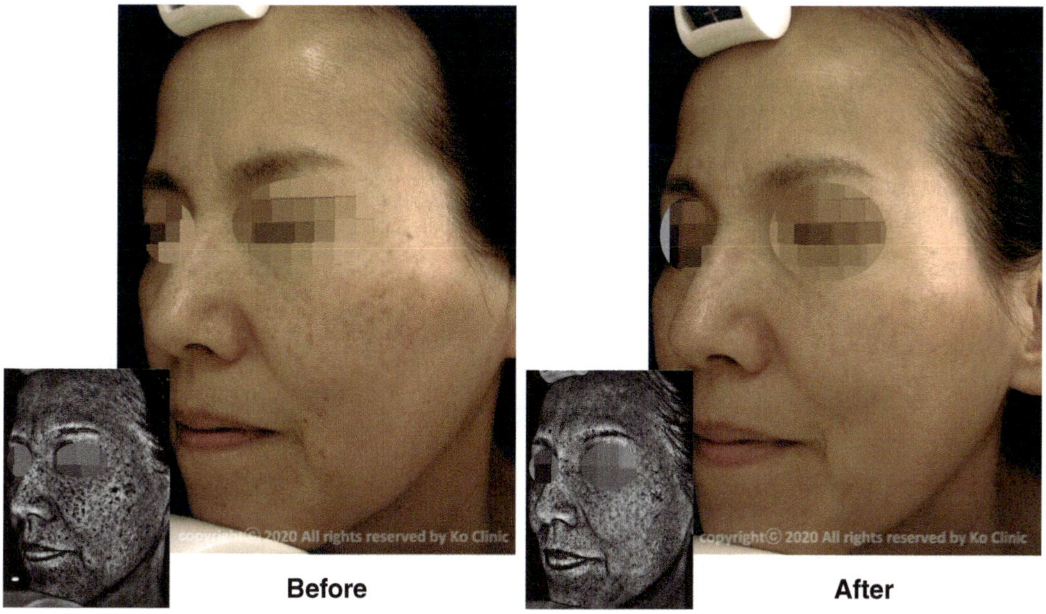

Fig. 6.4 Before and after 755 nm picosecond alexandrite laser in the treatment of pigment lesion. Laser used: Picowon, WONTECH Co. Ltd. Daejeon, Korea. Photos Courtesy of Ko Clinic, Japan

lesions is weak, light lesions is strong" (refer to Sect. 4.4 in Chap. 4). Since picosecond laser has a lower fluence for an appropriate response compared to Q-switched laser, the size of the vacuole caused by the shock wave in Q-switched laser is small. Therefore, in picosecond laser, the clinical end point of epidermal pigmentation is not whitening but "mild ash-gray." In dermal pigmentations, the clinical end point is set as "mild whitening," and in tattoo treatment, "whitening" is regarded as the clinical end point. Fluence should be adjusted to the corresponding clinical end point. Compared to Q-switched laser, picosecond laser has unclear clinical end point, making it difficult to set treatment standards.

Focusing method can also be used in picosecond lasers for dermal pigmentations such as ABNOM and tattoo treatment. However, the clinical end point of picosecond laser is unclear. Also, in picosecond alexandrite laser, the clinical end point cannot be identified immediately after laser irradiation due to tinted safety glasses, and thus focusing method is not used in picosecond alexandrite laser.

Similar to laser toning with Q-switched laser, laser toning can also be performed with picosecond alexandrite laser. The zoom handpiece of Picowon laser (WONTECH Co. Ltd. Daejeon, Korea) is designed to be collimated with a spot size greater than 7 mm. When using Picowon for laser toning, a spot size greater than 7 mm should be used because the handpiece should be at a distance from the skin during laser toning. The parameter is a spot size of 8 mm, 0.4 J/cm^2, 10 Hz, 1500 shots of the entire face with less than 500 shots per cheek. In the case of melasma patients, the number of shots should be reduced in half (750 shots of the entire face with less than 250 shots per cheek). If you want to increase the effect in patients with no melasma and reduce the number of shots for a quick treatment, increase the energy to 0.6 J/cm^2 and perform the treatment with a spot size of 7 mm and 10 Hz, less than 200 shots per cheek.

In epidermal pigmentations, treatment is performed at 2–4 intervals considering epidermal turnover. ABNOM is treated every 1–2 weeks or 4–8 weeks, and in case of Ota nevus or tattoo treatment, skin regeneration of the dermis is considered and treatment interval is every 8–12 weeks (refer to Sect. 5.8 in Chap. 5). Laser toning using picosecond alexandrite laser is performed every 2–4 weeks.

References

1. Karsai S, Bäumler W, Weiss C, Faulhaber J, Raulin C. Laser tattoo removal: do we already have picosecond lasers? J Dtsch Dermatol Ges. 2018;16(4):468–70.
2. Serup J, Bäumler W. Diagnosis and therapy of tattoo complications: with atlas of illustrative cases. Karger Medical and Scientific Publishers; 2017.
3. Niemz M. Laser-tissue interactions. Springer International Publishing; 2019.
4. Allemann IB, Goldberg DJ. Basics in dermatological laser applications. Karger Medical and Scientific Publishers; 2011.
5. Goldman MP. Cutaneous and cosmetic laser surgery. Philadelphia: Mosby Elsevier; 2006.
6. Raulin C, Karsai S. Laser and IPL technology in dermatology and aesthetic medicine. Heidelberg: New York; 2011.
7. Niemz MH. Laser-tissue interactions. New York: Springer; 2007.
8. Ho DDM, London R, Zimmerman GB, Young DA. Laser-tattoo removal—a study of the mechanism and the optimal treatment strategy via computer simulations. Lasers Surg Med. 2002;30(5):389–97.
9. Strauss M, Amendt PA, London RA, Maitland DJ, Glinsky ME, Lin CP, et al., editors. Computational modeling of stress transient and bubble evolution in short-pulse laser-irradiated melanosome particles. Laser-Tissue Interaction VIII; 1997: International Society for Optics and Photonics.

7 Long-Pulsed Nd:YAG Laser and Arrhenius Equation

7.1 Overview of Long-Pulsed Nd:YAG Lasers

Usually, only one wavelength comes out in one laser device, but lasers that can express multiple wavelengths in one laser device are being released recently. V-laser (WONTECH Co. Ltd. Daejeon, Korea) combines long-pulsed KTP laser (532 nm) and long-pulsed Nd:YAG laser (1064 nm) together to achieve 532 nm and 1064 nm wavelength in one laser device (Fig. 7.1). This chapter describes a long-pulsed Nd:YAG laser and will focus on 1064 nm wavelength.

1064 nm wavelength has a low absorption coefficient for all three major chromophores of the skin, melanin, hemoglobin, and water, so it is possible to treat deep in the dermis. The chromophore with the highest absorption coefficient is melanin, followed by hemoglobin and water. Look at the characteristics of 1064 nm long-pulsed Nd:YAG laser according to the chromophore. First, long-pulsed Nd:YAG laser is effective for hair removal because the absorption coefficient for melanin is higher than that of other chromophores. In particular, it has the longest wavelength compared to other hair removal lasers, so it can be safely used for hair removal for darker skin (refer to Sect. 2.7 in Chap. 2) [1]. Second, when heat is applied to hemoglobin, metHb is produced, which has a higher absorption coefficient than oxyHb and melanin at 1064 nm. Therefore, long-pulsed Nd:YAG laser can be used for vascular treatment. However, compared to PDL, there is a risk of side effects such as burns due to coagulation in the dermal layer around blood vessels. Finally, nonablative rejuvenation (NAR) can be attempted using water as a chromophore.

Unlike other lasers, in the long-pulsed Nd:YAG laser, the pulse duration can be selected. Short pulse duration and long pulse duration can be selected (Table 7.1). The short pulse duration is 0.3 ms, which is mainly used during genesis technique. The long pulse durations from 5 ms to 60 ms are also available.

There is a total of 8 spot size cartridges from 2 to 12 mm spot size, and the spot size can be adjusted by replacing the cartridge.

The epidermal cooling device uses a contact cooling method using a sapphire tip, and the skin temperature setting can be adjusted in a total of 4 steps (5, 10, 15, and 20 °C). Compared to other lasers, 1064 nm wavelength has the deepest photon penetration, so without epidermal cooling, there is a high risk of deep burns and scarring. Therefore, when using a long-pulsed Nd:YAG laser the cooling system should be checked.

J. D. Lee, M. J. M. Oh, *Lasers in Dermatology: Parameters and Choice*,
https://doi.org/10.1007/978-981-19-7568-4_7

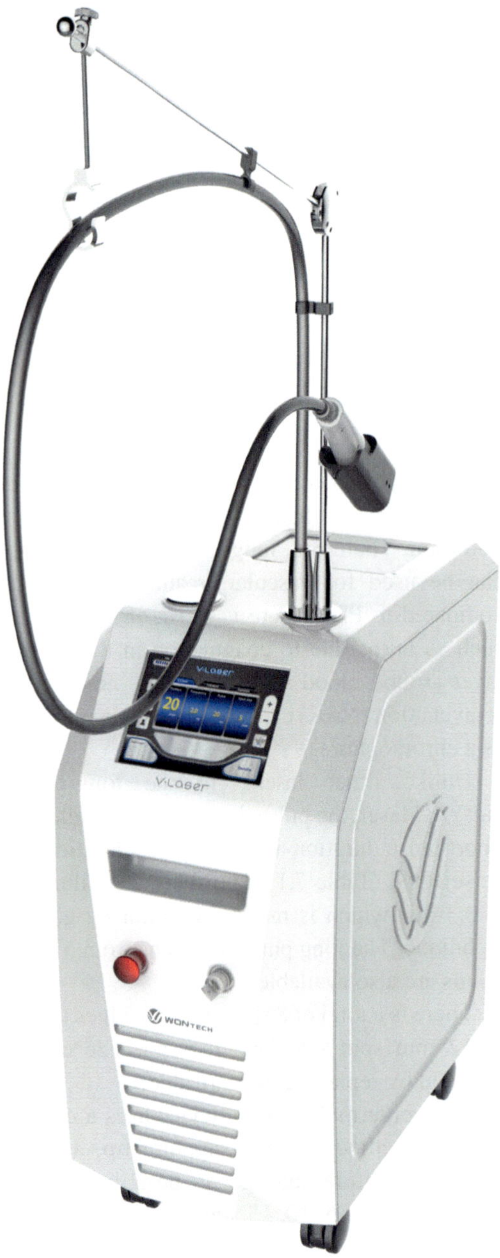

Fig. 7.1 Laser device combined with long-pulsed KTP laser and long-pulsed Nd:YAG laser together (V-Laser, WONTECH Co. Ltd. Daejeon, Korea)

Table 7.1 Specifications of long-pulsed Nd:YAG laser (V-Laser, WONTECH Co. Ltd. Daejeon, Korea)

Wavelength	1064 nm	532 nm	Genesis
Energy	50 J	10 J	4 J
Pulse duration	5 to 60 ms	1 to 40 ms	0.3 ms (300 μ)
Repetition rate	0.5 to 5 Hz	0.5 to 3 Hz	0.5 to 10 Hz
Spot size	2, 3, 4, 5, 6, 8, 10, 12 mm		
Cooling system	Sapphire window contact cooling (16 mm)		
Cooling temp.	5–20 °C		

7.2 Indications

The indications for long-pulsed Nd:YAG laser are laser hair removal, vascular treatment, and nonablative rejuvenation, as discussed above.

First, laser hair removal. The long-pulsed Nd:YAG laser is painful and the pulse duration cannot be reduced under 5 ms, so the effect is limited on thin hair. Because long-pulsed Nd:YAG laser has a longer wavelength than other hair removal lasers, it is the most appropriate laser for laser hair removal for darker skin. However, since Koreans do not have very dark skin (Fitzpatrick skin type VI), long-pulsed Nd:YAG laser is not absolutely necessary for hair removal purposes. For hair removal purposes, I mainly use long-pulsed alexandrite laser, which is less painful and effective even for thin hair.

Second, vascular treatment. With a pulse duration of 4 ms or more, metHb is generated [2]. This metHb is used for vascular treatment. The long-pulsed Nd:YAG laser can use a short pulse duration of 0.3 ms and a long pulse duration of 5 ms or more. Treatment of visible blood vessels is possible using a pulse duration of 5 ms or more, so it is difficult to treat diffuse erythema (TRT < 4.5 ms), where blood vessels are not visible by eye [3]. And because long-pulsed Nd:YAG laser has a high absorption coefficient of metHb at 1064 nm wavelength, and there is a risk of scarring at temperatures high enough to cause petechia, cautions should be taken with fluence control. Due to the long pulse duration it can also be used for vascular lesions with long TRT such as granuloma pyogenicum [4], venous lake [5], and senile hemangioma, and can also be used to remove warts [6].

Third, nonablative rejuvenation. For nonablative rejuvenation, there are methods A and B of the Arrhenius formula (refer to Sect. 7.3 in Chap. 7). Method A is a method that shortens a pulse duration and uses high energy, has a high risk of side effects and may result in severe pain. This is why I mainly use the genesis technique, which is a repetitive irradiation with a pulse duration of 0.3 ms (Method B of the Arrhenius equation).

7.3 Arrhenius Equation

When the photon of the laser meets the chromophore, temperature rises. Among the skin reactions caused by laser, coagulation, vaporization, carbonization, and melting occur in the photothermal effect. Among these phenomena, the Arrhenius equation is applied below 100 °C where no vaporization occurs. Here, we will only look at the meaning of the Arrhenius formula, not the Arrhenius formula itself. The Arrhenius formula has two meanings.

First, for tissue denaturation, not only temperature but also time is important. For example, the same tissue degeneration occurs at more than 1 s at 65 °C and at more than 10 s at 57 °C (Fig. 7.2). There is no absolute temperature for tissue degeneration or coagulation. Time as well as temperature must be considered. Therefore, various parameters exist for tissue degeneration below 100 °C.

Second, a threshold exists, and tissue degeneration does not occur if this threshold is not exceeded. We know that the treatment of epidermal pigmentation with IPL has no effect unless it exceeds a certain level of energy (damage threshold). There is also a threshold at which side effects occur. We know that when using a nonablative laser, if we increase the energy moderately, we can see the desired effect, but if we increase the energy a little more, scars due to burns occur (survival threshold). Calderhead gave rise to the concept of damage threshold and survival threshold by taking into account reversible and irreversible tissue damage including tissue denaturation and cell death (Fig. 7.3).

The purpose of nonablative rejuvenation (NAR) is collagen remodeling. Although there are several mechanisms of NAR, the mechanism by thermal injury with subsequent wound healing is considered to be the primary mechanism [9]. Although the exact mechanism is unknown, it is believed that thermal injury to the skin destroys collagen, resulting in recruitment and activation of fibroblasts for new collagen formation. This mechanism illustrates the paradox that in order for new collagen to form, collagen destruction must precede. On the other hand, Alexiades et al. observed that the effect of NAR increased as the

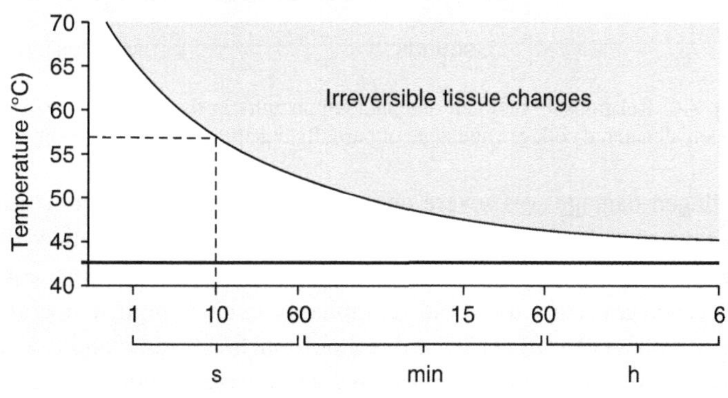

Fig. 7.2 Relationship between time and temperature in tissue damage. The threshold of tissue damage at each temperature depends on the laser energy and pulse duration. For a pulse duration of 1 s, 65 °C is the threshold, whereas for an irradiation time of 10 s, 57 °C is the threshold. Reproduced from [7]

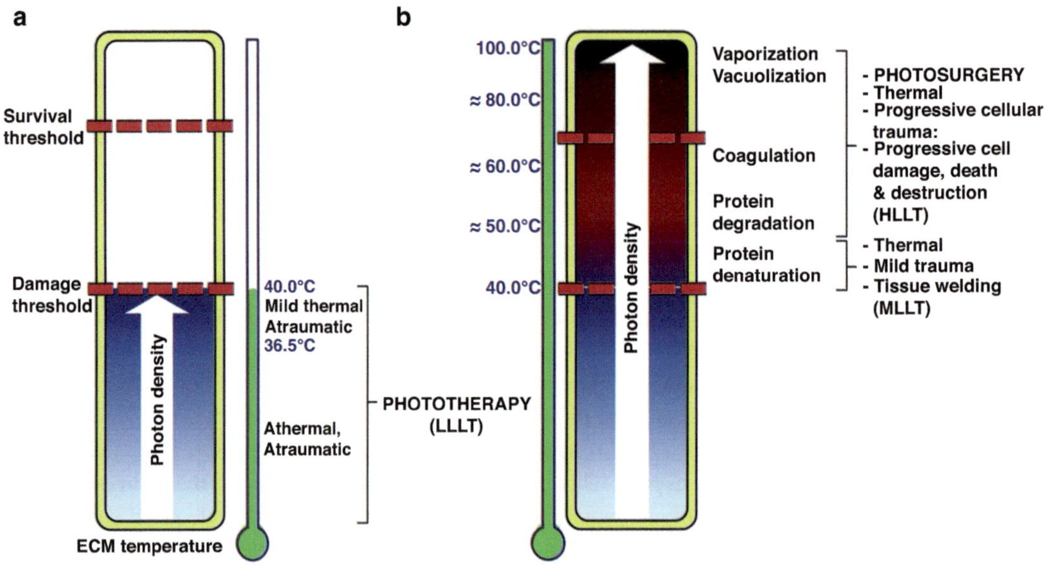

Fig. 7.3 Damage threshold and survival threshold. (**a**) reaction associated with low level light therapy (LLLT). (**b**) reactions associated with mid level laser treatment (MLLT) (reversible damage) and high-level light therapy (HLLT) (irreversible damage and cell death). Reproduced from [8]

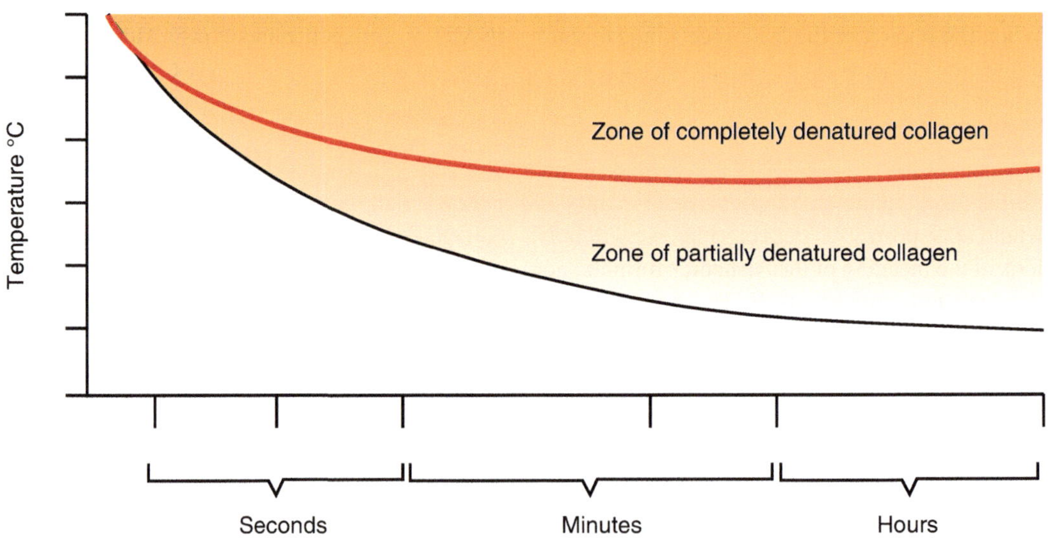

Fig. 7.4 Relationship between time and temperature in tissue damage. Zones can be divided into two: zone of completely denatured collagen and zone of partially denatured collagen. Modified from [7]

collagen damage was severe and the volume of denatured collagen increased (partially denatured collagen), but the effect decreased when it exceeded a certain threshold (completely denatured collagen) [10]. That is, thresholds such as damage threshold and survival threshold were found. So, I think in collagen denaturation, the Arrhenius equation will be like Fig. 7.4.

In conclusion, there are two methods for nonablative rejuvenation (NAR) applying the Arrhenius equation: Short exposure time and high temperature (method A) or long exposure time and low temperature (method B). These are summarized in Table 7.2.

Partial denaturation of collagen will be the same in both method: Short exposure time and

Table 7.2 Two methods for nonablative rejuvenation (NAR)

Method	Time and temperature	Therapeutic window	Drawback
A	Short time and high temperature	Narrow	Pain, side effect
B	Long time and low temperature	Wide	Long procedure time

high temperature (A) or long exposure time and low temperature (B). However, method A has a narrow therapeutic window. Therefore, it may not be effective or side effects such as scarring are likely. Also, severe pain is also a clinical problem. In contrast, method B can be implemented without worrying about side effects because of its wide therapeutic window. However, the procedure takes a very long time. For example, if the temperature is maintained at 45 °C, it takes at least 1 h for it to be effective. A typical example of method B is the genesis technique.

7.4 Drawbacks of Nonablative Lasers

Nonablative rejuvenation (NAR) has no downtime and few side effects compared to ablative rejuvenation. Despite these advantages, NAR has several disadvantages compared to ablative rejuvenation. Let's review the drawbacks of NAR.

First, NAR is significantly less effective than ablative rejuvenation [11]. Second, the results are not consistent. Some patients find it effective, while others do not. Third, despite topical anesthesia, there is considerable discomfort. Pain may be severe in method A. Fourth, the procedure time is the very long (15–20 min) for method B, so the operator is reluctant to perform the procedure. But if we shorten the procedure time, then it is less effective [9, 12]. Fifth, there is no clinical end point. The only visible symptom is erythema, but we do not know how long the erythema should last nor how red it should be. The next symptom observed on the skin is immediate epidermal whitening, which is not a clinical end point, but rather a warning end point that indicates scar formation. Therefore, when performing NAR, it is necessary to set the maximum energy, maximum number of shots, and maximum duration time in advance.

7.5 Fibroblasts in Papillary and Reticular Dermis

Wound healing can be divided into two types: reparative wound healing and regenerative wound healing. Reparative wound healing refers to wound healing in which wounds, such as burn scars, as they heal, leave scars and change into tissues without epidermal appendages such as hair follicles, eccrine glands, and sebaceous glands [13]. Examples of regenerative wound healing are newt (salamander)s and human fetuses. Newts are able to regenerate a fully functioning new leg after their original leg is cut off. Also, in the first trimester of pregnancy, even if the fetus gets wounded in the uterus they do not leave a scar. This kind of wound healing is called regenerative healing.

Through research, Ryan R. Driskell et al. revealed that fibroblasts in the papillary dermis and fibroblasts in the reticulated dermis have different origins and play different roles in the wound healing process. That is, fibroblasts in the papillary dermis are involved in regenerative healing, and fibroblasts in the reticular dermis are involved in reparative healing (Table 7.3).

In summary, if the damage is limited to the epidermis and the papillary dermis, regenerative healing takes place, which is the role of fibroblasts of the papillary dermis, and a completely new epidermis and papillary dermis is formed. On the other hand, if the reticular dermis is damaged, reparative healing takes place, which is the role of fibroblasts of the reticular dermis, thus scarring takes place.

Why does reparative healing take place, thus creating a scar, after the reticular dermis is damaged? I think the reason for this is because the most important function of the skin is barrier function: to protect our body from the outside world. When the damage is limited to the epidermis and the papillary dermis, the reticular dermis

Table 7.3 Comparison of fibroblasts of papillary and reticular dermis

	Fibroblast from papillary dermis	Fibroblast from reticular dermis
Wound healing	Regenerative	Reparative
Scarring	Without scarring	With scarring
Examples	Newts, salamanders Human fetus (first trimester)	Burn scar
Meaning	Esthetics	Survival
Ablative lasers	CO_2 laser resurfacing	CO_2 fractional laser
Nonablative lasers	Genesis technique Vascular laser	Needle RF Er:glass fractional laser

acts as a barrier, so there is no major problem in the barrier function even if regenerative healing takes place. But if the reticular dermis is damaged, reparative healing would be needed to rapidly recover barrier function despite the scarring.

We should choose a laser considering the differences in fibroblasts between the papillary and reticular dermis and the differences in wound healing. Which laser would be most effective? The most effective laser for skin regeneration is already known. The most effective laser for rejuvenation of papillary dermis is CO_2 laser resurfacing. Then what is the most effective laser for the reticular dermis? The damage to the reticular dermis should be limited as much as possible because reparative healing may cause scarring. However, collagen remodeling in the reticular dermis may be effective for elasticity, deep wrinkles, and scars. In other words, the reticular dermis may also be a treatment target. Considering the above, I think that fractional photothermolysis is the most appropriate method. Actually, CO_2 fractional lasers are known to be effective in treating scars.

I think the most effective method for NAR of papillary dermis is the genesis technique or the vascular laser. Also, I think that needle RF (fractional microneedle radiofrequency), an invasive bipolar radiofrequency method using a fine needle, is the most effective method for NAR of the reticular dermis.

It would be ideal if collagen was remodeled in both the papillary and the reticular dermis. Therefore, combination therapy is needed. The most effective method would be CO_2 laser resurfacing with CO_2 fractional laser treatment or pinhole method. A representative example is the scar sculpting technique presented by Dr. Lee Yong Soo [14]. Also, I think the most effective combination treatment in NAR is genesis technique followed by needle RF.

7.6 Parameters

As mentioned earlier, the indications for long-pulsed Nd:YAG laser are laser hair removal, vascular treatment (Fig. 7.5), and nonablative rejuvenation. I do not use a long-pulsed Nd:YAG laser for hair removal because I have a long-pulsed alexandrite laser. Therefore, the parameters of laser hair removal using long-pulsed Nd:YAG laser are not listed in Table 7.4.

First, let's look at the parameters for vascular treatment. If you have already purchased a laser, the wavelength among the three major laser parameters (wavelength, pulse duration, and fluence) has been determined, and you need to determine the pulse duration and fluence. Fluence is relatively constant regardless of pulse duration, so either refer to the fluence of the parameters provided by the company or use the fluence that has had a reaction, regardless of the pulse duration (refer to Sect. 10.5 in Chap. 10). Since most telangiectasias occurring on the face are thin blood vessels of 200 μm or less (TRT = 17.9 ms), I use 10 and 5 ms for the pulse duration. The clinical end point is considered "darkening" or "immediate disappearance." First, I irradiate the entire face lesion at 10 ms, 150 J/cm^2, and then return to the first treated lesion to exclude the heat accumulation effect. After reducing the pulse duration to 5 ms at the same fluence, nonresponsive lesions are irradiated (refer to Sect. 10.4 in Chap. 10). For lesions that still do not respond, I try increasing the fluence to 160 J/cm^2. If there is only one lesion, take enough time (at least 10 s) to exclude the heat accumulation effect

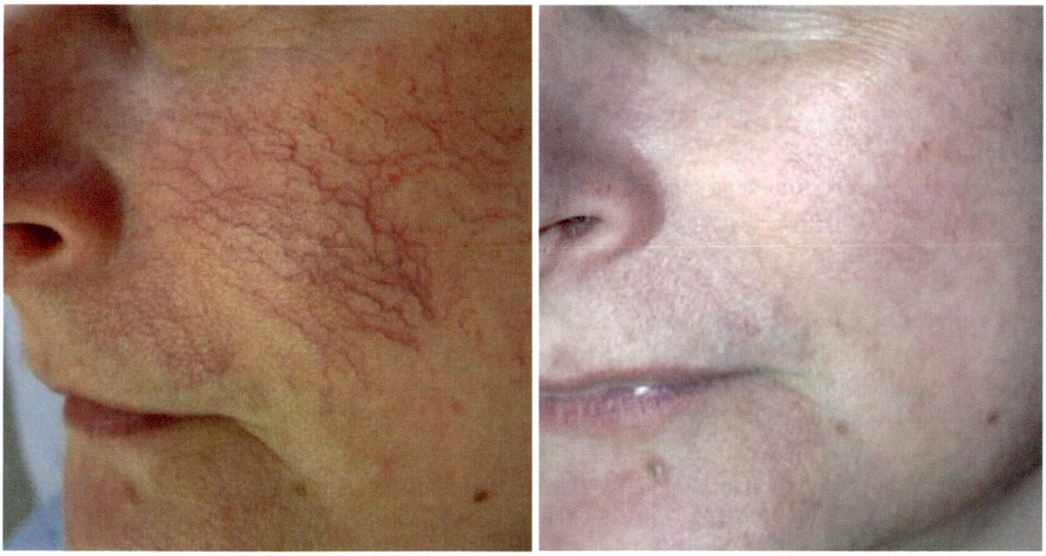

Fig. 7.5 Before and after long-pulsed Nd:YAG laser in the treatment of telangiectasia. Laser used: V-Laser, WONTECH Co. Ltd. Daejeon, Korea. Photos courtesy of Hugues Cartier, MD., France

Table 7.4 Parameters of long-pulsed Nd:YAG laser (V-Laser, WONTECH Co. Ltd. Daejeon, Korea)

Lesion	Spot size (mm)	Fluence (J/cm^2)	Duration (ms)	Frequency (Hz)	Temperature (°C)	Interval (week)
Telangiectasia	3–	150–160	5–10	1	15–20	4–6
Cherry angioma	3	150–160	5–10	1		4–6
Dark circle	5	>90	20–30	1		4–6
Vein	4–6	>150	20–30	1		4–6
Venous lake	5	>90	20–60	1		4–6
Warts	4	>220	20	1	5–15	4
Genesis	8	>7	0.3	10	Off	2
Tightening	10	35	30	1 (2–3 pass)	5	4–6
Acne, acne redness	5	80–100	10–15	1	5	2

after irradiation, and then as described above, first reduce the pulse duration and if there is still no response, try raising the fluence. Vessels that do not disappear even after 5 ms should be considered as vessels that cannot be treated with long-pulsed Nd:YAG laser and should not be treated any more. In particular, long-pulsed Nd:YAG lasers should never be stacked. Stacking is a method of irradiating once and irradiating once again if there is no reaction. But because the temperature rises before the heat dissipates, the risk of burns and scarring is very high. Also, if the handpiece is pressed hard on the skin, the blood vessels will disappear, and thus the handpiece should be lightly pressed. The largest spot size seems ideal when treating the dermis, but when treating blood vessels with a long-pulsed Nd:YAG laser, I use a spot size of 3 mm. Among the three factors involved in optical penetration depth (OPD), spot size, wavelength, and power density, the most important is wavelength. Long-pulsed Nd:YAG laser already has a deep OPD even if the spot size is not increased because of the long wavelength. Rather, it is an advantage to use a small spot size in the Nd:YAG laser [15]. First, the range of side effects is small even if side effects occur, and second, even if a small spot size requires higher energy than a large spot size, the total amount of energy is small, so the small spot size causes less pain than a large spot size. Therefore, it is safe to use a small spot size when treating blood vessels with a long-pulsed Nd:YAG laser. The disadvantage is that due to the small spot size, it takes a long time to treat the entire face.

For blue blood vessels such as dark circles, veins, and venous lakes, the spot size is increased to 4–6 mm because the blood vessels are thicker, and the pulse duration is also increased to 20–60 ms. As with telangiectasia treatment, it is irradiated at the standard fluence (dark circles and venous arcs are about 90 J/cm^2, and venous vessels about 150 J/cm^2) and 60 ms. If there is no response, it is irradiated at 40 ms, and if there is no response, it is irradiated at 20 ms. If there is still no response, fluence should be raised. Warts are irradiated with a 4 mm spot size, 20 ms, 220 J/cm^2, and the cooling temperature is lowered because the pain is severe. Treatments are performed at monthly intervals.

In nonablative rejuvenation (NAR), various parameters exist because the fluence varies according to the pulse duration as the Arrhenius formula is applied to the damage threshold. Therefore, the parameters presented for NAR are all different for each manufacturer. However, if you find a fluence that is between the damage threshold and the survival threshold at a specific pulse duration, all parameters will be effective. In genesis technique, if the spot size is larger than 10 mm, the skin temperature rises too quickly, so it is not suitable as the method B of the Arrhenius equation, which requires sufficient time. The spot size of 8 mm and the fluence of 7 J/cm^2 are frequently used. After repeated use of the laser, the output of the laser seems to have dropped, the fluence should be increased little by little. The handpiece should be placed at a distance of 1–2 cm from the skin, and since it takes too long to irradiate the entire face, irradiate 2500–2800 shots reducing the area and performing only on important parts such as nose, malar area, and cheeks for about 4–5 min. I do not think there is a clinical end point for NAR. Rather, I consider the patient's subjective hot sensation as a warning endpoint. To reduce the risk of burns, the handpiece should be moved more quickly or the fluence should be lowered so that the temperature rises gradually, and 2500–2800 shots could be achieved as much as possible. However, if the patient's subjective hot sensation continues, the genesis technique should be stopped.

As method A of the Arrhenius equation, there is a so-called "50/50 technique" (50 J/cm^2, 50 ms, 10 mm spot), which is a representative procedure for long-pulsed Nd:YAG laser [16]. However, I do not perform it frequently because of the risk of pain and side effects. If you want to try method A, reduce the pulse duration to 30 ms to reduce pain, lower the cooling temperature to the lowest level, and try with a fluence of 35 J/cm^2. It is essential to check whether the contact cooling is working well before the procedure, and close observation is needed to check whether there is a Nikolsky sign immediately after the procedure. I rarely use this method because I think that genesis technique alone has sufficient skin regeneration effect.

Because both inflammatory acne and erythema due to acne are made up of non-visible blood vessels, long-pulsed Nd:YAG laser cannot have a direct effect. However, if sufficient heat is delivered using NAR, the sebaceous glands can be damaged and I think it will help reduce inflammation. Therefore, for inflammatory acne (papules, pustules, nodules, cysts) and erythema due to acne, method A of the Arrhenius equation is used, irradiated only once with a 5 mm spot size at 1064 nm and 80–100 J/cm^2 at 10–15 ms.

References

1. Raulin C, Karsai S. Laser and IPL technology in dermatology and aesthetic medicine. Heidelberg: New York; 2011.
2. Niemz MH. Laser-tissue interactions. New York: Springer; 2007.
3. Lee W. Principles of IPL and its uses (Korean). Seoul: MDworld; 2008.
4. Hammes S, Kaiser K, Pohl L, Metelmann HR, Enk A, Raulin C. Pyogenic granuloma: treatment with

the 1,064-nm long-pulsed neodymium-doped yttrium aluminum garnet laser in 20 patients. Dermatol Surg. 2012;38(6):918–23.
5. Bekhor PS. Long-pulsed Nd:YAG laser treatment of venous lakes: report of a series of 34 cases. Dermatol Surg. 2006;32(9):1151–4.
6. Han TY, Lee JH, Lee CK, Ahn JY, Seo SJ, Hong CK. Long-pulsed Nd:YAG laser treatment of warts: report on a series of 369 cases. J Korean Med Sci. 2009;24(5):889–93.
7. Berlien H-P. Applied laser medicine. Springer Science & Business Media; 2003.
8. Calderhead RG, Vasily DB. Low level light therapy with light-emitting diodes for the aging face. Clin Plast Surg. 2016;43(3):541–50.
9. Goldman MP. Cutaneous and cosmetic laser surgery. Philadelphia: Mosby Elsevier; 2006.
10. Alexiades-Armenakas M, Newman J, Willey A, Kilmer S, Goldberg D, Garden J, et al. Prospective multicenter clinical trial of a minimally invasive temperature-controlled bipolar fractional radiofrequency system for rhytid and laxity treatment. Dermatol Surg. 2013;39(2):263–73.
11. Park SH, Yeo WC, Koh WS, Park JW, Noh NK, Yoon CS. Laser dermatology plastic surgery 2nd ed (Korean). Seoul: Koonja; 2014.
12. Wanner M, Sakamoto FH, Avram MM, Chan HH, Alam M, Tannous Z, et al. Immediate skin responses to laser and light treatments: therapeutic endpoints: how to obtain efficacy. J Am Acad Dermatol. 2016;74(5):821–33. quiz 34, 33
13. Woodley DT. Distinct fibroblasts in the papillary and reticular dermis: implications for wound healing. Dermatol Clin. 2017;35(1):95–100.
14. Lee Y. Scars and scarring: causes, types and treatment options. Nova Science Publishers, Inc.; 2013.
15. Christiansen K, Drosner M, Bjerring P. Optimized settings for Nd:YAG laser treatments of leg telangiectasias. J Cosmet Laser Ther. 2015;17(2):69–76.
16. Taylor MB, Prokopenko I. Split-face comparison of radiofrequency versus long-pulse Nd-YAG treatment of facial laxity. J Cosmet Laser Ther. 2006;8(1):17–22.

8 Pulsed Dye Laser (PDL) and Macropulse

8.1 Overview of PDLs

The 595 nm long-pulsed dye laser (PDL) has a lower absorption coefficient for hemoglobin than the previously released 585 nm PDL. In 595 nm, photons penetrate deeper than 585 nm and can treat thicker blood vessels. In addition, since the absorption coefficient for melanin is low, epidermal side effects can be reduced (refer to Sect. 2.7 in Chap. 2) [1]. The pulse duration of Vbeam Perfecta® (Candela Corp. Wayland, MA, USA) can be selected from a total of 8 pulse durations (0.45, 1.5, 3, 6, 10, 20, 30, 40 ms). The pulse duration other than 0.45 ms is a macropulse composed of subpulses (micropulses) (refer to Sect. 8.3 in Chap. 8, Table 8.1). A total of 8 subpulses are irradiated at a pulse duration of 3 ms or longer, and 4 subpulses are irradiated at 1.5 ms. In addition, because epidermal cooling is the most important strategy in vertical situations, DCD™ (dynamic cooling device) was installed to increase safety (refer to Sect. 1.14 in Chap. 1). Spray duration is the time during which DCD is sprayed before laser irradiation, and spray delay duration is the non-irradiation time between spray and laser irradiation. Therefore, the longer the spray duration and the shorter the spray delay duration, the better the cooling of the epidermis. Vbeam Perfecta® can adjust refrigerant cooling in three stages, and the spray duration/delay duration (ms) are 20/20, 30/20, and 40/20, respectively. Vbeam Perfecta® does not support postspray where refrigerant is sprayed after laser irradiation.

The spot size of Vbeam Perfecta® can be adjusted from 3 to 12 mm by replacing the cartridge (gauge) (Fig. 8.1). There is also a cartridge with an elongated spot size of 3X10mm to treat thin vessels. When the skin is pressed with diascopy, blood vessels constrict and blood disappears, leaving only melanin as the chromophore, enabling epidermal pigment treatment with PDL. There are also 7 mm PL and 10 mm PL cartridges (Pigmented Lesion Distance Gauge) specially manufactured for epidermal pigment treatment using this principle.

Table 8.1 Specifications of 595 nm long-pulsed dye laser (PDL) (Vbeam Perfecta®, Candela Corp. Wayland, MA, USA)

Laser type	Pulsed dye	
Wavelength	595 nm	
Pulse	0.45–40 ms	
Spot sizes (diameter) With maximum energy	3 mm–40 J/cm^2 5 mm–30 J/cm^2 7 mm–20 J/cm^2 10 mm–10 J/cm^2	12 mm–7 J/cm^2 3x10 mm–25 J/cm^2 7 mm PL–15 J/cm^2 10 mm PL–10 J/cm^2
Cryogen	Chemours HFC 134a US 20	
DCD™ spray duration	User adjustable range: OFF–100 ms	
DCD™ spray delay duration	User adjustable range: 10–100 ms	

J. D. Lee, M. J. M. Oh, *Lasers in Dermatology: Parameters and Choice*,
https://doi.org/10.1007/978-981-19-7568-4_8

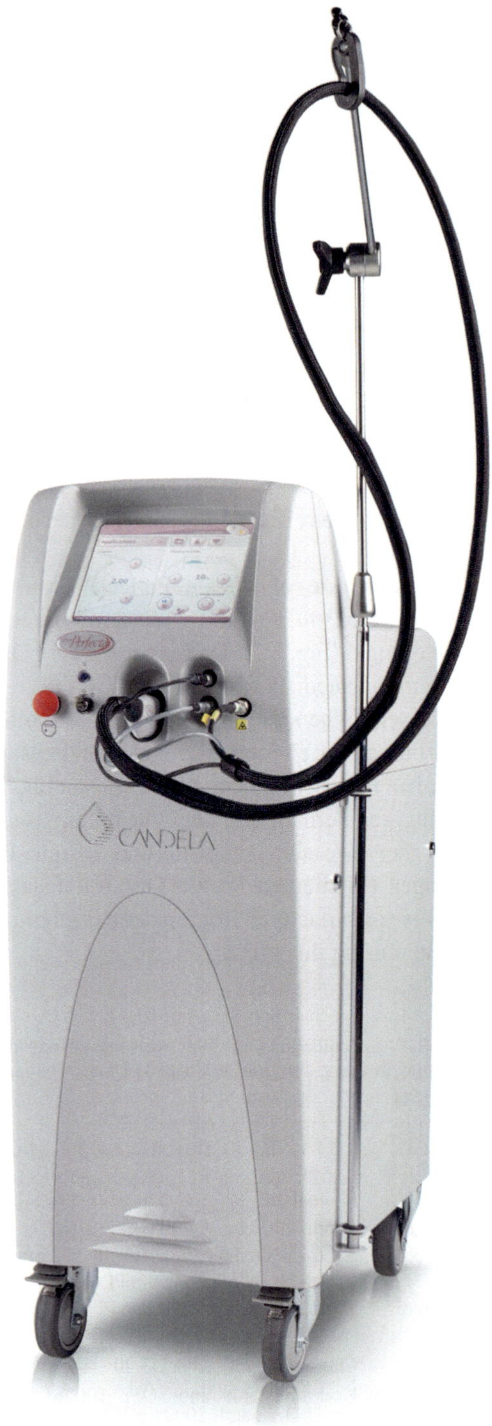

Fig. 8.1 Vbeam Perfecta® (Candela Corp. Wayland, MA, USA) implements various spot sizes and functions through cartridges

PDL is known as the treatment of choice in vascular therapy [1]. However, the biggest problem with PDL is not only the high purchase cost but also the high maintenance cost. Most of the consumables of Q-switched lasers and other long-pulsed lasers are flash lamps, which are external energy sources. However, in PDL, it costs to replace not only the flash lamp, which is an external energy source, but also the dye, which is the laser medium. Therefore, it is necessary to carefully purchase the laser considering the demand.

8.2 Indications

The indications for PDL can be divided into vascular diseases, skin regeneration, and other skin diseases (Table 8.2). Vascular diseases include telangiectasia, diffuse redness (erythema), rosacea, and vascular anomalies (hemangioma, pyogenic granuloma, and port wine stain) [2]. PDL acts on blood vessels to help regenerate the skin by collagen remodeling, which is effective for wrinkles. However, there are many other effective treatments for wrinkles, and PDL is not frequently used for the purpose of treating wrinkles because PDL has a high maintenance cost and risk of purpura. In addition, there are reports that PDL is effective on hypertrophic scars and keloids [3] and is also effective on red stretch marks, i.e., striae rubra [4]. When the skin is pressed with diascopy, blood vessels constrict and blood disappears, leaving only melanin, enabling epidermal pigment treatment with PDL

Table 8.2 Indications of PDL

Vascular lesions	Skin rejuvenation	Diseases
Diffuse redness Rosacea Acne Facial and leg telangiectasia Poikiloderma of Civatte Angiomas and spider angiomas Hemangiomas Port wine stains	Wrinkles Scars and stretch marks Benign pigmented lesions (Freckles, Sunspots)	Warts Psoriasis

[1]. However, there is a limit to reducing the pulse duration, and the cost of consumables is high compared to other lasers, so this is not frequently used. There are also reports that it is effective for skin diseases such as warts and psoriasis.

8.3 Macropulse

Macropulse is a method of irradiating several small pulses (subpulse, micropulse) in succession to make the pulse duration longer than the pulse duration of small pulses [1]. It is also called "Train pulse" because the connection of the pulses is like that of train. The representative laser of macropulse is PDL.

If the original pulse duration is 1.5 ms, the laser should be continuously irradiated for 1.5 ms (Fig. 8.2a), and the irradiation must be completed after 1.5 ms. This is called the "true long pulse" [6]. However, the actual PDL we use, V-beam, cannot produce a long pulse duration of 1.5 ms, but only 0.45 ms. So, 0.45 ms is irradiated three times consecutively (Fig. 8.2b) to increase the temperature for 1.5 ms, like a true long pulse.

The reason for creating macropulse was as follows. To produce a true long pulse, high power was required, but it was difficult to produce high power when long-pulsed laser was being developed. At this time, it was found that the same result could be achieved with irradiating multiple times instead of one time. Thus, a long-pulsed laser was created using macropulses that continuously collect and irradiate low-energy subpulses [7].

Then what is the difference between macropulse and true long pulse? First, the main difference is that it is difficult for macropulses to produce higher temperatures than true long pulses. During the break between subpulses, the temperature drops, resulting in a lower temperature than the true long pulse. However, this can act as an advantage, because of the lower temperature there are fewer side effects. We will review this in detail at Sect. 8.4 in Chap. 8.

Second, the characteristics of the subpulse remain [1]. For example, in the case of PDL, when a long pulse duration in milliseconds is made with macropulse, purpura should not occur due to photothermal effect. However, the characteristics of the subpulse of 0.45 ms remain and purpura occurs by photomechanical effect.

Third, even with the same type of laser, response and actual fluence may vary even if the same pulse duration and fluence are used. This is because the pulse duration and shape of the subpulse, fluence, and number of subpulse shots vary from manufacturer to manufacturer.

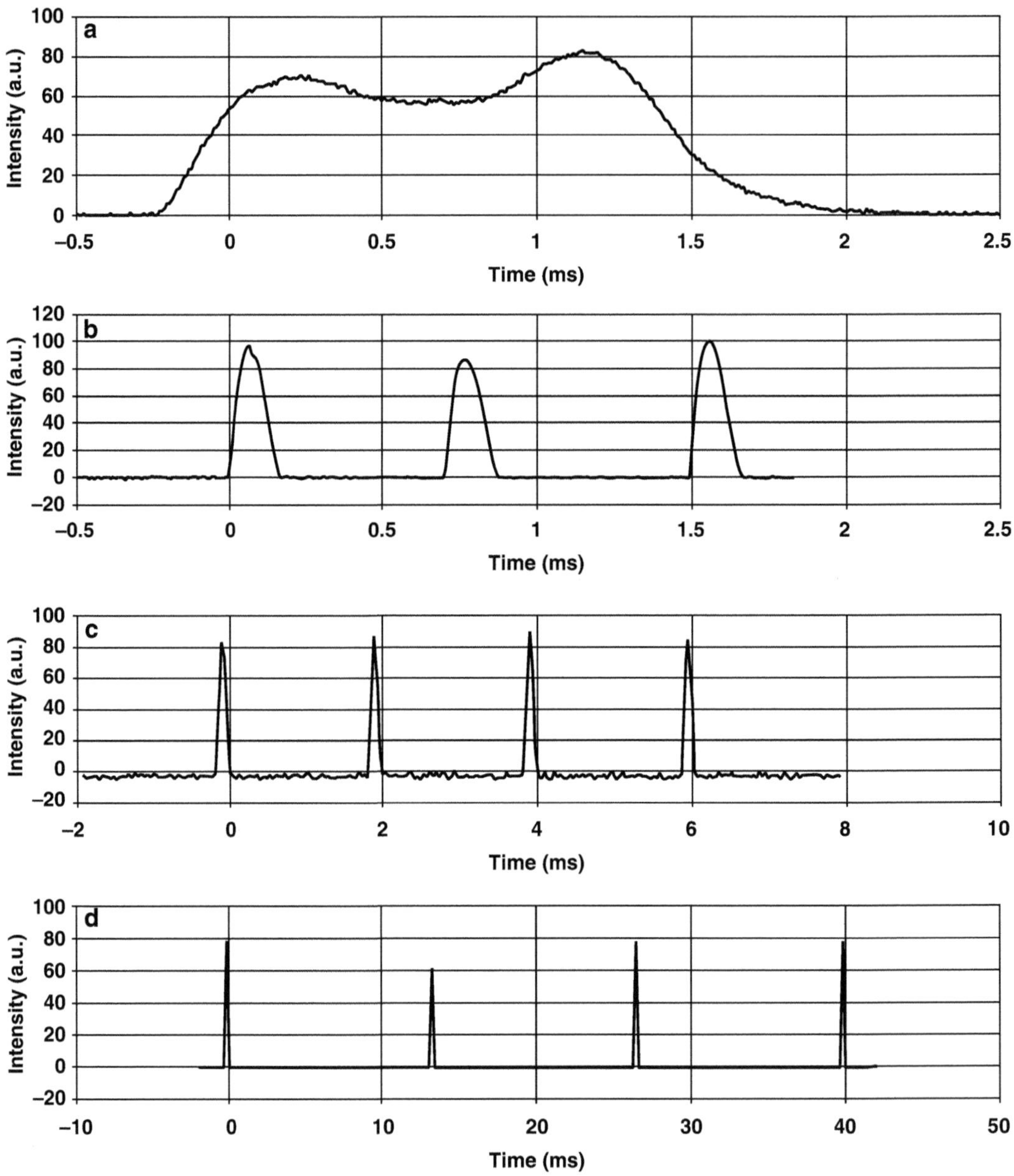

Fig. 8.2 Variety of pulse profiles. (**a**) ScleroPlus 1.5 ms, (**b**) V-Beam 1.5 ms, (**c**) V-Beam 6 ms, (**d**) V-beam 40 ms. Reproduced from [5]

8.4 Arrhenius Equation in Vascular Therapy

Now let's review vascular treatment based on Arrhenius equation (Fig. 8.3). At 33 ms, the coagulation temperatures for blood, arterial collagen, and bulk skin are 90.4 °C, 88 °C, and 70 °C, respectively. Therefore, according to the Arrhenius equation, if the temperature of the bulk skin rises, the arterial collagen or bulk skin will denature before the blood coagulates, which will cause side effects. One way to overcome this is by the theory of selective photothermolysis or the extended theory of selective photothermolysis

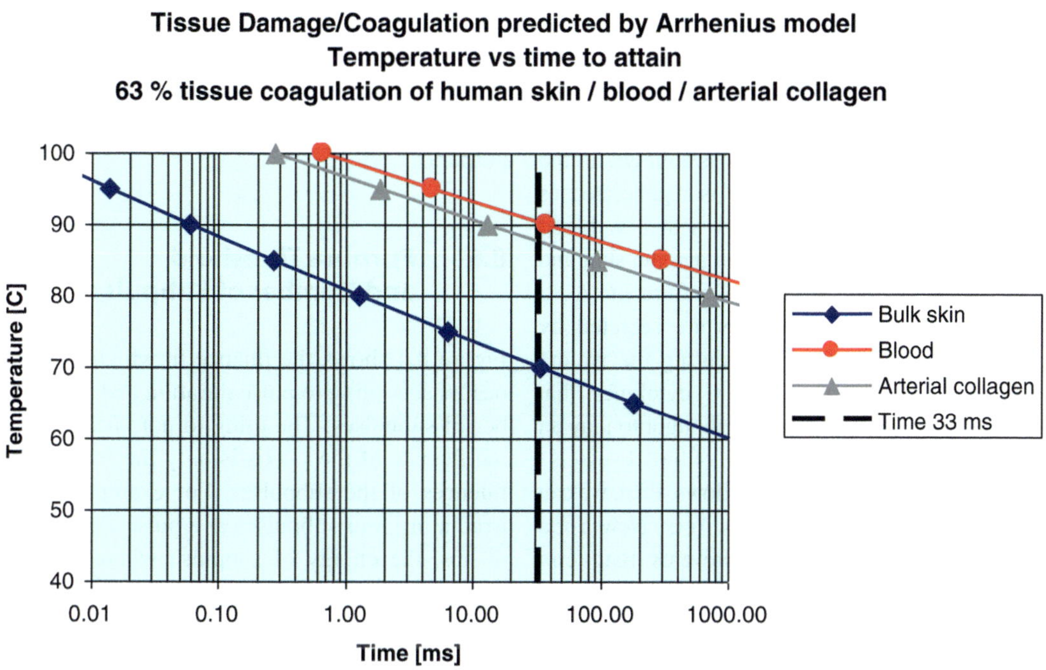

Fig. 8.3 Tissue denaturation temperature dependency versus time predicted by the Arrhenius model for bulk skin (blue), blood (red), and arterial collagen (gray). Reproduced from [8]

[8]. That is why TRT or TDT (thermal damage time) is of primary importance. Ultimately, however, tissue denaturation is based on Arrhenius equation. In this case, the important time is not the TRT, but the time at which 99% of the actual tissue degeneration occurs (t_{eden}, effective denaturation time).

For example, let's consider a PDL with a true pulse of 0.45 ms pulse duration. The pulse duration of 0.45 ms can treat blood vessels corresponding to a thickness of 30–100 μm. If the laser is irradiated with a true pulse with a pulse duration of 0.45 ms, blood vessels can be treated without purpura. However, considering the Arrhenius formula, the method of using high energy in a short pulse duration (method A) has a narrow therapeutic window (refer to Sect. 7.3 in Chap. 7). In addition, as the blood vessel bursts in temperatures over 100 ° C, purpura may occur, resulting in blood vessel recurrence (Fig. 8.3). On the other hand, in the method of using low energy in a long pulse duration (method B), due to the long pulse duration (e.g., 4.5 ms), 30–100 μm blood vessels corresponding to pulse duration of 0.45 ms are spared and cannot be treated due to thermal kinetic selectivity (TRT < PD) in the thermal phase of the optical thermal model. In summary, method B cannot treat blood vessels because of thermal kinetic selectivity. To overcome this, macropulse is used. When using a macropulse that irradiates low energy subpulses (0.45 ms) multiple times, photons are selectively absorbed in blood vessels of 30–100 μm (TRT ≥ PD), and because the subpulse is repeated and has a long pulse duration, blood vessels do not burst, and the therapeutic window can be broadened.

8.5 Repair and Re-Emergence of Blood Vessels

The paper mentioned above is based on the premise that the temperature of blood should not be above 100 °C because purpura should not occur. Why should there be no purpura during PDL?

After vascular laser treatment, the blood vessels regenerate, and symptoms recur.

Neovascularization occurs even after sclerotherapy for the treatment of varicose veins as well as after vascular lasers. This is very confusing, but there is still little research on this phenomenon [9].

The mechanism is assumed as follows. In the wound healing process, tissue is regenerated as the damaged tissue is replaced with new blood vessels. Vascular lasers also damage the skin and new blood vessels regenerate and recur. As a direct cause various cytokines are secreted by inflammatory cells generated during the wound healing process. Among them, cytokines that increase angiogenic factors are thought to play an important role in the recurrence of blood vessels.

Prevention methods are as follows. First, we can try Rapamune (Pfizer Inc., New York, New York, USA), a medication which prevents long-term rejection reaction in kidney transplant patients. Rapamune is known to inhibit cytokine production and there are some reports that it is effective for revascularization after laser treatment. Second, imiquimod is an immunomodulator which was used to prevent recurrence after laser on port wine stain (PWS), but the results were poor.

Considering the mechanisms of blood vessel regeneration and recurrence, I believe that shrinking blood vessels or creating intravascular coagulation to block blood vessels is a way to reduce blood vessel regeneration and recurrence, rather than rupturing blood vessels and developing inflammation. Therefore, the clinical end point should be darkening or disappearance, implying clot formation or vessel coagulation, not purpura.

8.6 Purpura Threshold and Number of Subpulses

Figure 8.4 shows the fluence in which purpura occurs according to pulse duration and the number of subpulses. The thing to note here is that the fluence of the y-axis is only the sum of the fluences of the subpulses. For example, when irradiating four subpulses at a pulse duration of 40 ms, the energy of subpulse where purpura starts to occur is 2.5 J/cm^2. There are four 2.5 J/cm^2 beams, so the instrument panel displays 10 J/cm^2.

The desired reaction is vessel contraction or vessel blockage due to intravascular coagulation without purpura. Therefore, energy that is lower than the purpura threshold should be irradiated. For example, the purpura threshold of PDL with eight subpulses at 20 ms is 16 J/cm^2 (Fig. 8.3). There are reports that blood vessels below 600 μm were successfully treated without downtime only with fluence of 9–10 J/cm^2 [10].

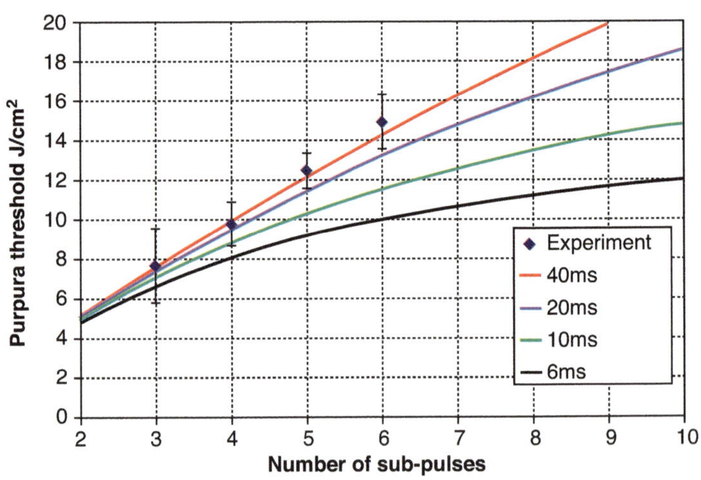

Fig. 8.4 Purpura threshold vs. number of subpulses. Reproduced from [9]

8.7 Parameters

The indications for PDL include vascular disease (Fig. 8.5), skin regeneration, and other skin diseases, as discussed above (Table 8.3).

First, let's look at the parameters of PDL for vascular disease. Since PDL uses macropulse composed of subpulses and subpulses do not change significantly depending on pulse duration, pulse duration is not adjusted according to the size of blood vessels. In PDL, the pulse duration of the macropulse means the time of the tissue denaturation process, i.e., the time in the Arrhenius equation.

According to the Arrhenius equation, there is a method using a high temperature for a short time (method A) and a method using a low temperature for a long time (method B) (refer to Sect. 7.3 in Chap. 7). Both methods have the same effect, but since method B has a wider therapeutic window, it is better to use a longer pulse duration than a shorter one. However, when a long pulse duration is used, the fluence required to produce the same effect is higher than that of the short pulse duration (Fig. 8.4), and the dye is consumed quickly. This is the reason why the pulse duration of 6 and 10 ms is frequently used. When there is no response of the blood vessels, treatment is attempted by reducing the pulse duration to 1.5 ms (four subpulses) or 0.45 ms (one subpulse) to rupture the blood vessels.

When treating the dermis with blood vessels, it is better to use the largest spot size possible (refer to Sect. 4.6 in Chap. 4). However, the larger the spot size, the faster the dye is consumed, so 7 or 10 mm spot size is usually used. However, for treatment of deep lesions or rapid treatment of large lesions such as port wine stains, the largest 12 mm spot size may be useful.

If the fluence is high, purpura may occur, which may have a significant impact on the patient's social life. Therefore, to prevent purpura, a fluence that does not cause purpura according to the pulse duration should be selected (nonpurpuragenic dose, Fig. 8.4). The clinical end point is regarded as "darkening," which appears due to the formation of a clot in the blood vessel, or "vessel disappearance," in which the vessel wall constricts. First, a test shot is performed on the lesion in an inconspicuous location. To find the appropriate fluence (1) the fluence should be gradually increased to find the fluence that shows the clinical end point or (2) the fluence should be reduced by 0.5 J/cm^2 from the fluence that causes purpura. If treatment is not successful, a fluence higher than the purpura threshold should be used to rupture the blood vessel (purpuragenic dose, Fig. 8.4). However, in this case, the blood vessel can burst

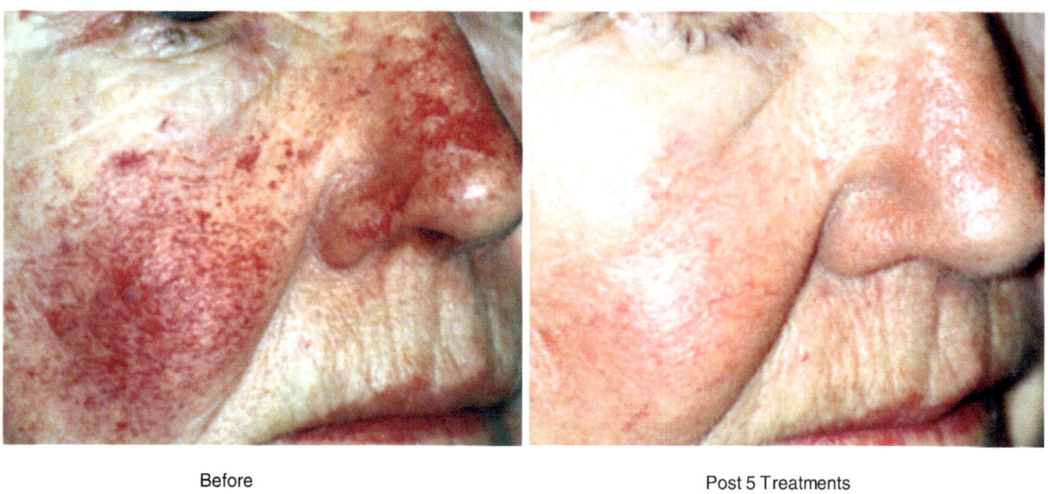

Fig. 8.5 Before and after PDL of rosacea patient. Laser used: Vbeam Perfecta® (Candela Corp. Wayland, MA, USA). Photos Courtesy of Ross Kaplan, MD

Table 8.3 Parameters of PDL (Vbeam Perfecta®, Candela Corp. Wayland, MA, USA)

Lesion	Spot size (mm)	Pulse width (ms)	Fluence (J/cm²)	DCD spray/delay	Interval (weeks)
Telangiectasia facial	5	6, 10, 20	7.5–12	30/20	4–6
	7	6, 10, 20	7–12		
	10	6, 10, 20	5.5–7.5		
	3x10	10	11–14		
Telangiectasia nasal	5, 7	10–40	8–12	30/20	4–6
	10		6.5–7.5		
	3 × 10		10–12		
Rosacea Diffuse redness	7	6, 10, 20	8–11	30/20	4–6
	10		5–7		
Port wine stains (PWS)	5	0.45	10–15	30/20	8–12
	7	1.5	8–12		
	10		4–4.75		
Poikiloderma of Civatte	10	10	5–6.5	30/20	4–6
Acne	7	6, 10	8–10	30/20	2–4
	10	3	4.5		
Cherry angioma Spider angioma	7	1.5	8–11.5	30/20	4–6
	10		5–10		
Venous lake	7	1.5	7–10	30/20	4–6
Hemangioma	7	1.5	6–10	40–20	2 weeks for neonate and infant/8–12 weeks for adult
	10		5–6		
Photo-rejuvenation Wrinkles	7	6–10	7	30/20	4–6
	10		6		
Hypertrophic scar Keloid	7	1.5, 3	10–13	Off	6–8
		10	9.5		
Striae	10	0.45	3–7	30/20	4–6
Scar	7	0.45, 1.5	7–8	30/20	4–6
	10		4–5		
Warts(facial)	5	1.5	9–9.5	30/20	2–3
Warts(non-facial)	5, 7	1.5	12–15	Off	2–3
Psoriasis	5	0.45, 1.5	6–8	Optional, may use 30/20	2–4
	7		4–8		
	10		3–8		

even with a short pulse duration, and to reduce dye consumption, the pulse duration should be reduced to 1.5 or 0.45 ms. Also, because purpura occurs, the patient should be informed in advance that a lot of bruising will persist for 10–14 days, which can affect social life.

Purpura is more likely to occur if the patient is taking medications that affect hemostasis, such as aspirin or anticoagulants, so thorough consultation with the patient before treatment is essential. For darker skin or recently tanned skin, the fluence should be lowered due to risk of hypopigmentation or post-inflammatory hyperpigmentation (PIH).

Because vascular treatment is a vertical situation, surface cooling is essential. Four- to six-week intervals are recommended when considering the skin regeneration of the dermis layer. However, in the case of port wine stains, treatment is performed every 8–12 weeks in consideration of sufficient skin regeneration. In acne, the size of the lesion is not large, and the skin is well moisturized due to much sebum production, so treatment every 2–4 weeks is possible.

If the diameter of the blood vessel is thin and shows a reticular pattern, or if the blood flow rate is fast and it recurs or does not disappear well, it can be treated by stacking method by lowering both pulse duration and fluence. The clinical end point is considered as an ambiguous state of purpura. For example, in reticulated telangiectasia that does not improve in 10 ms or 20 ms, the procedure is performed by stacking with a spot size of 10 mm, pulse duration 1.5 ms, 6.5–6.75 J/cm^2, DCD 30/20.

In patients with severe telangiectasia, if all blood vessels are treated at the first visit, the edema after the procedure may be severe, making daily life difficult. Thus, partial treatment is performed several times. (Published with kind permission of © Seung Choi MD. 2021. All rights reserved.)

Second, PDL can be used for hypertrophic scars, keloids, stretch marks, and postoperative wounds. As with vascular treatment, only the red lesion must be targeted because the purpose of PDL is to remove blood vessels in the scar. In the case of stretch marks, PDL is effective in red striae rubra but not effective in white striae alba without blood vessels. Recently, a method of irradiating PDL for scar prevention after stitch out is being studied [11, 12]. PDL usually attempted 2 weeks after stitch out.

Third, PDL may also be used for treatments of warts and psoriasis. However, it is not frequently used because of insurance issues and the maintenance cost of PDL.

References

1. Goldman MP. Cutaneous and cosmetic laser surgery. Philadelphia: Mosby Elsevier; 2006.
2. Allemann IB, Goldberg DJ. Basics in dermatological laser applications. Karger Medical and Scientific Publishers; 2011.
3. Gold MH, McGuire M, Mustoe TA, Pusic A, Sachdev M, Waibel J, et al. Updated international clinical recommendations on scar management: part 2--algorithms for scar prevention and treatment. Dermatol Surg. 2014;40(8):825–31.
4. Aldahan AS, Shah VV, Mlacker S, Samarkandy S, Alsaidan M, Nouri K. Laser and light treatments for striae distensae: a comprehensive review of the literature. Am J Clin Dermatol. 2016;17(3):239–56.
5. Kimel S, Svaasand LO, Cao D, Hammer-Wilson MJ, Nelson JS. Vascular response to laser photothermolysis as a function of pulse duration, vessel type, and diameter: implications for port wine stain laser therapy. Lasers Surg Med. 2002;30(2):160–9.
6. Kauvar A, Hruza G. Principles and practices in cutaneous laser surgery. CRC Press; 2005.
7. Park SH, Yeo WC, Koh WS, Park JW, Noh NK, Yoon CS. Laser dermatology plastic surgery 2nd ed (Korean). Seoul: Koonja; 2014.
8. Murphy M, Torstensson P. Thermal relaxation times: an outdated concept in photothermal treatments. Lasers Med Sci. 2014;29(3):973–8.
9. Raulin C, Karsai S. Laser and IPL technology in dermatology and aesthetic medicine. Heidelberg: New York; 2011.
10. Ross EV, Uebelhoer NS, Domankevitz Y. Use of a novel pulse dye laser for rapid single-pass purpura-free treatment of telangiectases. Dermatol Surg. 2007;33(12):1466–9.
11. Karmisholt KE, Haerskjold A, Karlsmark T, Waibel J, Paasch U, Haedersdal M. Early laser intervention to reduce scar formation—a systematic review. J Eur Acad Dermatol Venereol. 2018;32(7):1099–110.
12. Kent RA, Shupp J, Fernandez S, Prindeze N, DeKlotz CMC. Effectiveness of early laser treatment in surgical scar minimization: a systematic review and meta-analysis. Dermatol Surg. 2020;46(3):402–10.

9 Intense Pulse Light (IPL) and Extended Theory of Selective Photothermolysis

9.1 Overview of IPLs

Intense pulsed light (IPL) is light, and not a laser. Unlike laser, in IPL, there is no laser medium nor optical cavity, and only a flash lamp, which is an external energy source (pumping system), exists (Table 9.1). When electricity flows through the xenon gas of the flash lamp, a very bright, high-power light is generated [1].

Since IPL is light, it has the opposite characteristics to the four characteristics of laser: monochromaticity, coherence, collimation, and high intensity [2]. IPL's four characteristics are polychromaticity, incoherence, divergence, and low intensity. So, in IPL, various wavelengths from 500 to 1300 nm are irradiated at once (polychromaticity) [2]. And because of incoherence and low intensity, IPL cannot generate a pulse duration in nanoseconds like a Q-switched laser but has a pulse duration in milliseconds like a long-pulsed laser. Therefore, it shows a photothermal effect by using coagulation phenomenon. IPL also has an elongated flash lamp attached directly to the handpiece to reduce divergence. Therefore, IPL has a rectangular spot shape to use all the light of the elongated flash lamp. The spot size is larger than that of a laser (Fig. 9.1). Because IPL has a large spot size, it can be operated quickly. This is a great

Table 9.1 Specifications of IPL (Cellec V, Jeisys Medical Inc. Seoul, Korea)

Filters	420(S) / 500(S) / 530(S) /530(D) / 545(V) / 560 / 590 / 640 / 700
Fluence	1–60 J/cm^2
Pulse duration	1–60 ms
Delay time	1–60 ms
Lamp type	Xenon lamp
Spot size	40 mm × 10 mm

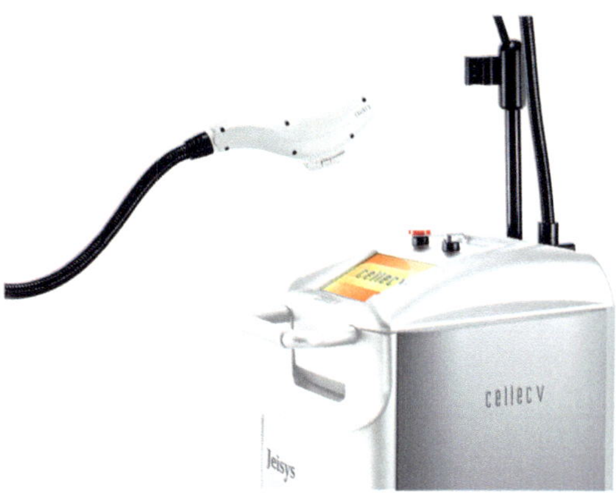

Fig. 9.1 IPL has a rectangular spot shape to use all the light of the elongated flash lamp. The spot size is larger than that of a laser (Cellec V, Jeisys Medical Inc. Seoul, Korea)

J. D. Lee, M. J. M. Oh, *Lasers in Dermatology: Parameters and Choice*,
https://doi.org/10.1007/978-981-19-7568-4_9

advantage when removing hair from a large area. However, because the spot size is large, side effects such as "tiger print" also occur (refer to Sect. 20.3.2 in Chap. 20). Recently, IPLs that additionally provide handpieces or filters to reduce spot size are being released. Cellec V (Jeisys Medical Inc. Seoul, Korea) provides "light guide" with a spot size of 15 × 9 mm.

In IPL, there can be one irradiation in one shot (single pulse), but there can also be two or three irradiations in one shot (multipulse). Also, the pulse delay time can be adjusted, so that various pulse sequences can be created.

The indications for IPL are various, such as acne treatment, vascular treatment, pigmentation treatment, laser hair removal, and nonablative rejuvenation. Thus theoretically, with only IPL and CO_2 laser purchase, all skin beauty problems may be solved. However, despite the many advantages of IPL, it is a very incomplete machine due to the non-uniformity of the raw spectrum, the ambiguity of the filter, the spectral shift (spectral shift refers to a phenomenon in which in the same IPL, when the electrical energy is high, short-wavelength light is irradiated, and when the electrical energy is low, long-wavelength light is irradiated [3]), and passive cooling. On the other hand, IPLs that reduce such imperfections and have a high output, are too expensive, so it has no major advantage compared to lasers. Therefore, it is important to purchase an IPL with high integrity, relatively high output, and low price.

9.2 Raw Spectrum and Indications

When no filter is used, the raw spectrum of the flash lamp shows a wavelength of 250 to 1400 nm, and the output is different for each wavelength. In general, the wavelength of the left ultraviolet region has high output, and the right near infrared region (750–1400 nm) has low output (Fig. 9.2). Because IPL has a wide spectrum, its indications vary from acne to vascular treatment, pigmentation treatment, laser hair removal, and nonablative rejuvenation. However, since IPL does not have the same far-infrared wavelength (>3000 nm) as the CO_2 laser or Er:YAG laser, ablative rejuvenation cannot be performed.

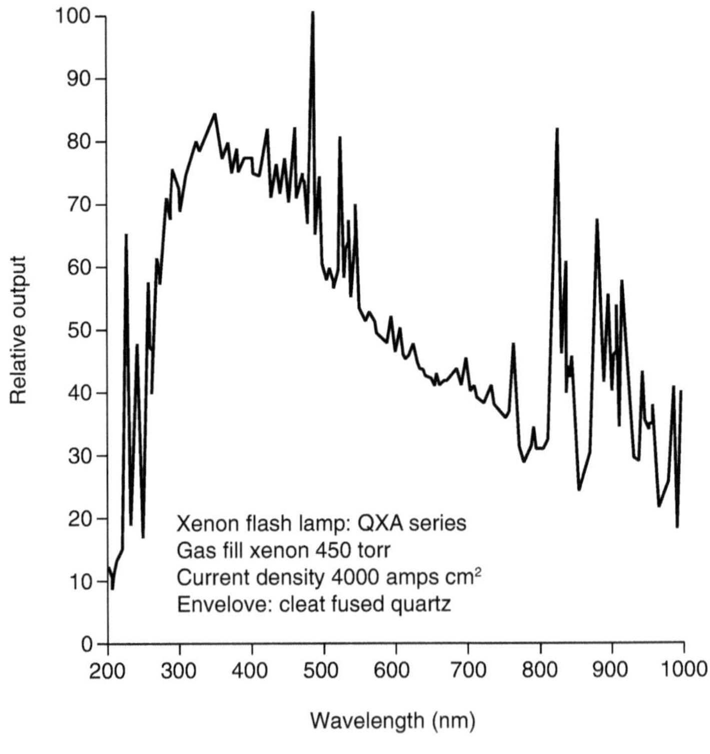

Fig. 9.2 Raw spectrum of xenon flash lamp. It can be seen that the output is mainly located in the ultraviolet region. Reproduced from [4]

In addition, since the raw spectrum of IPL is biased toward the ultraviolet region, and wavelengths over 950 nm is filtered by a water filter, the absorption coefficient of mid infrared (1400–3000 nm) is lowered. Thus, high power is required to perform nonablative rejuvenation using mid-infrared rays. But if high output is used, the energy of 500~600 nm wavelengths may be too high, and side effects may occur. Therefore, it is difficult to see the effect of nonablative rejuvenation using mid-infrared rays with IPL.

However, by using the 500~600 nm wavelengths of IPL, a nonablative rejuvenation effect can be seen either by (1) transferring heat to blood vessels to indirectly heat water in the dermis to achieve collagen remodeling or (2) to produce collagen through the wound healing process by generating cellular mediators and growth factors [5]. For the same reason, the output of the wavelength corresponding to the optical window (600–1200 nm), which is the wavelength range suitable for laser hair removal or dermal pigment treatment, is also low. Thus, it is difficult to see the effect of laser hair removal in low-cost IPLs with low output. In addition, epidermal cooling is important in vertical situations such as laser hair removal, but in the case of IPL, there is an elevated risk of side effects because passive cooling does not provide sufficient cooling. And since IPL cannot create a pulse duration of nanoseconds, it cannot treat dermal pigmentations or tattoos. Therefore, I think the indications for IPLs are only acne treatment, vascular treatment, epidermal pigmentation treatment, and nonablative rejuvenation.

9.3 Optical Filter

IPL can control the spectrum according to the purpose of treatment by using various filters on the raw spectrum. First, a water filter is used to remove wavelengths of 950 nm or more, which is a wavelength with a high absorption coefficient of water, and then the optical filter is used to remove ultraviolet rays and some visible rays harmful to the skin [1]. For example, if a 640 nm filter is selected, light with a wavelength range of 640–950 nm is emitted.

In addition, IPL can control the spectrum with various optical filters for one therapeutic purpose. For example, various optical filters such as 530 nm, 560 nm, and 590 nm can be used for vascular treatment (Fig. 9.3, Table 9.2). The key

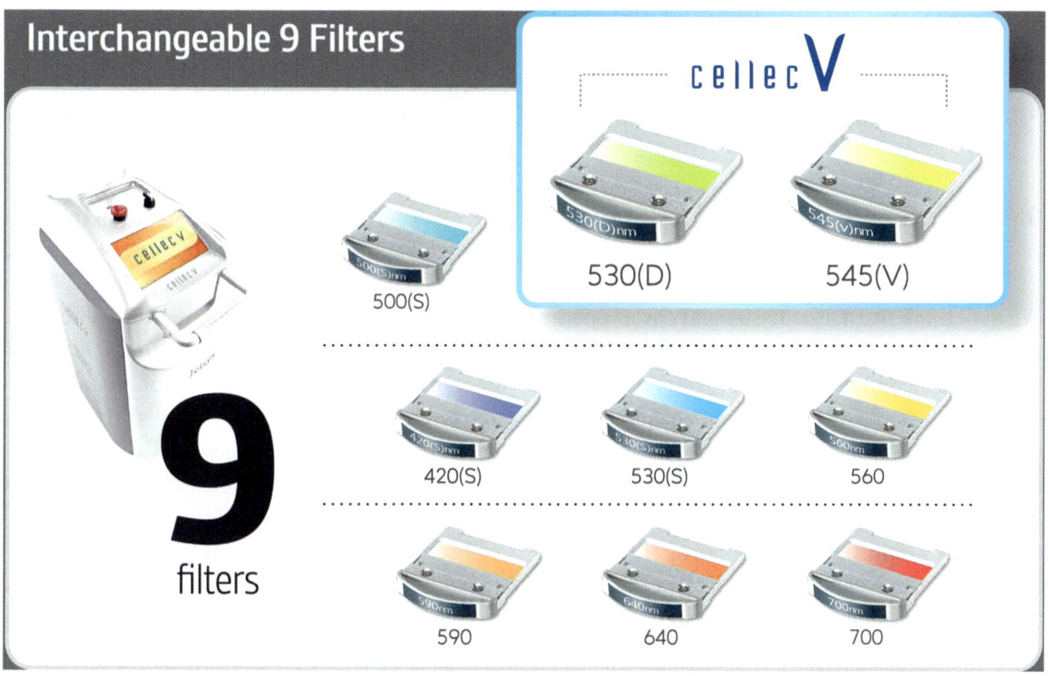

Fig. 9.3 Various optical filters of IPL (Cellec V, Jeisys Medical Inc. Seoul, Korea)

Table 9.2 Various optical filters and indications. (Cellec V, Jeisys Medical Inc. Seoul, Korea)

Filter	Range	Indications
420(S)nm Tip	420–600 nm	Acne, photoshower mode
500(S)nm Tip	500–600 nm	Facial telangiectasia
530(S)nm Tip	530–600 nm	Facial telangiectasia
530(D)nm Tip	530–650 nm, 900 nm~	Rosacea, diffuse erythema
545(V)nm Tip	545–800 nm	Freckle, lentigo
560 nm Tip	560–950 nm	Freckle, lentigo, facial telangiectasia, cell toning mode, photoshower mode
590 nm Tip	590–950 nm	Freckle, lentigo, melasma, facial telangiectasia
640 nm Tip	640–950 nm	Melasma
700 nm Tip	700–950 nm	Hair removal, photoshower mode

Table 9.3 Chromophore and target cell of laser hair removal

Location	Chromophore	Target cell
Bulge region	Hair shaft	Follicular stem cell
Hair bulb	Hair matrix	Hair germ cell

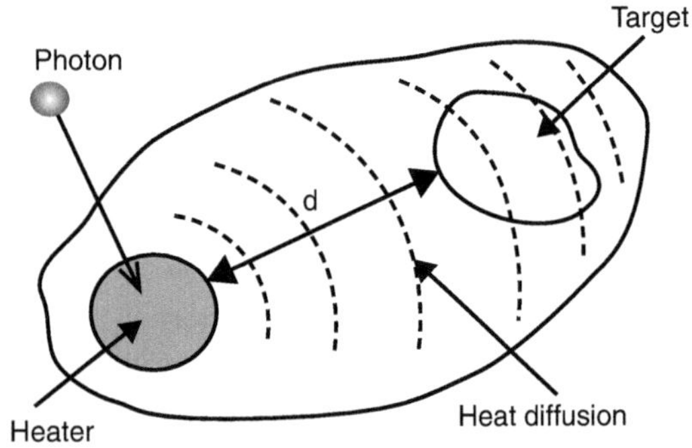

Fig. 9.4 General structure of biological target tissue with space separation between target and absorber (heater). Reproduced from [7]

point here is that the appropriate fluence for each optical filter is different. In the 530 nm optical filter, all wavelengths from 530 nm to 600 nm corresponding to blood vessels are irradiated, and a low fluence should be applied because short wavelength shows high output. On the other hand, since only the wavelength of 590 nm to 600 nm is irradiated with the 590 nm optical filter and has only a low output, higher fluence than the 530 nm optical filter should be applied.

9.4 Extended Theory of Selective Photothermolysis

We may think that target tissue and chromophore (component of the skin that absorbs photons) match, but in real practice, however, target tissue and chromophores often do not match [6]. An example is a laser hair removal. The target tissues of laser hair removal are hair germ cells and follicular stem cells in the hair bulb and hair bulge, respectively, and the chromophores are the hair matrix and hair shaft, respectively (Table 9.3). Hair germ cells and follicular stem cells do not have melanin.

Extended theory of selective photothermolysis (extended theory) is a theory that damages target tissues when chromophores and target tissues do not match [7]. In the previously mentioned example of laser hair removal, irradiation with the laser raises the temperature of the hair shaft, the chromophore, and the temperature is transferred to the follicular stem cells through heat diffusion and the cells are destroyed. Extended theory is a principle that indirectly damages the target tissue through heat diffusion from the heat generating chromophore (heater) (Fig. 9.4). Therefore, thermal relaxation time (TRT) described in selective photothermolysis does not apply to extended theory, but instead thermal damage time (TDT) is applied. TDT is defined as the time it takes from the heat generating chromophore (heater) to the temperature at which the outermost layer of the target tissue is damaged through thermal diffusion. By definition, TDT is longer than TRT (TDT > TRT) and pulse duration (PD) must be between TDT and TRT (TDT ≥ PD > TRT).

Then what are the conditions for the extended theory to be applied? One laser text describes that extended theory applies to “non-uniformly absorbing target structure” [6]. The three major

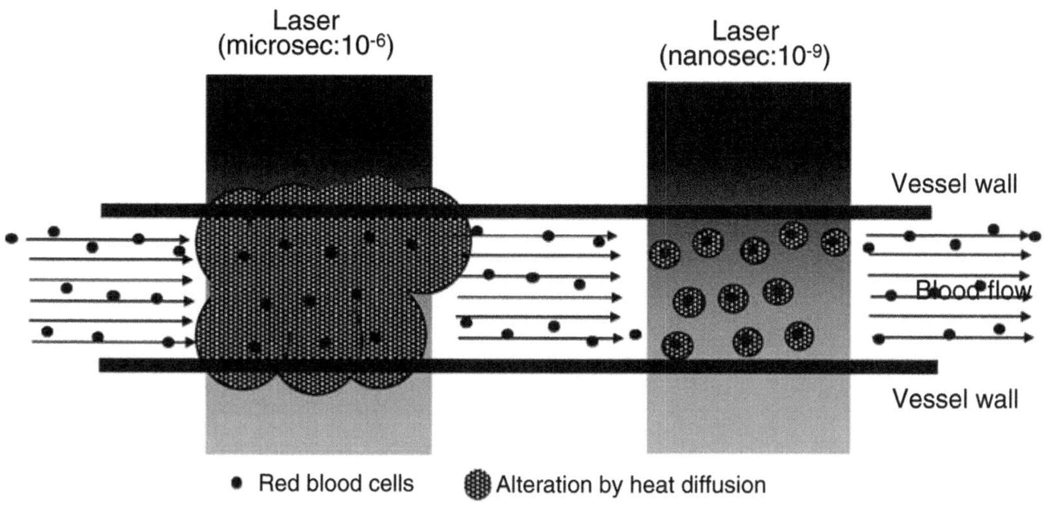

Fig. 9.5 A schema showing the difference in the treatment of vascular lesions between long (microsecond) and short (nanosecond) pulsed lasers. Nanosecond pulsed lasers can injure red blood cells, but not vessel walls, resulting in no effect to vascular lesions. However, microsecond pulsed lasers can injure not only red blood cells, but also vessels walls. Reproduced from [8]

chromophores of the skin are melanin, hemoglobin, and water. Since water is uniform to the skin, extended theory does not apply, but melanin and hemoglobin may not be uniform.

For example, RBC in blood vessel is uniform, but the blood vessel is composed of blood and vascular endothelial cells, so the entire blood vessel is not uniform [8]. Irradiating a 532 nm Q-switched laser with a 10 ns pulse duration targeting an RBC with a TRT of 2–5 μs could damage the RBC but will not result in treatment of blood vessels (Fig. 9.5). Therefore, vascular therapy is possible only by irradiating pulsed dye laser (PDL) with pulse duration corresponding to TDT (or TRT of the entire blood vessel) in which heat is transferred to the vessel wall, not with pulse duration corresponding to chromophores (hemoglobin and RBC). In the case of vessels with a TRT of 1.2–4.8 ms, a 450 μs 585 nm PDL corresponding to microseconds and not nanoseconds should be used to achieve the desired effect. The same applies to melanin. Melanin in the melanosomes may be uniform, but melanocytes or keratinocytes with melanosomes, or the basal layer in which the keratinocytes are situated are not uniform.

Therefore, extended theory is applied to laser hair removal, vascular treatment, and epidermal pigment treatment using long-pulsed laser. IPL has pulse durations of milliseconds, and extended theory is applied in IPL treatment. Therefore, the target tissue of IPL in pigmentation treatment is the epidermis and not melanosome, and the target tissue of IPL in vascular treatment is the capillaries or erythema and not the hemoglobin. In addition, TRT of the epidermis, basal layer, capillaries, and hair follicles as we know it is written as TRT, but it means TDT if the exact concept is considered (Table 1.8).

9.5 Meaning of Multipulse

The biggest difference between IPL and laser parameters is that multipulse is possible in IPL. Except for PDL, no laser has the same pulse sequence as the multipulse of IPL. Even IPL, unlike PDL, can control both pulse duration and pulse delay time. However, there are still many controversies about the meaning of multipulse in IPL. The meaning of multipulse in IPL can be considered from three aspects.

First, the multipulse of IPL acts like the macropulse of a vascular laser (refer to Sect. 8.3 in Chap. 8). The reason for using macropulse in vascular therapy is that purpura can occur when the temperature exceeds 100 °C, so a short pulse duration cannot be used for high energy. Also, if a long pulse duration is used for low energy, small blood vessels are spared in the thermal phase of the optical thermal model due to thermal kinetic selectivity, which makes treatment impossible. For the same reason, multipulse in IPL is used for vascular therapy. Conversely, multipulse has no meaning other than its use for vascular therapy.

Then, what is the difference between IPL's multipulse and PDL's macropulse? The subpulse of PDL usually has a pulse duration of less than 450 us, and the subpulse of IPL usually has a pulse duration of 2 ms or more. Therefore, blood vessels smaller than those corresponding to TRT of 2 ms cannot be treated. Because the subpulse of PDL has a short pulse duration, it can treat blood vessels corresponding to a TRT of less than 2 ms. Conversely, purpura occurs easily in PDL because subpulse is very short, while purpura is less common in IPL because subpulse of IPL is more than 2 ms.

Second, the simultaneous treatment at the same time by multipulse can be considered [5]. For example, if the first and second pulse durations are 2.4 and 8 ms, respectively, and the delay time is 20 ms, small blood vessels can be treated with the first irradiation, 2.4 ms, and large blood vessels can be treated simultaneously with the second irradiation, 8 ms. Similarly, in pigmentation treatments, small pigmentations can be treated first, and large pigmentations can be treated later. However, this method is not consistent with thermal kinetic selectivity (TKS) (refer to Sect. 10.4 in Chap. 10). According to TKS, it is safe to treat large tissues first and then small tissues later. Usually, when setting the multipulse parameter of IPL, the first pulse is shorter than the second pulse. This is against TKS. In addition, in TKS, the tissue that responded to the first irradiation should not be irradiated with the second irradiation, and only the nonresponsive tissue should be irradiated. But since the multipulse of IPL is irradiating twice at the same spot, the temperature of the responsive tissue rises further and there is a risk of side effects. Also, as opposed to macropulse, single pulse treatment requires high fluence in a short time (Method A of Arrhenius equation). In this case, the temperature may rise up to 100 °C, resulting in purpura and side effects. Therefore, I think IPL should not be used for the simultaneous treatment effect of multipulse.

Third, the three stages of optical thermal model are optical phase, thermal phase, and tissue denaturation process (refer to Sect. 2.3 in Chap. 2). Among these, the tissue denaturation process is a process in which the optical properties of the tissue are changed [9]. For example, the lentigo turns brown in response to IPL. In the tissue denaturation process, the absorption coefficient of the tissue is usually increased, and if it is repeatedly irradiated using this phenomenon, the absorption coefficient becomes higher and can be raised to a higher temperature. Since the multipulse of IPL also corresponds to repeated irradiation, the absorption coefficient will be higher. Factors that increase the absorption coefficient through repeated irradiation in vascular therapy are known to be metHb production, clot production, and increased blood flow [1, 10]. Since the first irradiation of IPL is usually less than 4 ms, the generation of metHb is not significant (absorption coefficient rises by metHb when it has a long pulse duration of at least 4 ms [11]). Therefore, when treating blood vessels, the absorption coefficient will slightly increase due to clot formation or increased blood flow, rather than a sudden increase in absorption coefficient of metHb. However, when treating pigmentations, the absorption coefficient increases due to coagulation, and repeated irradiation increases the temperature to an extremely high temperature, which can cause side effects. Therefore, IPL's multipulse is not meaningful in pigmentation treatment. I think that multipulse should not be used for pigmentation treatment.

I think that the multipulse of IPL is a method using the macropulse concept and tissue denaturation process. Moreover, I think that the multipulse of IPL uses the tissue denaturation process more than the macropulse concept. IPL has lower output compared to laser. Therefore, it is thought that IPL uses multipulse to take advantage of the increased absorption coefficient in the tissue denaturation process to overcome the low output.

9.6 Parameters

The indications for IPL are acne treatment, vascular treatment, epidermal pigmentation treatment, and nonablative rejuvenation (Table 9.4).

First, in the case of acne treatment, an optical filter of 420(s)nm is used. The 420(s)nm optical filter is useful for acne because a part of the Soret band and most of the Q band are irradiated (Fig. 9.6). However, high fluence should not be used because melanin absorption is very high. Because the purpose of phototherapy for acne is to eventually create much singlet oxygen, it is safe to lower the fluence and irradiate it several times. I use IPL for photodynamic therapy (PDT) using methyl aminolevulinate (MAL) and proceed with the following protocol. After incubating the MAL for 30 minutes, LED is applied for 10 min, then IPL is irradiated on the entire face with one pass using IPL's 420 nm optical filter and the acne is re-irradiated 1–2 times. The ultrasound gel is not applied, and the IPL is placed about 1 cm from the skin, so that the patient does not feel much pain. I do not use ultrasound gel when using IPL in acne patients, as I often experience worsening acne when IPL is applied after applying ultrasound gel. Although there is no clinical end point, if the patient feels pain, it is considered as a warning end point and the area is not irradiated further, or the procedure is completely stopped. Treatments are performed at least 2 weeks apart.

Table 9.4 Parameters of IPL (Cellec V, Jeisys Medical Inc. Seoul, Korea)

Indications	Filter (nm)	Pulse duration 1st, 2nd (ms)	Pulse delay (ms)	Fluence (J/cm²)
Acne	420(S)	2.4–2.8/5.0–5.4	20–40	≥9
Rosacea, diffuse erythema	530(D)	8.8		14–20
Facial telangiectasia	560 or 590	2.4/4.4	20	25–27
Lentigo, freckle	560 or 590	4.0		≥18
Cell toning	560	0.7	0.3	15–20 (10 shot)
PhotoShower (PDT)	420(s)			3 (3 Hz)
PhotoShower (rejuvenation)	560			5 (3 Hz)
	700			4 (3 Hz)

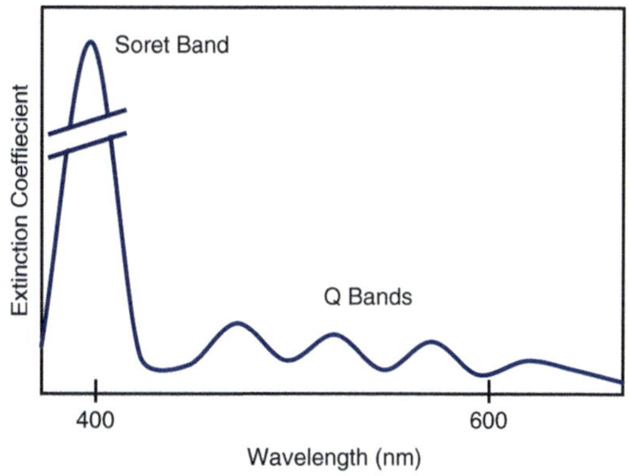

Fig. 9.6 Photoexcitation spectrum of protoporphyrin. Soret band and Q bands are observed. Reproduced from [1]

Second, in case of erythema or telangiectasia, it is safe to use the longest wavelength possible among the 500~600 m wavelengths for the optical filter (590 nm optical filter is safer than 560 nm). Triple pulse is good if the output is stable, but most IPLs use double pulse because the output decreases as the pulse increases. In case of telangiectasia, the clinical end point is "darkening" in which blood clots form or "disappearance" in which blood vessels disappear. Even though the clinical end point does not appear, re-irradiating immediately can cause burns due to heat accumulation effect. Thus, re-irradiation with higher fluence should be performed after a sufficient period of time (30 s to 2 min [12]). Cold ultrasonic gel is used to cool the epidermis. The treatment interval should be 8–12 weeks regarding dermis regeneration, but I sometimes set the treatment interval to 4 weeks because I think that when blood vessels are treated partially, there is not much problem with skin regeneration in 4 weeks.

Third, in case of epidermal pigmentation treatment, a single pulse should be used. A filter with a long wavelength of 640 nm is safe, but it is difficult to produce a high fluence enough to coagulate a pigmented lesion because of its low output, so most use a filter with a wavelength of 500~600 nm. In the case of 500~600 nm wavelengths, keep in mind that side effects may occur and the fluence should be carefully controlled. 590 nm filter should be used before the 560 nm because the longer the wavelengths, the safer they are. Since fluence is relatively constant regardless of pulse duration, refer to the fluence of the parameters provided by the company or use the fluence that has had a reaction as a reference regardless of pulse duration (refer to Sect. 10.5 in Chap. 10). In the case of pulse duration, since it is based on the epidermis, and not melanosomes, according to extended theory of selective photothermolysis, it is first treated with 10 ms for seborrheic keratosis (TRT 10–1000 ms), and then treated sequentially while reducing pulse duration to 6 ms and 4 ms (refer to Sect. 10.7 in Chap. 10). The clinical end point is regarded as "darkening" or "delay perilesional erythema" (Fig. 9.7). When treating dermis such as erythema or nonablative rejuvenation, a cold gel should be used to cool the epidermis, but in the case of epidermal pigmentation treatment, using a gel at room temperature is more useful because it keeps the fluence constant and does not increase the fluence unnecessarily. Cell toning is a method similar to the repeat pulse method of the 532 nm Q-switched Nd:YAG laser (refer to the Sect. 5.6 in Chap. 5). This enables epidermal pigmentation treatment by repeatedly irradiating and slowly raising the temperature. However, the repeat pulse method of Q-switched Nd:YAG laser controls only three variables: frequency,

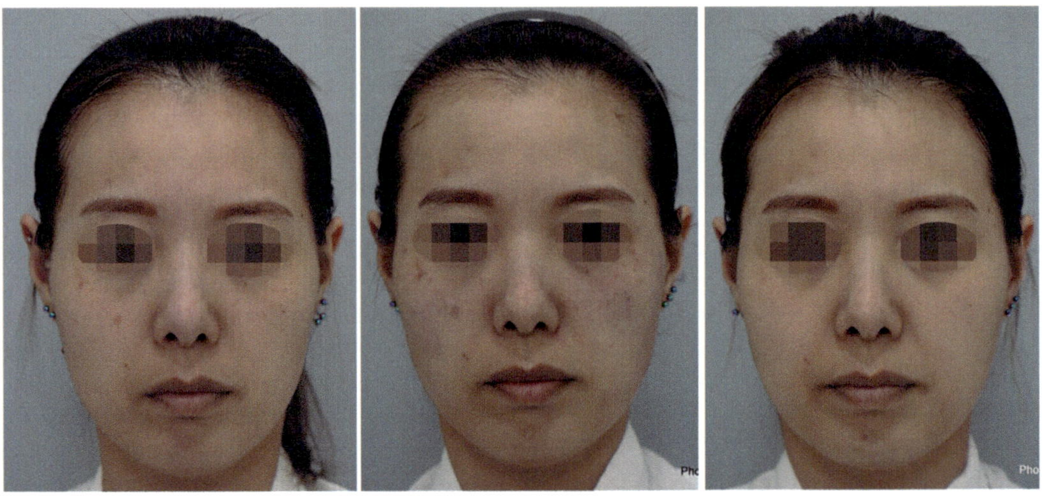

Fig. 9.7 Treatment of lentigo by IPL. Left: Before treatment, Middle: Immediately after treatment, Right: After treatment. (Photos Courtesy of Je Hyeok Lee, MD, Dr. BOM clinic, Seoul, Korea. System used: Cellec V, Jeisys Medical Inc. Seoul, Korea)

pulse count, and fluence. On the other hand, cell toning is much more complicated because it must control pulse duration in addition to these three variables. To simplify the parameters, I fixed the parameters to pulse duration 0.7 ms, pulse delay 0.3 ms, and fluence 15 J/cm^2, and adjusted the number of shots only to 10, or 8, or 12, and if the effect is insufficient, fluence should be raised from 15 to 16 J/cm^2 and then the number of shots should be readjusted. In principle, the treatment interval should be at least 4 weeks, which is the epidermal turnover, but since the epidermis damage is usually focal in epidermal pigmentation treatment, I sometimes perform it every 2 weeks.

Fourth, I think that Photoshower has the same mechanism as genesis technique. Therefore, I think it is important to repeat the irradiation for a long time like genesis technique. However, if the patient feels too much heat, I think of it as a warning end point. In this case it is important to move the handpiece faster, widen the area, or lower the fluence to treat for as long as possible (Method B of Arrhenius equation). The face should be divided into zones and 3–5 passes per zone should be performed. Because this is a nonablative rejuvenation, there is no clinical end point, but if the patient feels pain, it should be regarded as a warning end point and the procedure should be performed in another zone, or the fluence should be lowered or the procedure should be stopped. Cool ultrasonic gel is used to cool the epidermis, and the procedure is performed every 2 weeks.

References

1. Raulin C, Karsai S. Laser and IPL technology in dermatology and aesthetic medicine. Heidelberg: New York; 2011.
2. Allemann IB, Goldberg DJ. Basics in dermatological laser applications. Karger Medical and Scientific Publishers; 2011.
3. Park SH, Yeo WC, Koh WS, Park JW, Noh NK, Yoon CS. Laser dermatology plastic surgery 2nd ed (Korean). Seoul: Koonja; 2014.
4. Samotaev N, Vasilyev V, Malkin E, Gromov E, Belyakov V, Golovin A, et al. System for synchronous detection trace of explosives and drags substances on human fingers. Procedia Eng. 2015;120:1050–3.
5. Goldman MP. Cutaneous and cosmetic laser surgery. Philadelphia: Mosby Elsevier; 2006.
6. Goldman MP. Lasers and energy devices for the skin. [S.I.]: Taylor & Francis; 2013.
7. Altshuler GB, Anderson RR, Manstein D, Zenzie HH, Smirnov MZ. Extended theory of selective photothermolysis. Lasers Surg Med. 2001;29(5):416–32.
8. Watanabe S. Basics of laser application to dermatology. Arch Dermatol Res. 2008;300(Suppl 1):S21–30.
9. Mordon S, Brisot D, Fournier N. Using a "non uniform pulse sequence" can improve selective coagulation with a Nd:YAG laser (1.06 microm) thanks to Met-hemoglobin absorption: a clinical study on blue leg veins. Lasers Surg Med. 2003;32(2):160–70.
10. Myhill J, Bäumler W, Hennings L, Bearden ED, Buckmiller LM, Shafirstein G. The interaction of broadband intense pulsed light (IPL) and skin during a multi-pulse application. Med Laser Appl. 2008;23(2):71–8.
11. Welch AJ, Gemert MJCv. Optical-thermal response of laser-irradiated tissue. Dordrecht: London; 2011.
12. Hammes S, Kaiser K, Pohl L, Metelmann HR, Enk A, Raulin C. Pyogenic granuloma: treatment with the 1,064-nm long-pulsed neodymium-doped yttrium aluminum garnet laser in 20 patients. Dermatol Surg. 2012;38(6):918–23.

10 Long-Pulsed Alexandrite Laser and Thermal Kinetic Selectivity

10.1 Overview of Long-Pulsed Alexandrite Lasers

Lasers usually have one wavelength in one device, but recently, complex wavelength lasers that can produce multiple wavelengths in one device are being released. Nobleen laser (FineMEC Co. Ltd. Seoul, Korea) combines long-pulsed alexandrite laser and long-pulsed Nd:YAG laser and has 755 nm wavelength and 1064 nm wavelength in one device (Fig. 10.1). In this chapter I will describe long-pulsed alexandrite laser and focus on the 755 nm wavelength.

The chromophore of 755 nm wavelength includes melanin and hemoglobin, but the absorption coefficient for hemoglobin at 755 nm wavelength is much lower than that of melanin. Therefore, if the fluence is increased to treat blood vessels with a long-pulsed alexandrite laser, the risk of epidermis damage is high. So, in Caucasians, long-pulsed alexandrite laser may be used for vascular treatment [1], but in Asians, melanin is the target chromophore and long-pulsed alexandrite laser is mainly used for epidermis pigmentation treatment and laser hair removal.

The pulse duration of the long-pulsed alexandrite laser is in milliseconds, and laser hair removal is possible by the extended theory of selective photothermolysis, and by controlling the pulse duration targeting the epidermal layer, it is possible to treat epidermal pigmented lesions

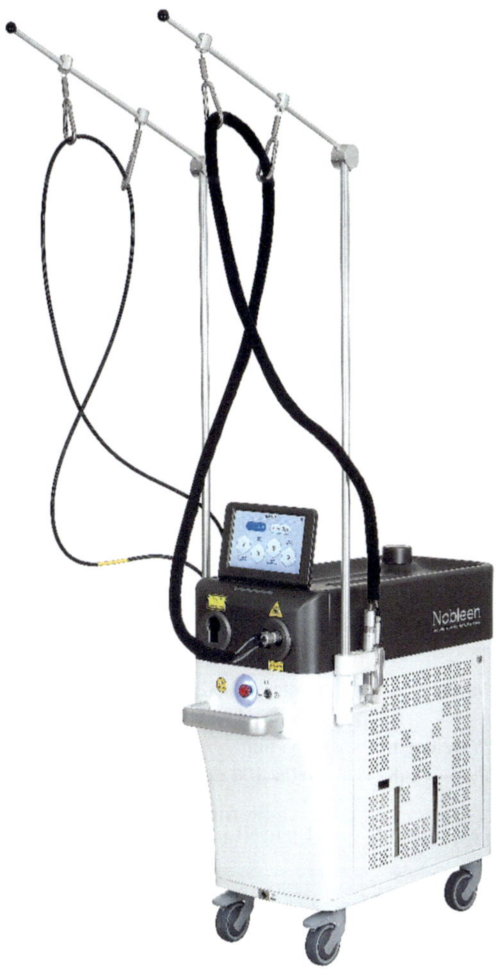

Fig. 10.1 A complex wavelength laser combining long-pulsed alexandrite laser and long-pulsed Nd:YAG laser (Nobleen, FineMEC Co. Ltd. Seoul, Korea)

J. D. Lee, M. J. M. Oh, *Lasers in Dermatology: Parameters and Choice*,
https://doi.org/10.1007/978-981-19-7568-4_10

of various depth (refer to Sect. 9.4 in Chap. 9). The pulse duration of the long-pulsed alexandrite laser may be reduced to 0.1–0.2 ms, which is the shortest among long-pulsed lasers (Table 10.1). The shortest pulse duration is the biggest advantage of long-pulsed alexandrite laser. Compared to other millisecond long-pulsed lasers or IPLs, it can remove thinner hair, and it can treat light colored lentigines.

Recently, lasers equipped with fractional handpieces on Q-switched lasers or long-pulsed lasers are emerging. I believe that using a fractional handpiece at the wavelength where the water is not a target and where scattering occurs is not suitable for fractional photothermolysis. Fractional photothermolysis does not irradiate the entire skin, but instead irradiates laser beams here and there and leaves normal tissue between the beams, reducing the side effects by quickly regenerating the necrotic tissues from normal surrounding tissues. However, in the wavelength at which scattering occurs, not only is the laser irradiated where the beam is irradiated, but also absorption occurs even in parts that are not irradiated due to scattering. This is why I believe that fractional handpiece at the wavelength at which scattering occurs is not suitable for fractional photothermolysis, but rather has the effect of only (1) lowering energy and (2) smaller spot size and shallower penetration depth and (3) strong energy may be irradiated where the laser is directly irradiated increasing the possibility of side effects. This is why I do not use the fractional handpiece on a long-pulsed alexandrite laser.

Table 10.1 Specifications of Nobleen laser with both long-pulsed alexandrite laser and long-pulsed Nd:YAG laser (FineMEC Co. Ltd. Seoul, Korea). RCS: rapid cooling system (dynamic cooling device)

Module	Long-pulsed alexandrite & Nd:YAG laser	
Wavelength	755 nm	1064 nm
Pulse width	0.08–100 ms	0.08–300 ms
Output energy	Up to 80 J	Up to 100 J
Repetition rate	1–20 Hz	
Spot size	2, 3, 5, 7, 10, 15, 20 mm	
Fractional hand piece (Optional)	15 mm spot size (130 dots, 400 μm dot size)	
Beam delivery	Lens coupled optical fiber with handpiece	
Skin cooling system	Selective RCS gas cooling/air cooling (external)	

For epidermal cooling, evaporative cooling, which is a cooling method using a refrigerant, or convective cooling using cold wind can be used in this laser. The pros and cons of each are as follows. Evaporative cooling has a strong cooling effect, with less side effects and less pain but there are maintenance costs. Convective cooling is effective and inexpensive when treating large areas such as arm and leg laser hair removal, but it is difficult to apply to the face because the patients have difficulty breathing when it is used near the patient's nose. I use a rapid cooling system (RCS), because I mainly do laser hair removal on small areas such as the face and armpits.

10.2 Indications

The long-pulsed alexandrite laser is used for treating epidermal pigmentation (refer to Sect. 4.3 in Chap. 4) and laser hair removal as described above. Because long-pulsed alexandrite laser has a pulse duration in milliseconds, it is not effective for treating dermal pigmentation with cells with microsecond TRT (refer to Sect. 10.4 in Chap. 10). The TRT of a tattoo can be in milliseconds if the tattoo particles are small but agglomerated. Therefore, a long-pulsed alexandrite laser should not be irradiated onto a tattoo as it can cause side effects such as scarring. Congenital and acquired melanocytic nevi and seborrheic keratosis may be treated with a long-pulsed alexandrite laser by adjusting to millisecond TRT. However, in the case of melanocytic nevi removal, if heat is applied to the melanocytic nevi cells located in the dermis, there is a possibility that side effects such as burns may occur due to damage around the dermis. I treat seborrheic keratosis by ablative laser such as a CO_2 laser or Er:YAG laser, which has a higher absorption coefficient for water than a long-pulsed alexandrite laser. Because the TRT of the seborrheic keratosis has a wide range of 10–1000 ms, it is difficult to match the pulse duration, and the seborrheic keratosis has a histologically moist basal layer [2], so it is rather safe because it is difficult to damage below the basal layer with an ablative laser. I irradiate the entire seborrheic keratosis with a CO_2 laser, peel it off with gauze (demo-epidermal sliding effect), irradiate it again and peel it off repeatedly until the moist basal layer appears [3]. In addition, long-pulsed alexandrite laser can be used for the treatment of trichostasis spinulosa [4, 5]. Trichostasis spinulosa is a disease that clinically looks like black spots on hair follicles. Histologically, trichostasis spinulosa is a skin disease in which hair follicles are filled with vellus hair masses and keratin plugs. It usually occurs in nose or forehead and is also found in body [2].

The mechanism of removing epidermal pigmentations by long-pulsed alexandrite laser and IPL is based on the extended theory of selective photothermolysis. The epidermal pigmentation is removed by increasing the epidermal turnover of the epidermis through the photothermal effect that coagulates the epidermal pigment using a pulse duration of milliseconds.

10.3 Laser Selection for Epidermal Pigment Treatment

The most problematic complication for Koreans in epidermal pigmentation treatment is post-inflammatory hyperpigmentation (PIH). Long-pulsed lasers have a lower PIH incidence than Q-switched lasers or ablative lasers such as CO_2 lasers. In one paper, it was described that when epidermal pigmented lesions were treated with CO_2, Q-switched, and long-pulsed lasers, 50%, 10%, and 1% PIH occurred, respectively [6, 7]. Long-pulsed laser has the fewest side effects, but they had to be repeated several times.

Chan et al. found that treatment of lentigines with 532 nm Q-switched and 532 nm long-pulsed lasers were equally effective. But 532 nm Q-switched lasers had a higher risk. Also when 755 nm Q-switched alexandrite lasers and long-pulsed alexandrite lasers were compared, the results showed that both had the same effect, but the Q-switched laser had 22% PIH and long-pulsed lasers 6%. Finally, they concluded that long-pulsed alexandrite lasers are safe [8]r.

Long-pulsed lasers also generate PIH, but the incidence is lower than other lasers, and above all, even if PIH occurs, it is not as intense as PIH generated by Q-switched lasers or ablative lasers and disappears quickly. However, it is difficult in long-pulsed lasers to remove all the pigments at once, repeated treatment is required, and 100% disappearance of the epidermal pigment is not possible.

IPL also exhibits a similar effect to the long-pulsed alexandrite laser. However, the advantage of long-pulsed alexandrite laser compared to IPL is as follows. First, it can reduce the pulse duration by 0.1–0.2 ms, so it can treat even epidermal pigments that cannot be treated with IPL. Second, while IPL has shortcomings such as non-uniformity of raw spectrum, ambiguity of filter, and spectral shift (refer to Chap. 9), long-pulsed alexandrite laser has high accuracy and produces the same effect every time, i.e., high reproducibility. Third, since long-pulsed alexandrite laser does not use ultrasound gel unlike IPL, changes in lesions can be observed immediately after laser irradiation, and there is no acneiform eruption caused by ultrasound gel. Above all, the procedure is convenient because there is no need to use the ultrasound gel.

10.4 Thermal Kinetic Selectivity (TKS)

Thermal kinetic selectivity (TKS) is a theory applied to determine pulse duration when large and small target tissues coexist. It is a theory that is deviated from the selective photothermolysis theory [9].

Let's see Fig. 10.2. Since TRT is proportional to the square of the diameter, large tissues will have a longer TRT (T_2), and small tissues will have a shorter TRT (T_1) ($T_1 < T_2$). If the pulse duration (PD) is between TRTs of large and small tissues ($T_1 < PD < T_2$), large tissues will be damaged because large tissues ($PD < T_2$) are

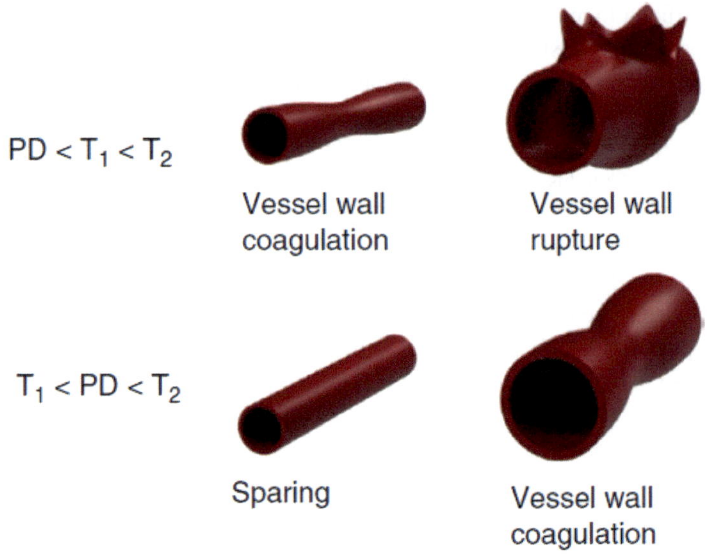

Fig. 10.2 Two tissues in the skin (1 and 2), T_1, T_2: thermal relaxation times (TRT) of 1 and 2, respectively. PD: pulse duration (Published with kind permission of © Jin Kwon Cho 2019. All rights reserved)

TRT > PD according to theory of selective photothermolysis. The problem is with small tissues. In the case of small tissues (T_1 < PD), because TRT < PD, according to theory of selective photothermolysis, surrounding tissues should become damaged and have side effects (refer to Sect. 1.11 in Chap. 1). In practice, however, side effects do not occur; rather, small tissues are preserved without any effect. The theory that explains this phenomenon is thermal kinetic selectivity.

When TRT < PD, if the pulse duration is long enough, the temperature of small tissues does not rise further but cools down during irradiation. Why did the phenomenon deviate from the theory of selective photothermolysis? There are three ways to lose heat in tissues: heat conduction, heat convection caused by blood flow, and heat radiation [6]. Heat conduction, which transfers heat to the surroundings, is the main method of heat dissipation. However, if the pulse duration is long enough, small tissue cools down due to the latter two phenomena (heat convection and heat radiation). It is as if water is poured down slowly into a bucket with holes and it doesn't fill up. For example, during the treatment of large tissues as in vascular therapy, small tissues such as melanosomes show no change. Also, during laser hair removal, even without epidermal cooling, pulse durations longer than the epidermal TRT (1–10 ms) such as 30 ms do not damage the epidermis. TKS is also applied to a variety of situations.

Then, at what pulse duration does TKS occur? I believe that TKS occurs at long pulse durations of milliseconds. In particular, I think it is a phenomenon that occurs in the photothermal effect below 100 °C.

Let's think about pulse duration in large and small tissues again. In the situation (T_1 < PD< T_2), large tissues are treated while small tissues are preserved. On the other hand, if the pulse duration (PD) is shorter than the TRTs of small tissues (PD < T_1 < T_2), both large and small tissues will be treated because TRT > PD (selective photothermolysis). In this case, temperatures of large tissues can rise to temperatures that are too high, causing side effects (Top right figure in Fig. 10.2) [9]. Therefore, (T_1 < PD < T_2) is safer than (PD < T_1 < T_2). Then how do we treat small tissues? After removing large tissues first with PD < T_2, the pulse duration should be reduced, less than the TRT of the small tissue (PD < T_1), and the small tissues can be removed sequentially.

In conclusion, in long pulse durations of milliseconds, it is safe to remove large tissues first, and small tissues later. Therefore, if the clinical end point does not appear at a low fluence, the fluence should be adjusted by increasing it to a high fluence, while the pulse duration should be adjusted by reducing the pulse duration from long to short.

10.5 Relation Between Fluence and Pulse Duration

How should fluence be changed according to pulse duration? We reviewed the equation that showed the relationship between fluence and pulse duration (τ_p) (refer to Sect. 4.4 in Chap. 4). However, since the pulse duration is part of the denominator under the exponential function, it is difficult to know the correlation between fluence and pulse duration at first glance. But if you put numbers in the equation, you can see that pulse duration and temperature are inversely related. Conversely, fluence and pulse duration are proportional if the temperature is the same.

Trafeli et al. used long-pulse alexandrite laser to measure the fluence of similar clinical end points, i.e., the same tissue response, depending on the pulse duration [10]. At 40 ms, when there is no refrigerant cooling, the fluence is a bit peculiar, but if we ignore this, two conclusions can be drawn. First, pulse duration and fluence are proportional. In other words, to see the same effect, fluence should be increased to increase pulse duration and fluence should be lowered to shorten pulse duration. Second, pulse duration and fluence are proportional, but there is no significant difference in fluence. Thus, if there is a clinical end point that is appropriate for a particular fluence at a given pulse duration, there is no need to adjust fluence whether the pulse duration is reduced or increased. Of course, in order to safely perform the procedure, it would be better to reduce the fluence when reducing pulse duration.

10.6 Permanent Hair Removal or Reduction

Although in private practice, physicians use the term "permanent hair removal" to explain to patients as if laser hair removal results in a lifelong permanent hair eradication, permanent hair loss is currently not possible [6]. To be precise, the term "permanent hair reduction" should be used instead of the term "permanent hair removal."

Permanent hair reduction refers to a long-term, stable reduction of the number of hairs that grow back after a number of laser hair removals. The term "long-term" refers to the time of more than one hair cycle [6]. If hair does not grow during one hair cycle, it is unlikely that it will grow afterwards. So permanent hair reduction can be defined as a condition in which the number of hairs that grow back decreases during the period of 4 to 12 months or more, which is the hair cycle excluding the scalp [3]. The U.S. Food and Drug Administration (FDA) also states that permanent hair removal does not refer to complete hair loss, in which all hair is lost [11].

There are two major factors that affect the subjective satisfaction of patients undergoing laser hair removal. First, the number and rate of regrowing hairs, and second, the thickness and color of the regrowing hairs [6]. Patients may misunderstand that when they receive laser hair removal, the term "permanency" means that hair will not ever grow again. Fortunately, laser hair removal reduces the number and proportion of hair that grows again, slows hair growth and hair becomes thinner and brighter in color like vellus hair. Most patients are satisfied with the result, but a small number of patients may complain that they did not receive "permanent" hair removal (to be exact, complete hair loss). I therefore recommend that the pre-procedure explanation to the patient must be explained in more detail. This is how I explain: "Laser hair removal is treated by an indirect method of transferring heat from hair bulb to stem cells. With tweezers, 100 hairs are gradually reduced to 90, 80, and 70 hairs. But this is not so in lasers. 100 stem cells are reduced to 90, 80, and 70 stem cells, resulting in hair becoming thinner and some hair may disappear in this process. However, after five laser hair removal sessions, the number of hairs is significantly reduced and becomes thinner like vellus hair, so most patients are satisfied."

10.7 Parameters

As mentioned earlier, the indications for long-pulsed alexandrite laser are laser hair removal, trichostasis spinulosa, and epidermal pigmentation. I also use it for the treatment of melasma (Table 10.2).

First, laser hair removal and treatment of trichostasis spinulosa. It is known that a pulse duration of 30–40 ms is clinically appropriate for laser hair removal regardless of the laser. However, 3 ms is also said to be effective in most cases [12]. The long-pulsed alexandrite laser has a short pulse duration of 3–5 ms as a true pulse, and this short pulse duration is also effective for laser hair removal. However, if the fluence is slightly high, side effects such as folliculitis occur easily (Method A of Arrhenius equation, refer to Sect. 7.3 in Chap. 7). Rather, I think that overlapping irradiation with a short pulse duration is more effective for thin hair due to the macropulse-like effect of the vascular laser (method B of Arrhenius equation, refer to Sect. 8.4 in Chap. 8). So, in case of philtrum laser hair removal, I lower the fluence to 7–8 J/cm^2 and irradiate it with 50% overlap at 1 Hz. When treating the dermal layer, the larger the spot size, the deeper the photons enter, and the epidermis is well protected (refer to the Sect. 4.6 in Chap. 4), and because the procedure is completed quickly, the largest spot size of 20 mm is used for laser hair removal. Laser hair removal is a typical procedure without a clinical end point. In procedures without clinical end points, we have no choice but to determine fluence empirically. The procedure must be repeated for several times to find the fluence that is effective without side effects. Epidermal cooling is the most important strategy in laser hair removal. (refer to Sect. 1.14 in Chap. 1). Therefore, the laser physician should not neglect to check cooling system. Laser hair removal requires precooling as well as postcooling in cooling because overlapping parts exist [3]. However, since Koreans have relatively bright faces, in the case of vellus hairs on women's faces, epidermis cooling is not usually needed. Laser hair removal is performed at intervals of 1–2 months, and at least 5 treatments are recommended. For thick hair such as armpits or calves, patients are satisfied with 5 to 8 treatments, but thin hair such as women's philtrum is less effective in laser hair removal, so 10 treatments or more may be needed. In the case of men's beard laser hair removal, although the hair is thick, possibly due to the effect of strong male hormones, the effect of laser hair removal is low, so it is necessary to perform more than 10 treatments to see the effect. In addition, in the case of laser beard hair removal for men, pain during the procedure is severe, and it takes up to 20–30 treatments to reduce to the point where there is almost no hair. Even with many laser beard hair removals, it is not possible to completely avoid shaving, so sufficient consultation with the male patient is required before laser beard hair removal.

Long-pulsed alexandrite laser can be used to treat trichostasis spinulosa. The exact pathogen-

Table 10.2 Parameters of long-pulsed alexandrite laser (Nobleen, FineMEC Co. Ltd. Seoul, Korea). RCS: Rapid cooling system (dynamic cooling device)

Indications	Spot size (mm)	Pulse width (ms)	RCS precooling	RCS postcooling	Fluence (J/cm^2)
Hair (fine)	20	3	6	6	6–12
Hair (medium)	20	5	6	6	7–12
Hair (thick)	20	10	6	6	8–11
Trichostasis spinulosa	10	3	6	6	14–18
	7	0.5	6	6	15–17
Freckle, lentigo	10	3	X	X	15, 20
	10	1	X	X	15, 20
	5	0.3	X	X	15, 20
	5	0.2	X	X	12–14
	3	0.1	X	X	12–13
Melasma	7	0.2–0.3	X	X	7–8

esis of trichostasis spinulosa is not known, but an abnormal follicular unit is thought to be the cause. In other words, the entrance to the follicle is blocked due to follicular keratosis in the follicular infundibulum or abnormal angulations of the isthmus with respect to the infundibulum, so small telogen hairs cannot come out [5]. Therefore, the treatment of trichostasis spinulosa is not possible by laser hair removal. It is possible by mechanical hair follicle destruction through hair follicle damage or vaporization, so the fluence is increased by 2 times.

Second, treating epidermal pigmentation (Fig. 10.3). When treating epidermal pigmentations such as freckles or lentigo, in patients who do not have melasma and are unlikely to develop PIH, "strong treatment" is performed with energy of 20 J/cm^2 or more for a quick effect, and if there is melasma or PIH is likely to occur, "weak treatment" is performed with an energy of 15 J/cm^2 or less (refer to Sect. 2.9 in Chap. 2). The clinical end point of "strong treatment" is based on the "popping sound" that appears during the procedure and the "immediate erythema" that appears immediately after the procedure. However, the fluence that removes the epidermis is not suitable. The clinical end point of "weak treatment" is based on "delayed perilesional erythema" in which erythema appears on the initial irradiation site after irradiating the epidermal pigmentations on the entire face. The epidermal pigmentation of the entire face is first irradiated with a pulse duration of 3 ms, and when returning to the first irradiation site, if the pigmentation is non-responsive, the pulse duration is reduced to 1 ms and irradiated it again. It is then reduced again from 0.3 ms to 0.2 or 0.1 ms and only the non-responsive pigmentation is irradiated. The reason for the treatment by gradually reducing the pulse duration is because of the thermal kinetic selectivity. Also, the reason the fluence is lowered little by little each time the pulse duration is decreased is that fluence and pulse duration are proportional if the reaction temperature is the same (refer to Sect. 10.5 in Chap. 10). As for the spot size, if the face tone is not very dark, the largest spot size possible should be used for quick procedure. If the face tone is dark, a small spot size of 3 or 5 mm should be used so that it does not stand out even if "relative" hypopigmentation, in which the treated area turns brighter than the surrounding normal skin, occurs (refer to Sect. 20.3.2 in Chap. 20). Although epidermal cooling is used for the purpose of protecting the epidermis while treating the dermal layer, epidermal cooling is not very helpful when treating the epidermis. Although it is a procedure that does not require local anesthesia, I apply anesthetic cream to reduce PIH by reducing blood vessels and also to reduce pain in sensitive patients. The anesthetic cream is occluded for 20 min and then laser treatment is performed. In principle, the treatment interval should be at least 4 weeks, which is the epidermal turnover, but since epidermis damage is local rather than general, I sometimes perform the procedure every 2 weeks.

Third, melasma treatment. Melasma can be considered as an epidermal pigmentation and the epidermal pigmentation laser can be used. However, unlike epidermal pigmentations, caution should be taken during melasma treatment because "active melanocytes" cause PIH or side effects that worsen melasma during laser treatment (refer to Sect. 18.3 in Chap. 18). Therefore, the safest laser for epidermal pigmentations should be used. The long-pulsed alexandrite laser is the safest among laser-tissue interactions because it uses coagulation among the photothermal effects, and it has the longest wavelength among long-pulsed lasers (long-pulsed Nd:YAG laser is not used for epidermal pigment treatment) and is the safest in terms of wavelength (refer to Sect. 2.7 in Chap. 2). However, "strong treatment" of melasma with the same fluence as epidermal pigmentation treatment has a high risk of side effects, so I perform "weak treatment" of 15 J/cm^2 with pulse durations of 3 ms and 1 ms, and 7–8 J/cm^2 with a pulse duration of 0.3 ms. This is about half of the fluence used for treating epidermal pigmentation. I also perform only one pass to avoid overlap. Also, I consider the clinical end point as "delayed perilesional erythema which occurs usually when patients are finished with their face pack and ready to go home". Using a long-pulsed alexandrite laser for melasma does not

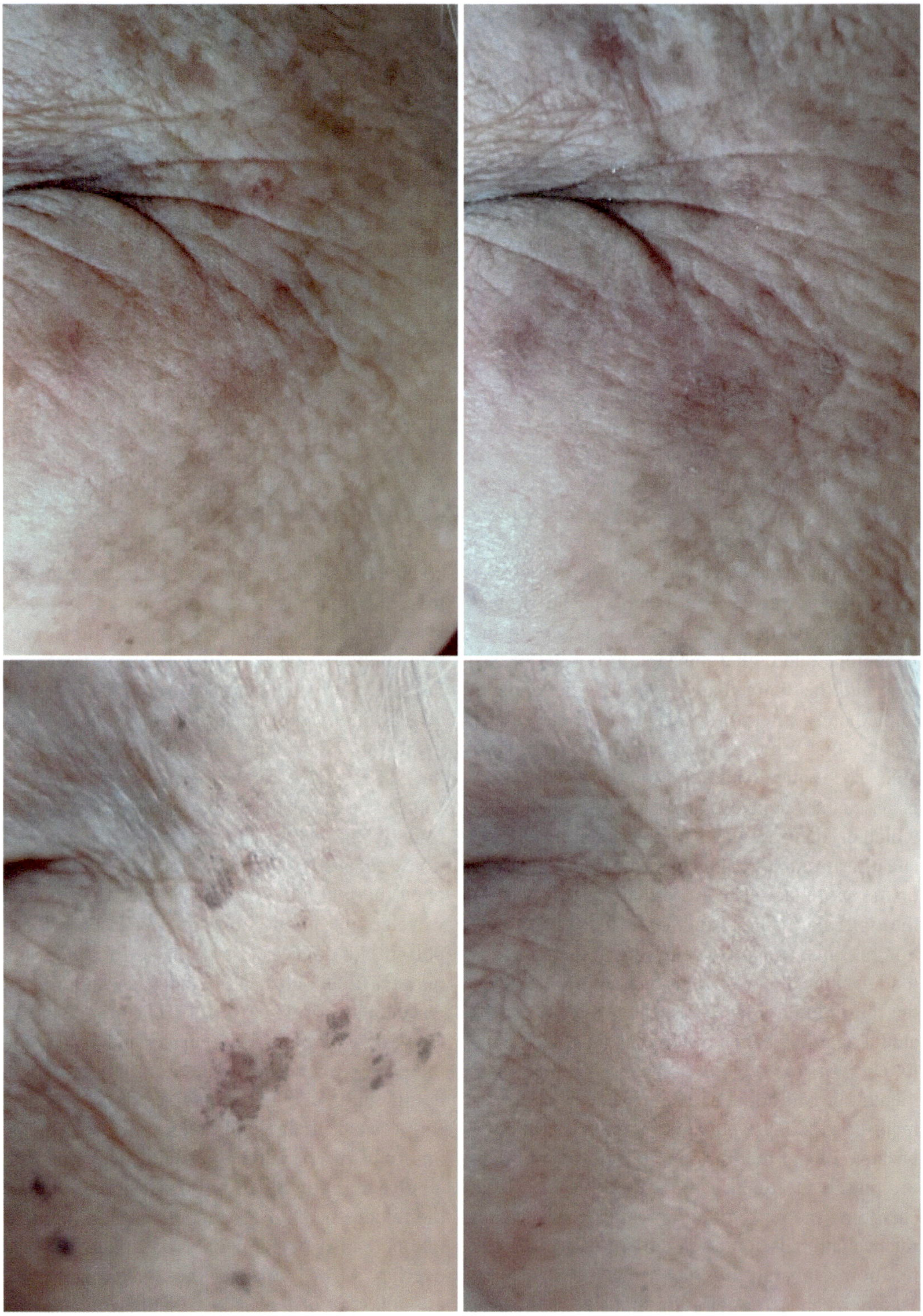

Fig. 10.3 Photographs before and after 755 nm long-pulsed alexandrite laser in the treatment of epidermal pigmented lesions. Top left: before treatment. Top right: immediate after treatment. Bottom left: 7 days after treatment. Bottom right: 1 month after treatment. Laser used: Nobleen, FineMEC Co. Ltd. Seoul, Korea

eliminate 100% of melasma but shows a very rapid improvement. The procedure can be repeated every 4 weeks in consideration of epidermal turnover. However, I usually only use the long-pulsed alexandrite laser once for melasma treatment. Because with repeated treatment with the same parameters, the lesions already responding to the corresponding parameters will all disappear with the first treatment, so there will be no response to the second treatment. In addition, the parameters can be changed, but the pulse duration cannot be changed because the shortest pulse duration is usually used as a parameter in the first treatment, and higher fluence can have side effects during melasma treatment. Therefore, I usually use the long-pulsed alexandrite laser only once for melasma treatment. After that, laser toning using Q-switched Nd:YAG laser is mainly used.

References

1. Ross EV, Meehan KJ, Domankevitz Y, Trafeli JP, Annandono J, Jacoby M. Use of a variable long-pulse alexandrite laser in the treatment of facial telangiectasia. Dermatol Surg. 2010;36(4):470–4.
2. Textbook compilation committee in Korean Dermatological Association. Text book of dermatology 6th edition (Korean). Seoul: Daehanuihak; 2014.
3. Lee JD, Lee JK, Oh MJM. Principles and choice of laser treatment in dermatology. Singapore: Springer; 2020.
4. Badawi A, Kashmar M. Treatment of trichostasis spinulosa with 0.5-millisecond pulsed 755-nm alexandrite laser. Lasers Med Sci. 2011;26(6):825–9.
5. Toosi S, Ehsani AH, Noormohammadpoor P, Esmaili N, Mirshams-Shahshahani M, Moineddin F. Treatment of trichostasis spinulosa with a 755-nm long-pulsed alexandrite laser. J Eur Acad Dermatol Venereol. 2010;24(4):470–3.
6. Allemann IB, Goldberg DJ. Basics in dermatological laser applications. Karger Medical and Scientific Publishers; 2011.
7. Kauvar A, Hruza G. Principles and practices in cutaneous laser surgery. CRC Press; 2005.
8. Hruza GJ, Tanzi EL. Lasers and lights. Edinburgh: Elsevier; 2018.
9. Goldman MP. Lasers and energy devices for the skin. [S.I.]: Taylor & Francis; 2013.
10. Trafeli JP, Kwan JM, Meehan KJ, Domankevitz Y, Gilbert S, Malomo K, et al. Use of a long-pulse alexandrite laser in the treatment of superficial pigmented lesions. Dermatol Surg. 2007;33(12):1477–82.
11. Goldberg DJ. Laser hair removal. London: Informa Healthcare; 2008.
12. Park SH, Yeo WC, Koh WS, Park JW, Noh NK, Yoon CS. Laser dermatology plastic surgery 2nd ed (Korean). Seoul: Koonja; 2014.

Er:YAG Laser and Residual Thermal Damage (RTD)

11

11.1 Overview of Er:YAG Lasers

The wavelength of Er:YAG laser (2940 nm) has an absorption coefficient 10 times higher than that of the CO_2 laser (10,600 nm) [1] (Table 11.1). The pulse duration (PD) of Er:YAG laser is 250 μs (250–350 μs), this is the sum of subpulses similar to the macropulse of PDL (pulsed dye laser). The subpulse of Er:YAG laser is less than 1 μs. The beam profile of Er:YAG lasers is Gaussian mode, such as that of the CO_2 laser. However, unlike the CO_2 laser, by turning the handpiece, the spot size can be easily adjusted from 1 to 6 mm in 1 mm increments. Although there are differences between laser companies, in general, if the handpiece is lifted from the skin, the spot size increases and the power density decreases (defocusing), so the defocusing method can be used like the CO_2 laser (refer to Sect. 4.5 in Chap. 4). Unlike CO_2 laser, the Er:YAG laser causes rapid vaporization and the smoke spreads widely obscuring the view of the procedure. Therefor an assistant must suction the smoke with a smoke evacuator from the side. Some Er:YAG lasers have a built-in smoke evacuator enabling direct suction of the smoke into the handpiece, resulting in clear visualization of the remaining tissue after ablation, thus a quick and accurate procedure is possible (Fig. 11.1).

Table 11.1 Specifications of Er:YAG laser (MCL30 Dermablate, Asclepion Laser Technologies GmbH, Jena, Germany)

Laser type	Er:YAG laser
Wavelength	2940 nm
Pulse energy on skin	Up to 1.5 J
Fluence on skin	1–100 J/cm^2
Frequency	1–20 Hz
Handpiece	1–6 mm VarioSpot, TEAM technology
Smoke evacuation	Integrated, laser-synchronous

J. D. Lee, M. J. M. Oh, *Lasers in Dermatology: Parameters and Choice*,
https://doi.org/10.1007/978-981-19-7568-4_11

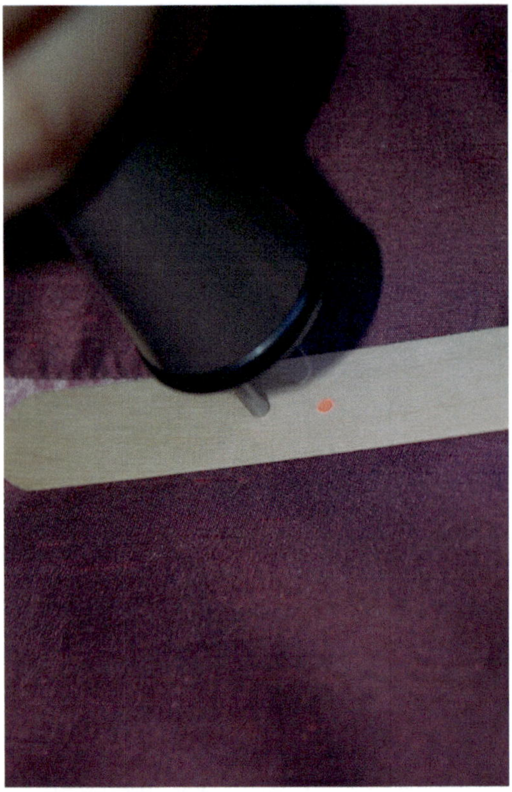

Fig. 11.1 Er:YAG lasers with suctioning properties have the advantage of observing ablation in real time

11.2 Indications

Typical lasers used for ablative rejuvenation include CO_2 lasers and Er:YAG lasers with high absorption coefficient of water. Since the skin contains 70–80% water, the Er:YAG laser can be applied to any situation that requires ablation from the surface of the skin towards the dermis.

First, it is used to remove acquired melanocytic nevus and can be applied to the treatment of various skin nevi and tumors, including epidermal nevus, seborrheic keratosis, sebaceous hyperplasia, ectopic sebaceous gland, syringoma, soft fibroma, etc.

Second, it can also be applied to epidermal and dermal melanocytic lesions (refer to Sect. 4.3 in Chap. 4). Er:YAG lasers can be used to treat epidermal melanocytic lesions, such as freckles, lentigo, and nevus spilus. However, in the case of dermal melanocytic lesions such as Nevus of Ota or Acquired bilateral nevus of Ota-like macules (ABNOM), and tattoos and congenital melanocytic nevus it should not be used because ablative procedures may cause scarring, but instead a procedure called pinhole method can be used. However, since the spot size of the CO_2 laser is smaller than the Er:YAG laser, which allows for precise procedures, I mainly use a CO_2 laser when performing pinhole therapy.

Third, because collagen remodeling occurs due to ablation, it has an effect on enlarged pores, scars, wrinkles, and elasticity. This is called ablative rejuvenation. However, ablative rejuvenation has severe side effects and a long downtime, so fractional lasers using fractional photothermolysis are more commonly used (Er:YAG fractional laser). However, since CO_2 lasers are more effective in skin regeneration than Er:YAG lasers, I use CO_2 fractional lasers when skin regeneration is needed.

11.3 Mechanism of Ablative Rejuvenation

Although the mechanism of ablative rejuvenation can be thought of as vaporizing skin tissue, it is not. When energy accumulates in the skin in a very short time and the water temperature rises, vaporization occurs, increasing the volume of the water and increasing the pressure. At 300 °C, the water rises to 1000 atm. As the water pressure increases in the tissue, the water in the tissue is exploded due to the pressure difference with the atmosphere, and the skin tissue is removed by explosive removal. The mechanism of ablative rejuvenation is not to vaporize all skin tissue, but to use water to forcibly eject skin tissue from the surface [1]. Therefore, ablative rejuvenation should be described as "cutting" or "digging" rather than "burning" (Fig. 11.2).

Therefore, ablation due to vaporization removes not only the target tissue but also surrounding tissues, causing damage to the surrounding tissue resulting in side effects. CO_2 lasers are known to have the highest side effects in treating epidermal pigments than long-pulsed lasers or Q-switched lasers [3].

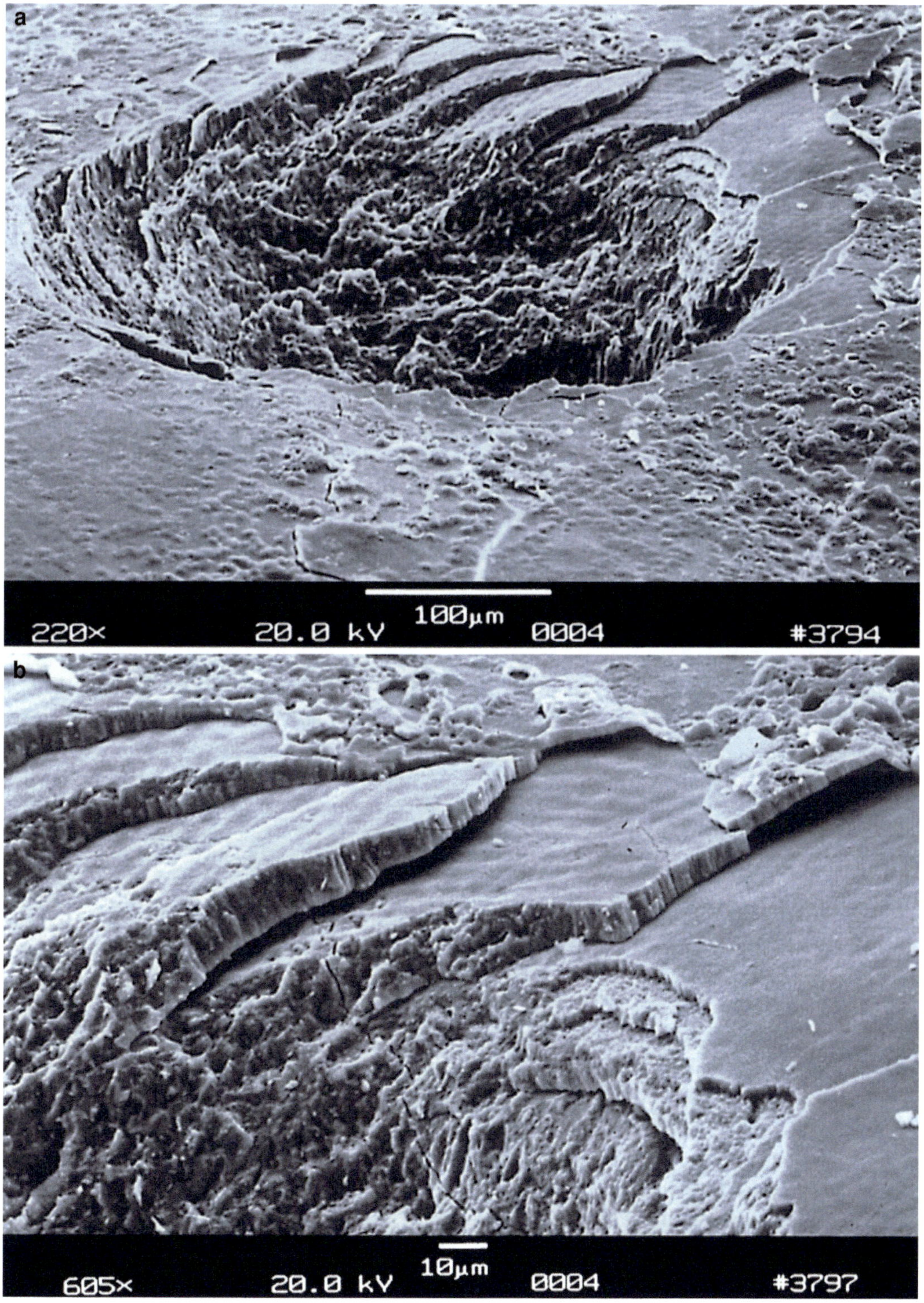

Fig. 11.2 (**a**) Human tooth vaporized by 20 pulses from an Er:YAG laser (pulse duration: 90 µs, pulse energy: 100 mJ, repetition rate: 1 Hz). (**b**) Enlargement showing the edge of ablation. Reproduced from [2]

11.4 Water Vaporization Threshold

In order to remove the tissue by water vaporization and explosion (explosive removal), the energy must be higher than the energy for the water to vaporize. Energy needed for water vaporization in the epidermis is known to be 2500 J/cm^3. Therefore, more than 2500 J/cm^3 of energy is required to remove epidermal tissue. In contrast, the energy needed for water vaporization in the dermis is 4300 J/cm^3, which is about twice the energy needed for the epidermis [1]. The reason for this is because of the high tensile strength of the collagen fibers in the dermis. If the dermis is treated with the energy needed for water vaporization for the epidermis, ablation will not occur. It will only cause dry skin, which will make the area of residual thermal damage (RTD) become larger, which is likely to cause side effects. Therefore, when treating the dermis, it is necessary to increase the energy twice as much as the energy used for the epidermis.

The energy needed to vaporize water (*Ev*) is known as the following equation:

$$E_{\mathrm{v}} = \mathrm{fluence} \times \mu_{\mathrm{a}}$$

The absorption coefficient of water of a CO_2 laser is 500 cm^{-1}, so if we substitute this into the formula:

$$\mathrm{Fluence} = 2500/500 = 5\left(\mathrm{J/cm^2\ in\ CO_2\ laser}\right)$$

At least 5 J/cm^2 of energy is required when using the CO_2 laser for ablative rejuvenation. In contrast, vaporization does not occur below 5 J/cm^2. This is called the water vaporization threshold of the CO_2 laser [1]. Since the absorption coefficient of Er:YAG laser is 10 times higher than that of CO_2 laser, it is known that the vaporization threshold of water in Er:YAG laser is 0.5–1.5 J/cm^2, which is 10 times lower. Therefore, the Er:YAG laser needs to use at least 1 J/cm^2 of energy for vaporization to occur.

11.5 Residual Thermal Damage (RTD)

Ohshiro presented the laser apple concept in 1995 [5]. The laser apple concept is that not all photons irradiated with ablative laser are used for ablation, but some are absorbed in the remaining tissue, elevating temperature and influencing tissue response. The remaining tissue shows a series of temperature-dependent bioreactions in tissue [6]. As shown in Fig. 11.3, when CO_2 laser is irradiated on the skin most photons are irradiated on the skin surface making the temperature highest. As we go deeper into the skin, there are fewer photons resulting in lower temperatures.

The thermal reactions of skin tissue are as follows:

>100 °C: vaporization
>60 °C: coagulation
>55 °C: protein degradation
>40 °C: protein denaturation.

Ohshiro assumed that irreversible damage occurs over 40 °C. Residual thermal damage (RTD) refers to the tissue that has not been vaporized and has been irreversibly damaged. RTDs are not normal tissue and is eventually discharged out of the skin. This means that RTDs are eventually removed later.

For example, when removing melanocytic nevus by CO_2 laser, even if we take care to remove the nevus only and do not remove surrounding tissue, the surrounding tissue is damaged anyway because of RTDs. These tissues are eventually removed, resulting in undesirable side effects. That is why, when removing nevus, we should not try to remove them all at once but should rather leave a little bit of nevus tissue behind. If there are remnant nevus tissue, it can be removed later. This is why I perform nevus removal at least two times, with intervals in between.

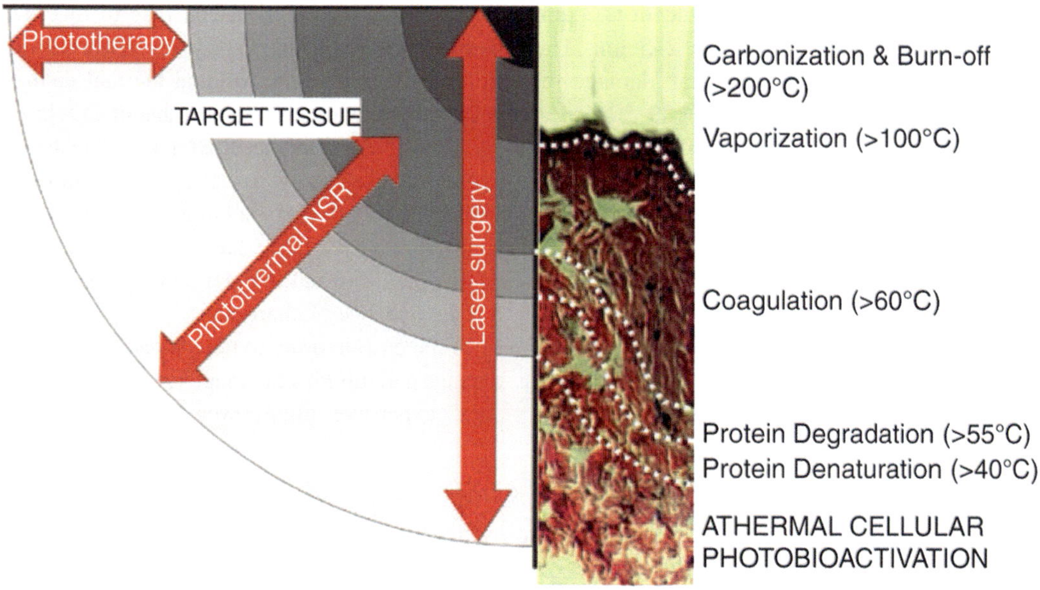

Fig. 11.3 Laser apple concept of Ohshiro. Histological changes of skin according to the temperature after irradiation with CO_2 laser. Reproduced from [4]

11.6 Thermal Relaxation Time (TRT) in Ablative Laser

$$\delta = \frac{1}{\mu_a}$$

δ: the wavelength dependent optical penetration depth of light, or the depth at which there is attenuation to 37% of the surface value (37% = 1/*e*, where *e* = 2.7, the base of the natural logarithm).

μ_a: absorption coefficient.

If we know the absorption coefficient, we can substitute this in the equation above, and calculate the optical penetration depth [1]. For example, the absorption coefficient of water in a CO_2 laser is 500 cm^{-1}. The optical penetration depth is calculated to be 20 μm. This is consistent with the actual ablation depth of 20–60 μm [1].

$$\mathrm{TRT} = d^2 / g\kappa$$

g: geometric factor, κ; thermal diffusivity.

In CO_2 laser, the diameter *d* in the TRT formula is the depth of penetration which is 20 μm. g is a geometric factor, and since skin is on a plane it is 4. The thermal diffusivity constant κ is about 1.3×10^{-3} cm^2/s. If we substitute these in the equation above, the TRT is approximately 800 μs. Therefore, the pulse duration of the CO_2 laser should be 800 μs or less, approximately 1 ms or less [1].

Since the absorption coefficient of the Er:YAG laser is 10 times that of the CO_2 laser, the optical penetration depth is 10 times lower resulting in 2 μm and the actual penetration depth is known as 2–5 μm. If this is put into the TRT formula, it should be 8 μs or less, and the PD of the Er: YAG laser should be about 10 μs or less.

In summary, the pulse duration for CO_2 laser should be less than 1 ms when the fluence is at least 5 J/cm^2. In this case, the optical penetration depth is 20 μm, and the actual ablation depth is 20 to 60 μm. The residual thermal damage is known to be 3–4 times the optical penetration depth [7], and the actual residual thermal damage depth is about 60–100 μm. On the other hand, the pulse duration for Er:YAG laser should be less than 10 μs when the fluence is at least 1 J/cm^2. In this case, the optical penetration depth is 2 μm, and the actual ablation depth is 2–5 μm. The actual depth of residual thermal damage of Er:YAG laser is known to be about 20–50 μm.

11.7 Er:YAG Laser

Although the PD of Er:YAG laser is known to be 250 μs, the subpulse is 1 μs, showing not only photothermal effect but also photomechanical effect. Thus, tissue particles are removed at supersonic velocities because of the more explosive pressure than CO_2 lasers. Due to this phenomenon, the skin is pushed down when using Er:YAG lasers and the residual thermal damage is 20–50 μm, which is less than that of CO_2 lasers [1] (Fig. 11.4). On the other hand, due to the explosive pressure, there are more hemorrhage with Er:YAG lasers. In summary, Er:YAG lasers compared to CO_2 lasers have shallower ablation depths, less residual thermal damage, and therefore less chance of charring.

In the past, in order to reduce residual thermal damage and minimize damage to surrounding tissues, expensive high-power CO_2 lasers drew

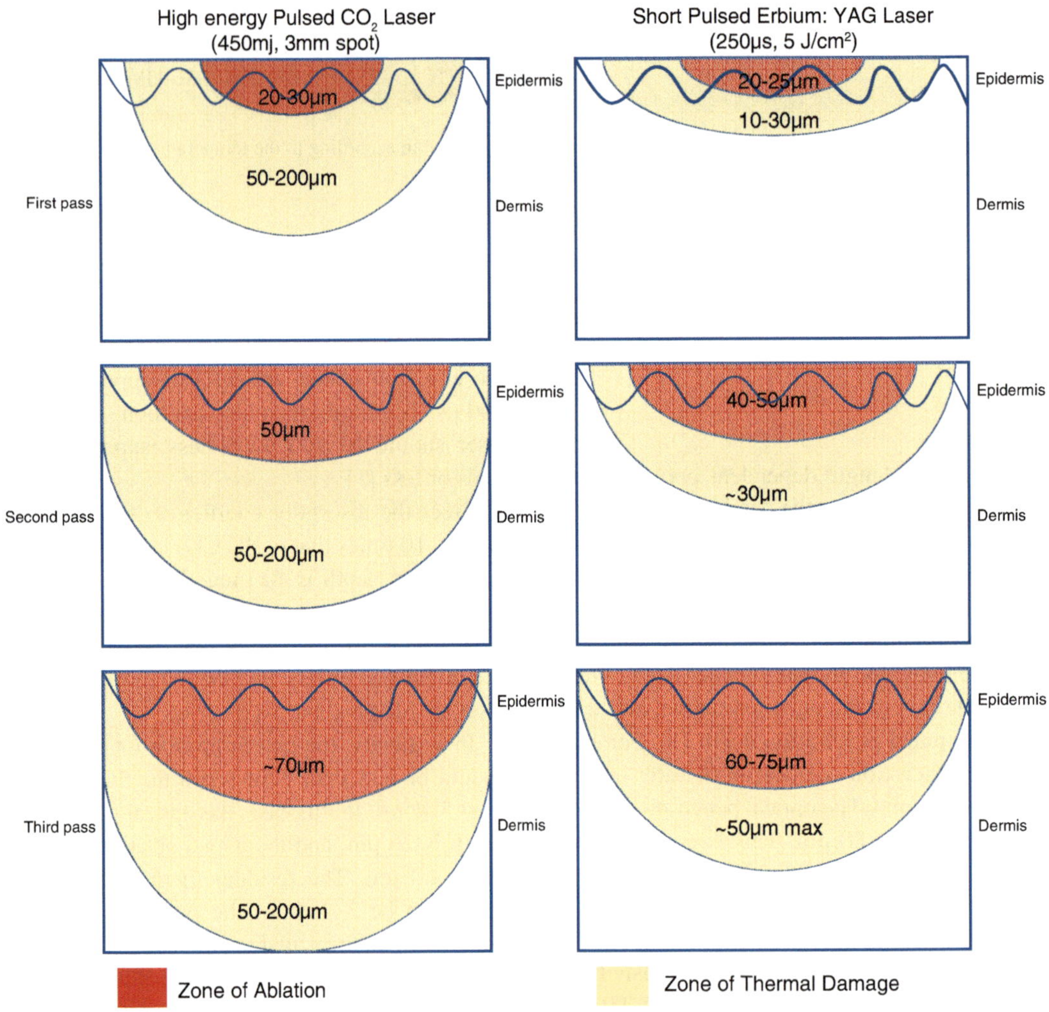

Fig. 11.4 Comparison between the depth of ablation by CO_2 laser and Er:YAG laser and the depth at which residual thermal damage occurs. When the energy of the Er:YAG laser is increased so that the depth is the same as the CO_2 laser, there is much less residual thermal damage. Reproduced from [8]

attention in the ablative laser market. However, with the introduction of Er:YAG lasers with much less residual thermal damage, the market for ablative laser is now divided into Er:YAG laser and low-power CO_2 laser.

11.8 Pros and Cons of Er:YAG Laser

The followings are the pros and cons of Er:YAG laser.

1. The depth of RTD in Er:YAG laser is much less than that of CO_2 laser, which means less side effects and faster wound healing.
2. Er:YAG laser has a shallow penetration depth, allowing precise depth adjustment.
3. Due to less RTD and explosive pressure, bleeding occurs very well in Er:YAG lasers. The disadvantage is that this makes deep ablation difficult, but the advantage is that it may be safe because ablation beyond the papillary dermis (where with blood vessels are) is difficult. However, with pulse stacking, it is possible to go deeper than the papillary dermis.
4. The depth of ablation and RTD is shallow in Er:YAG lasers. Thus, unlike CO_2 lasers, skin shrinkage and skin elasticity effect are minimal, resulting in inferior effect on wrinkles compared to CO_2 lasers.
5. Due to the nerve coagulation effect of RTD, there are less pain during CO_2 lasers, unlike Er:YAG lasers which do not have this effect and are more painful during the procedure.
6. Er:YAG lasers are loud due to photomechanical effects.
7. CO_2 lasers cost little to maintain because the pumping system is electricity, but Er:YAG lasers cost much more because the pumping system is a flash lamp, which requires replacement costs and is expensive to purchase.

11.9 Depth of Ablation and RTD

What is the relationship between fluence, ablation depth, and the depth of RTD? Ross et al. biopsied pig skin after CO_2 laser exposure of 10 J/cm^2 [7]. Since CO_2 is a Gaussian beam, it has the highest fluence (20 J/cm^2) in the middle. The middle portion is the deepest, indicating that ablation depth is the deepest in the middle. The center is the most depressed, showing the deepest ablation. Therefore, we can see that the higher the fluence, the deeper the ablation depth.

From the end of the laser beam to the center, the RTD area initially becomes a little thicker, but after it reaches 3 J/cm^2 (this fluence probably corresponds to the vaporization energy of water in pig skin) the thickness is relatively constant. i.e., when the energy is lower than the water vaporization threshold, higher fluence increases the depth of RTD, but when it is higher than the water vaporization threshold, the depth of RTD is relatively constant.

11.10 Calculation of Depth of Ablation and RTD in Er:YAG Laser

What is the depth in which tissue can be removed without causing scarring? There is no known data regarding this, but I think there would be no problem ablating to the papillary dermis because the papillary dermis heals through regenerative wound healing (refer to Sect. 7.5 in Chap. 7). The thickness of the epidermal layer is known to be about 100 μm, and the thickness of the papillary dermis is known to be about 150–300 μm. That is, tissue can be removed without causing scarring up to 250–400 μm.

Er:YAG laser can remove most pigmentations in the dermoepidermal junction or upper dermis and junctional nevi through 4–10 passes of fluence 5.2–14.4 J/cm^2 [9]. Let's see if this parameter is correct. My parameter for the Er:YAG laser is 6 J/cm^2 and less than 8 passes when treating epidermal pigmentation or junctional nevi. The water vaporization threshold for the Er:YAG laser is about 1 J/cm^2. The fluence of 6 J/cm^2 is 6 times this, so the penetration depth should be about 12–30 μm, which is 6 times the depth of penetration which is 2–5 μm. Eight passes will add up to 96–240 μm and adding up 20–50 μm of RTD will result in 120–290 μm. Ten passes will result in 140–350 μm. Therefore, I use 6 J/cm^2

with Er:YAG laser and perform a maximum of eight passes and stop when the target tissue is ablated. But for very deep nevi up to 10 passes may be performed.

11.11 Spot Size in Ablative Laser

Which spot size should be used in ablative lasers? The use of small spot sizes results in remnant tissues, because the results are irregular and uneven (Fig. 11.5). Poor hemostasis is also a problem because bleeding from blood vessels larger than the spot size cannot be stopped. The use of large spot sizes results in a smoother, more even ablation of tissues. Therefore, small spot sizes should be used to make incisions, and large spot sizes should be used to remove nevi or for skin rejuvenation [1]. But if the spot size is larger the power density decreases, and longer pulse duration is needed to achieve the same effect. This may result in the risk of increasing residual thermal damage area and charring, and eventually scarring. To avoid this, ablative laser with a high output must be used or the spot size should be adjusted according to the output.

In Chap. 1 "Scattering and spot size (Sect. 1.6)" we reviewed that as the spot size becomes larger, the optical penetration depth (OPD) becomes deeper. But the ablation depth is the same even though the spot size increases (Fig. 11.5). What is the reason for this phenomenon? The reason that the OPD becomes deeper as the spot size becomes larger, is due to scattering. Since scattering is almost nonexistent in far-infrared lasers, the OPD is determined by the absorption coefficient regardless of the spot size change. Therefore, if the laser is a far-infrared laser of the same wavelength, the ablation depth is the same regardless of spot size.

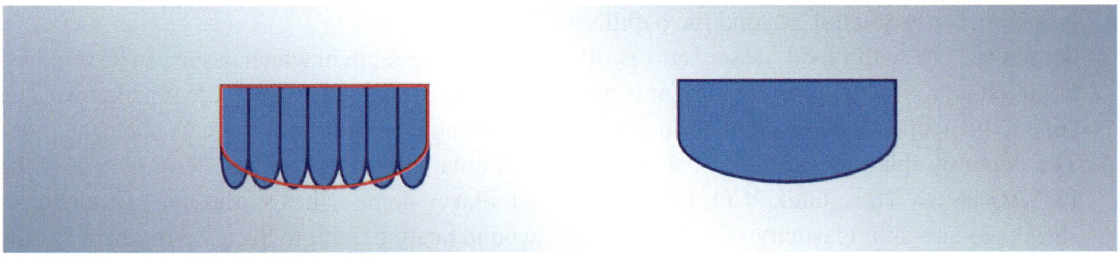

Fig. 11.5 Difference in spot size in ablative lasers. When small spot sizes are used to remove the same volume of tissue (e.g., nevi, depicted as red boxes), some tissues are remained while some are excessively removed (left)

11.12 Parameters

The Er:YAG laser has a fixed wavelength and PD among the 6 parameters of the laser, and since epidermal cooling is not required, only the spot size, fluence, and frequency (Hz) may be adjusted. In particular, frequency should take into account the number of total passes, not just for the purpose of controlling the time between irradiations. That's why I use 4 Hz, so that I can count the number of passes and also for quick procedure. The spot size should be adjusted to the size of the lesion, but since most lesions such as melanocytic nevus and lentigo are 2–3 mm, I mainly use a 2 mm spot size.

As we have seen, the indications for Er:YAG laser are, first, melanocytic nevus, epidermal nevus, and benign tumors. Second, epidermal pigmentation such as lentigo or freckles. Third, for ablative rejuvenation. But since CO_2 fractional lasers are safe and more effective than Er:YAG laser, I do not use Er:YAG lasers for ablative rejuvenation (Table 11.2).

As seen above, for junctional nevus I use 6 J/cm^2 with Er:YAG laser and perform a maximum of 8 passes and stop when the target tissue is ablated. But for very deep nevus up to 10 passes may be performed. The remaining nevus are removed with a CO_2 laser or CO_2 laser pinhole. Considering skin regeneration, the following procedure is performed after 3 months, and if there are any remaining nevus, they are removed again in the same way.

Since compound nevus and intradermal nevus are indistinguishable from normal skin in the case of nevus cells without black pigmentations, they should be ablated only up to a depth of 250 to 400 μm, which is a depth that does not cause scarring. However, because the depth cannot be accurately measured visually, nevus removal is stopped at a position approximately 0.5 mm lower than the height of the surrounding skin. Pinhole method is then performed with a CO_2 laser. If there are any remaining nevus at intervals of 3 months, they are removed again in the same way.

The pinhole method uses a small spot size with the CO_2 laser, which allows for precise procedures, but it is not possible to quickly eliminate large lesions. That's why I use the pinhole method with the Er:YAG laser for congenital melanocytic nevus [10]. The spot size is set at 2 mm, so that it does not overlap and is performed dense as possible to the depth at which the pigmentation is ablated and repeated every 3 months.

Table 11.2 Parameters of Er:YAG laser (MCL30 Dermablate, Asclepion Laser Technologies GmbH, Jena, Germany)

Indications	Spot size (mm)	Fluence (J/cm^2)	Technique	Remarks
Junctional nevus	2	6	Stacking or paintbrush	≤8–10 pass in stacking
Compound and intradermal nevus	2–3 according to lesion size	6	Stacking or paintbrush	To a depth of 0.5 mm lower than surrounding skin
Congenital melanocytic nevus (small)	2	6	Stacking (pinhole method)	Continue treatment until no more pigment is visible
Epidermal nevus	2–3 according to lesion size	6	Stacking or paintbrush	To a depth of 0.5 mm lower than surrounding skin
Xanthelasma palpebrarum	2–3	6	Stacking	Requires ablation of the complete lesion
Freckles or small lentigines	1–3 according to lesion size	6	Stacking or paintbrush	≤8 passes in stacking

In the case of epidermal nevus, which protrudes in the form of a wart above the surface of the skin, the spot size is set to match the size of the lesion, and the laser is irradiated until the position is approximately 0.5 mm lower than the height of the surrounding skin.

Xanthelasma palpebrarum is removed with a spot size 2–3 mm until the yellow lesion is completely removed. I warn the patient in advance that if the size of the xanthelasma palpebrarum is small, the skin may be slightly depressed and if it is large, it may leave scars, although not severe.

In cases such as epidermal pigmented lesions, such as freckles and lentigo, several passes are performed at 6 J/cm^2 using a spot size of 1–3 mm to match the size of the lesion, and if the pigment is removed before 8 passes, the procedure is discontinued. Even if the pigment remains, only 8 passes are used.

References

1. Goldman MP. Cutaneous and cosmetic laser surgery. Philadelphia: Mosby Elsevier; 2006.
2. Niemz M. Laser-tissue interactions. Springer International Publishing; 2019.
3. Kauvar A, Hruza G. Principles and practices in cutaneous laser surgery. CRC Press; 2005.
4. Nouri K. Lasers in dermatology and medicine: dermatologic applications. Springer International Publishing; 2018.
5. Ohshiro T. The laser apple: a new graphic representation of medical laser applications. Laser Therapy. 1996;8(3):185–90.
6. Omi T, Numano K. The role of the CO2 laser and fractional CO2 laser in dermatology. Laser Ther. 2014;23(1):49–60.
7. Ross EV, McKinlay JR, Anderson RR. Why does carbon dioxide resurfacing work? A review. Arch Dermatol. 1999;135(4):444–54.
8. Riggs K, Keller M, Humphreys TR. Ablative laser resurfacing: high-energy pulsed carbon dioxide and erbium:yttrium-aluminum-garnet. Clin Dermatol. 2007;25(5):462–73.
9. Baba M, Bal N. Efficacy and safety of the short-pulse erbium:YAG laser in the treatment of acquired melanocytic nevi. Dermatol Surg. 2006;32(2):256–60.
10. Chung BY, Han SS, Kim BW, Chang SE, Lee MW. Effective treatment of congenital melanocytic nevus and nevus sebaceous using the pinhole method with the erbium-doped yttrium aluminium garnet laser. Ann Dermatol. 2014;26(5):651–3.

CO_2 Fractional Laser and Fractional Photothermolysis

12

12.1 Overview of CO_2 Fractional Lasers

CO_2 fractional lasers are ablative fractional lasers because they are based on a 10,600 nm CO_2 laser (Table 12.1). Recently, CO_2 fractional lasers have emerged that can use a single beam by replacing the fractional handpiece with a surgical handpiece (Fig. 12.1). When replaced with a surgical handpiece, it can be used for melanocytic nevus removal, seborrheic keratosis removal, incision, hemostasis, pinhole method, etc. Since this chapter deals with CO_2 fractional lasers, I will limit my discussion to procedures using fractional handpieces.

In U-Pulse laser (SNJ Co. Ltd. Seoul, Korea), the pulse duration varies depending on the pixel energy: approximately 5 mJ, the pulse duration is 200 μs, the 40 mJ is 800 μs, and the 300 mJ is 8000 μs (8 ms). The TRT of water on the CO_2 laser is 800 μs or less (refer to Sect. 11.6 in Chap. 11). Therefore, the U-Pulse laser must use energy of 40 mJ or less. Scanning sizes can be used up to 20 × 20 mm, and variety of shapes may be used, including squares, triangles, and circles. Square shapes are mainly used. The beam pattern can use standard, alternate, random, scatter, etc., but standard or random pattern is mainly used.

Table 12.1 Specifications of CO_2 fractional laser (U-Pulse, SNJ Co. Ltd. Seoul, Korea)

Wavelength	10,600 nm
Mode	FRX (fractional)/CO_2 (surgical)
Max. power	100 W
Pixel energy	5–300 mJ
Scan area	1 × 1–20 × 20 mm
Density	0.1–2.0 mm/Overlap:1–10
Laser shape	Square, Rectangle, Triangle, Circle
Beam pattern	Standard, Alternate, Random, Scatter

Some fractional lasers adjust the treatment density in units of "%" or "spots/cm^2," while U-Pulse lasers adjust the treatment density by the distance (mm) between beams. That is, the shorter the distance between beams, the higher the treatment density, and the longer the distance, the lower the treatment density. The distance between beams may be adjusted from 0.1 mm to 2.0 mm. Usually, based on 1.0 mm, less than 1.0 mm is used to increase treatment density, and more than 1.0 mm is used to lower treatment density. The U-Pulse laser can set the number of overlaps and can overlap up to 10 passes.

J. D. Lee, M. J. M. Oh, *Lasers in Dermatology: Parameters and Choice*,
https://doi.org/10.1007/978-981-19-7568-4_12

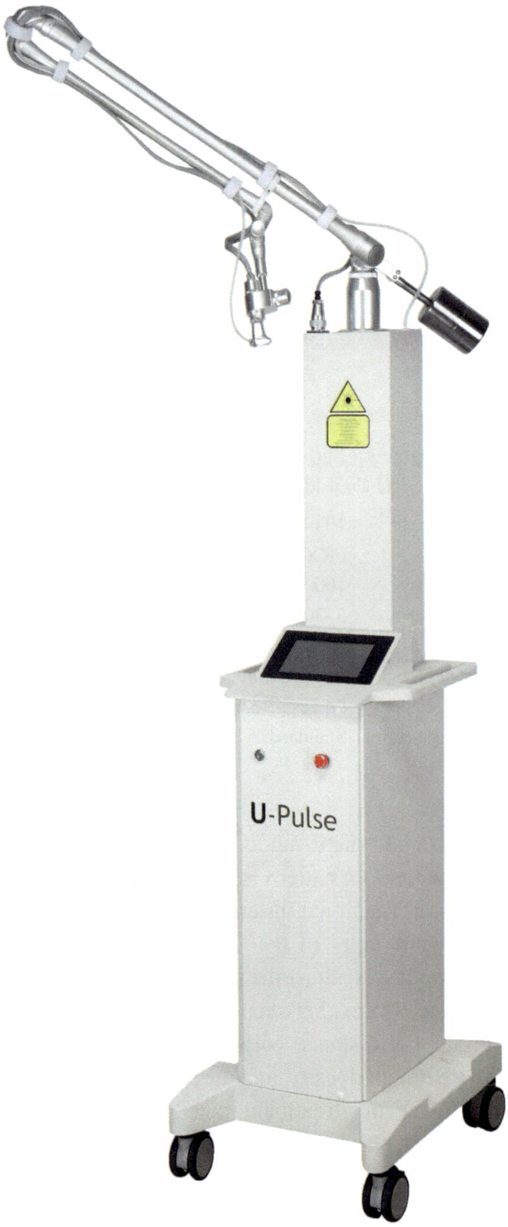

Fig. 12.1 CO_2 fractional lasers have emerged that can use a single beam by replacing the fractional handpiece with a surgical handpiece (U-Pulse, SNJ Co. Ltd. Seoul, Korea)

12.2 Indications

Indications for CO_2 fractional lasers are "large pore, scar, wrinkle, tightening," as are indications for ablative rejuvenation (Table 12.2). In particular, it is known to be more effective than other non-ablative lasers or non-ablative fractional lasers or vascular lasers in atrophic acne scars. It is reported to be effective against hypopigmentation such as striae alba [1] and vitiligo [2], and when used with lower energy, it is reported to be effective on hypertrophic scars and keloids [3].

Table 12.2 Indications of CO_2 fractional laser

Skin rejuvenation	Scars
Large pore	Acne scar
Fine wrinkle	Striae distensae
Skin tightening	Hypopigmentation (vitiligo)
	Hypertrophic scar and keloid

Since fractional lasers can be used in dermal pigmentation treatment by melanin shuttles, I also use them in conjunction with Q-switched lasers in the treatment of tattoo treatments [4] or nevus of Ota [5] (refer to Sect. 12.5 in Chap. 12).

12.3 Laser Resurfacing

Peeling the entire skin is called skin resurfacing or ablative rejuvenation. There is chemical, physical, and laser methods. Chemical methods include peeling using phenol, and physical methods include dermabrasion using sandpaper or grinder. Lasers include laser resurfacing using CO_2 lasers or Er:YAG lasers. Among the three methods, the easiest to control and with the most consistent results is laser resurfacing. In addition, laser resurfacing is known to be the most effective among ablative rejuvenation because it causes collagen regeneration by reversible thermal damage as well as neocollagenesis by the wound healing process.

Laser resurfacing is not only effective for acne scars, but also for facial tone, skin texture, collagen contraction and remodeling, and skin elasticity, making the skin look 10 years younger. Laser resurfacing using a CO_2 laser improves atrophic acne scars by 43–80% (average 66.8%) [6], and scars are known to improve gradually up to 18 months after the procedure. However, laser resurfacing requires general anesthesia and needs closed dressing such as a mask, which makes social life difficult and requires hospitalization.

In addition, side effects are so severe that erythema, edema, and oozing occur, and complications such as inflammation, milia, and PIH are not uncommon. Erythema lasts from 1 to 6 months. This is why laser resurfacing is seldom used these days.

12.4 Comparison of Rejuvenation Methods

In the past decades, ablative rejuvenation using CO_2 lasers has been recognized as the gold standard for skin resurfacing [7]. However, due to serious side effects such as long downtime and scarring, and long PIH duration especially in Koreans the procedure is not as popular as it used to be.

This is why nonablative rejuvenation, which has less side effects, has been developed. But nonablative rejuvenation is much less effective. This brings us to the recently developed fractional laser. Fractional lasers have fewer side effects than ablative rejuvenation but are more effective than nonablative rejuvenation. The first fractional laser to be developed was 1550 nm Er:glass laser, which did not induce ablation but only coagulation (which is why it is called nonablative fractional rejuvenation). This fractional laser was thought to lack efficacy, and hence the use of CO_2 laser, for ablative fractional rejuvenation. Fractional rejuvenation with a CO_2 laser or an Er:YAG laser is called ablative fractional regeneration (Fig. 12.2).

As we go through the history of lasers and consider the reasons why lasers were developed, the effects and the side effects of each laser can be understood.

Ablative rejuvenation > ablative fractional rejuvenation > nonablative fractional rejuvenation > nonablative rejuvenation

The order of effectiveness is as above. The reverse order will be the ones with the least adverse effects. Currently, ablative fractional laser (AFL) is considered as the gold standard for skin resurfacing.

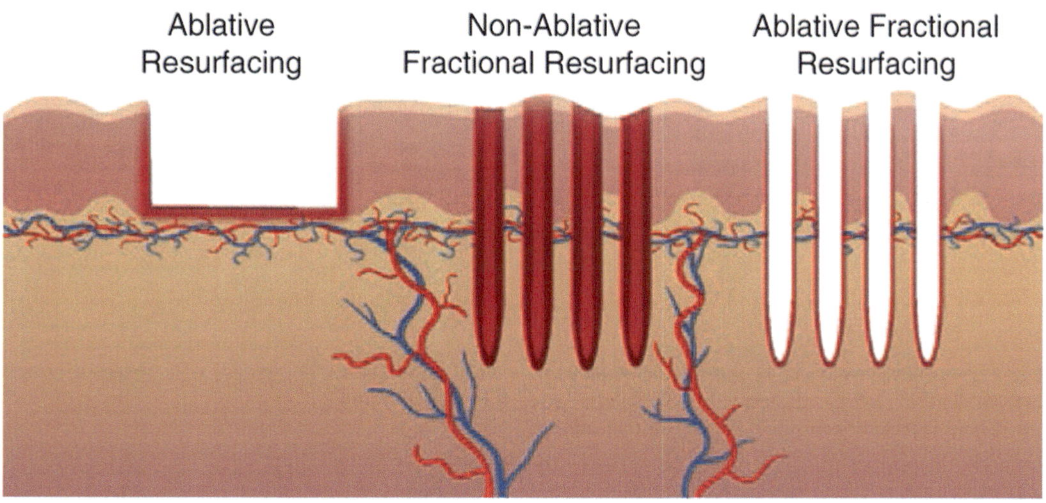

Fig. 12.2 Comparison of penetration depth and residual thermal damage of ablative and fractional rejuvenation. Reproduced from [8]

12.5 Fractional Photothermolysis and Melanin Shuttle

Fractional lasers do not irradiate the entire skin, but instead irradiate parts of the skin, leaving normal tissue between the beams, so that the regeneration of the tissue from the normal tissues is faster, reducing side effects (fractional photothermolysis) [9].

The area irradiated with fractional laser beam is called the microscopic treatment zone (MTZ), and the tissue that is irradiated, necrotized, and is pushed out of the skin is called microscopic epidermal necrotic debris (MEND) (Fig. 12.3). Since MEND contains not only epidermal keratinocytes but also melanin in keratinocytes, laser texts often refer to them as "melanin shuttle" [5]. Although the term MEND includes "epidermal," it also includes dermal tissue because fractional laser beam reaches the dermal layer and may also include dermal melanin pigmentations. Therefore, fractional laser can theoretically be applied to both epidermal and dermal pigmentation treatments. The CO_2 pinhole method can also be used for pigmentation treatment in place of fractional lasers because the melanin shuttle concept is applied.

Fractional lasers are used for dermal pigmentation treatment rather than epidermal pigmentation treatment. It is especially used for tattoo removal. However, because ablative fractional lasers do not have a deep penetration depth, they must increase their energy or overlap (stacking). Still, there are limitations, so I use the CO_2 pinhole method, not the CO_2 fractional laser, when treating blue nevus and tattoo.

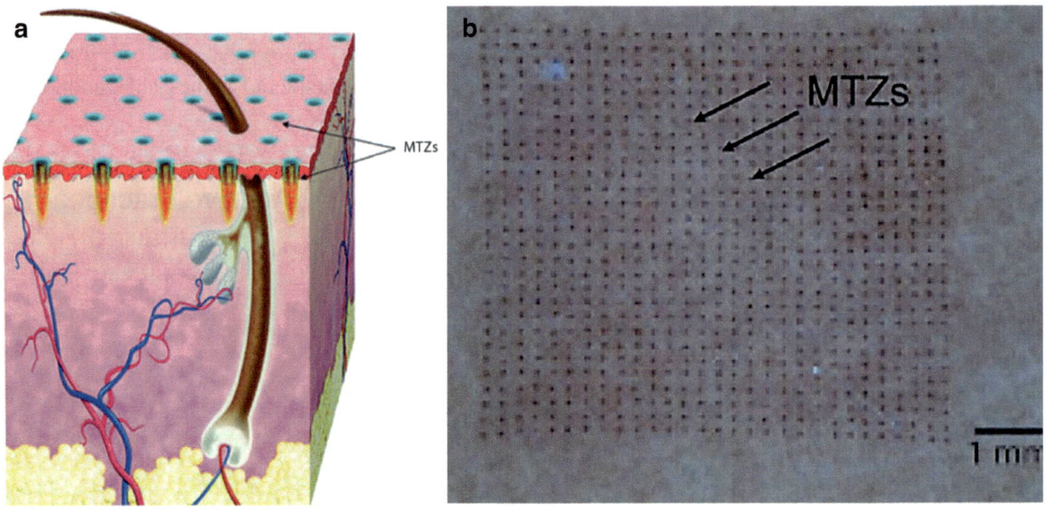

Fig. 12.3 (**a**) Schematic picture of fractional photothermolysis depicting MTZs surrounded by unharmed tissue. (**b**) Clinical picture depicting MTZs surrounded by unharmed tissue. *MTZs* microscopic treatment zones. Reproduced from [5]

12.6 Relationship Between Treatment Density and Side Effects

Patient satisfaction and procedure results in fractional lasers are associated with high energy, but the risk of side effects is associated with high treatment density, i.e., irradiating the beam densely [7]. Several papers also indicate that treatment density, rather than energy, is an important factor in PIH. In one paper, the total treatment density was lowered (the number of passes - 1 pass means one full-face treatment - was reduced to four passes rather than the eight) and the treatment session was increased from three to six times and the incidence of PIH in Asians has decreased from 18.2% to 6% [10]. In other words, lowering the treatment density reduces side effects, while increasing energy and increasing the number of treatments result in better effects.

In ablative fractional laser (AFL) 1 pass is generally recommended, and 1 pass is known to be effective in scar treatment and skin rejuvenation of Asians.

12.7 Parameters of Fractional Lasers

There are four major factors that influence the outcome of fractional laser treatment [11] (Table 12.3). First, it is the ratio of the fraction where the fractional laser is irradiated and the fraction that is not irradiated. The higher the proportion of the irradiated area, the greater the efficacy and the greater the likelihood of side effects.

Table 12.3 Factors that affect the results of fractional laser procedures and their corresponding parameters

Points to consider in parameters	Parameters in fractional laser
Percentage (cross-section area) of skin ablated	Density
Diameter of the individual microwounds	Spot size and energy per MTZ
Depths of the individual injuries	Energy per MTZ
Ratio of ablation of coagulation	Kinds of fractional laser (laser medium)

The parameter of the fractional laser that determines this ratio is "treatment density." Sometimes "%" is used, or "spot/cm^2" is used as well. Of the two units, "%" is a more accurate unit because in "spot/cm^2" treatment density varies depending on the fluence and the spot size of the beam.

Second, as described earlier, the ratio may vary depending on the diameter of the MTZ. The parameter corresponding to this is also the spot size of the beam, but the diameter of the MTS also varies depending on the energy. That is, the higher the energy per MTZ, the wider the diameter of the MTZ.

Third, the depth of MTZ also influences the outcome. Depending on the depth of the MTZ, different effects can be seen. If the depth of the MTZ is shallow, it can have an effect on pigments, skin tones, skin textures, etc., and if the depth of the MTZ is deep, it can also have an effect on moderate wrinkles and acne scars [11]. If the depth of MTZ is deeper, it is more effective but the likelihood of side effects is also high. Therefore, the depth should be determined according to the effect desired by the operator. The corresponding parameter is energy per MTZ.

Finally, it is the ratio of ablation and coagulation. The parameter corresponding to this is the laser wavelength (medium), i.e., the type of laser. It is known that CO_2 fractional lasers have an ablation:coagulation ratio of 70:30, which is most effective. Both Er:YAG fractional laser (90:10) and nonablative fractional laser (0:100) are known to be less effective than the CO_2 fractional laser.

To sum up the above from the laser physician's point of view, first, the medium of the fractional laser is typically CO_2, Er:YAG, Er:glass, and the most effective laser is the CO_2 fractional laser. Second, the energy per MTZ determines the diameter of the MTZ. Before taking into account the diameter, the energy suitable for the depth of the MTZ is selected, according to the indications. The problem is that if the energy is high, the diameter of the MTZ will widen, which increases the risk of side effects, so when increasing the energy to treat a deeper area, the treatment density should be lowered. Third, treatment density (MTZ) is associated with the likelihood of side effects. Treatment density should be lowered to reduce side effects, but in this case multiple sessions are needed because the treatment area is small. I increase the treatment density by taking into account the indications and the patient skin type because if the depth of the MTZ is limited to the papillary dermis, no serious side effects such as scar appear (refer to Sect. 12.8 in Chap. 12). Fourth, the spot size affects the diameter of the MTZ and determines the ratio of the irradiated area and the unirradiated area. However, since the smaller the spot size, the fewer side effects, and because lasers with the lower output can make the spot size small, I think small spot size is better than large. I adjust the proportion of the irradiated area only by treatment density alone, and do not change the small spot size.

12.8 FAST Method

The most effective treatment for collagen remodeling is ablative rejuvenation (laser resurfacing) with CO2 laser, but it is currently not well performed due to the recovery period, side effects, and complications. Therefore, at present the CO_2 fractional laser, which is an ablative fractional laser, is known as the gold standard. So what are the parameters of the CO_2 fractional laser that make it the most effective and least prone to side effects?

Schweiger et al. treated acne scars by a new method using CO_2 fractional laser [12]. Only areas with scars were treated, normal areas were not treated. In addition, parameters that increase both energy and treatment density were used (high energy, high density). The authors of the paper define this method as "Focal Acne Scar Treatment" and call it the "FAST method." All six patients treated with the FAST method had significant posttreatment improvement ranging from 40% to 70% as estimated by the treating doctor and the patient at 4 weeks post treatment. Patient satisfaction was high following FAST method. Temporary post-inflammatory hyperpigmentation was seen in two patients but resolved after a single 1550 nm Er:glass fractional laser treatment. Schweiger et al. concluded that the FAST method is more effective, the recovery was faster, and there were no permanent side effects compared with whole face fractional CO_2 laser resurfacing.

In principle, the treatment density should be reduced in fractional lasers to reduce side effects, and energy should be increased to increase the effectiveness (high energy, low density) [10]. On the other hand, laser resurfacing is a way to increase treatment density. In my opinion, a more effective and safer treatment is possible if these two are combined: the treatment density and the energy must both be increased, but only the scars should be treated, leaving the normal tissue intact, i.e., "The fractional laser should be used fractionally." The paper above defines this as the FAST method. I use the CO_2 fractional laser to increase the treatment density with enough energy to damage the papillary dermis, and treat the scar by irradiating it with an area of 5×5 mm.

12.9 Parameters

If we calculate the TRT of water on the CO_2 laser, the pulse duration should be 800 μs or less. So the energy in the U-Pulse laser should be used less than 40 mJ because the corresponding energy of the pulse duration less than 800 μs in the U-Pulse laser is 40 mJ. The higher the energy, the greater the amount of tissue vaporized, so the deeper the penetration depth and the wider the diameter of the MTZ. In addition, the higher the energy, the longer the pulse duration, so the wider the residual thermal damage. Therefore, even if the spacing between beams is the same, increasing the energy widens the diameter of the MTZ and increases the treatment density, so the treatment density must be lowered by widening the gap between beams. Conversely, if the energy is low, the penetration depth is shallow and the diameter of the MTZ is reduced, so shortening the gap between beams does not become a problem. In addition, lower energy reduces the pulse duration, so there is less residual thermal damage resulting in fewer side effects. Laser shape can be chosen from a variety of shapes, and although theoretically the shape should be chosen in regard to the shape of the lesion, in practice the squares are often chosen (Table 12.4).

Ablative lasers, Q-switched lasers, and picosecond lasers can use epidermal cooling devices to alleviate pain in patients, although epidermal cooling does not affect the outcome of the procedure [13]. Most ablative lasers are not equipped with a cooling device, so ice-cube is usually used before and after the procedure, or a cold fan, i.e., convective cooling. When using a cold fan, blowing the wind towards the nose makes it difficult for the patient to breathe, so the wind direction should be directed from the patient's forehead to the chin, and the patient should breathe through the mouth.

Table 12.4 Parameters of the CO_2 fractional laser (U-Pulse, SNJ Co. Ltd. Seoul, Korea). SK: seborrheic keratosis

Indications	Energy (mJ)	Density (mm)	Scanning size (mm)
Skin rejuvenation (T zone, front cheek, nasolabial folds)	10–12	0.8–1.0	20 × 20
Skin rejuvenation (forehead, periorbital, side of face)	10–12	1.0–1.2	20 × 20
Large pore (T zone, front cheek, nasolabial folds)	14–24	0.8–1.0	20 × 20
Large pore (forehead, periorbital, side of face)	14–20	1.0–1.2	20 × 20
FAST method	18–22	0.8	≤5 × 5
Deep boxcar scar	24–40	1.2–1.4	≤5 × 5
Hypertrophic scar	20–40	1.0–1.2	≥5 × 5
SK	5	0.2	≥5 × 5
Skin booster	5	0.7–0.8	20 × 20

Indications for CO_2 fractional lasers include skin rejuvenation such as large pore, wrinkle, and tightening, drug infiltration with skin booster and scar treatment (Fig. 12.4). Most CO_2 fractional laser procedures are performed after applying topical anesthesia (occlusive dressing 20 to 40 minutes) to reduce pain.

The parameters of skin rejuvenation are as follows. For a quick procedure, set the scanning size to a maximum of 20 x 20 mm. In the case of the nose and the front cheek, the skin is thick, and the skin is well regenerated, thus the distance between the beams can be decreasing by 0.8–1.0 mm for increasing treatment density. When performing procedure on the forehead,

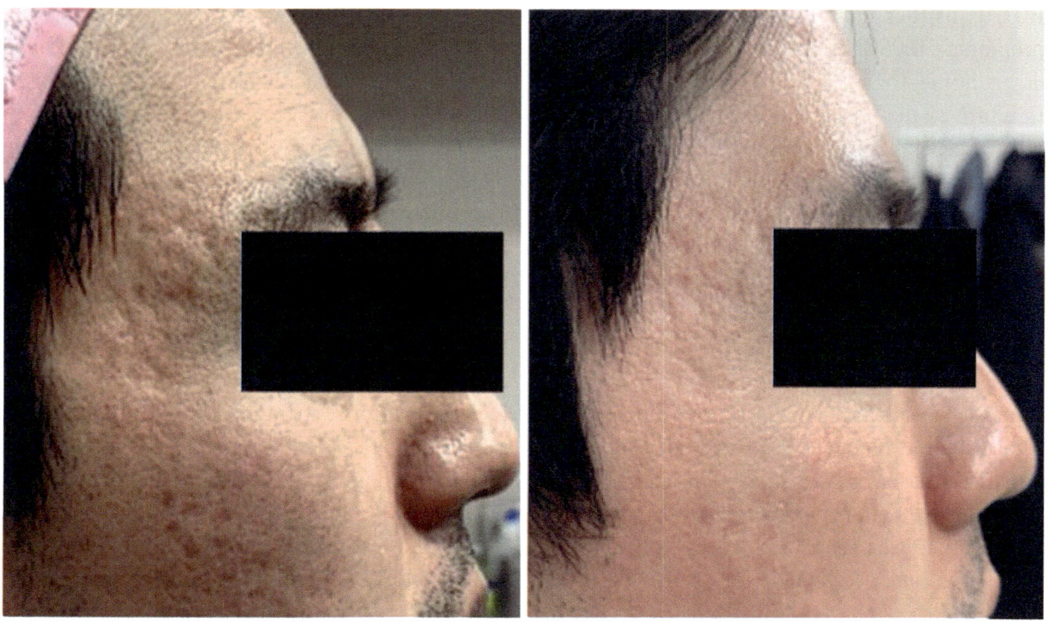

Fig. 12.4 Photographs before and after treatment of atrophic acne scar with CO_2 fractional laser. Left: Before the procedure, Right: 7 months after the 3 laser procedures. Laser used: U-Pulse laser (SNJ Co. Ltd. Seoul, Korea)

periorbital, or chin line, i.e., the side of face, treatment density should be lowered to 1.0–1.2 mm. In the case of forehead, the entire area is not treated, only the glabella, the upper eyebrows, and some wrinkle areas are treated, and the upper eyelid is not treated. The reason for this is that in the case of the forehead and upper eyelids, the swelling is severe, resulting in a longer downtime. Depending on the indications, the treatment depth should be different, because the higher the energy, the greater the amount of ablation and the deeper the penetration depth. This is why the energy should be increased to more than 14–20 mJ for large pores and scars and lowered to 10–12 mJ for small pores and skin rejuvenation. The interval between treatment is 4–8 weeks, taking into account the epidermal turnover when only the epidermis and some papillary dermis are treated. When treatment depth involves the papillary dermis and reticular dermis, skin regeneration is taken into account and intervals of 8–12 weeks, or more are needed. However, if erythema remains, I postpone the procedure because I think skin regeneration has not been completed. I have frequently experienced acneiform eruption after CO_2 fractional laser, and in order to reduce the risk of PIH, I instruct the patient to apply clobetasol propionate 0.05%, a group 1 steroid, 3 times a day at home, for a total of 6 times for 2 days, and to return to the hospital if erythema or swelling is severe or itching, papules and pustules occur after 2 days.

In the case of atrophic acne scars, the FAST method is performed for rolling scars or for shallow boxcar scars. In the FAST method, the distance between beams is reduced to 0.8 mm to increase treatment density. In this case, PIH and erythema may occur, so the patient should be informed in advance of the risk of side effects. The principle of the FAST method is to use a "fractional laser fractionally," so it does not treat areas other than atrophic acne scars. In the case of a deep boxcar scar, the energy is raised to 24–40 mJ and overlapped to remove the deep fibrous tissue and irradiated twice. However, not all fibrous tissue should be eliminated, since the skin with fibrous tissue is a poorly regenerated area (refer to Sect. 17.2 in Chap. 17). By increasing the distance between beams to 1.2–1.4 mm, the treatment density is lowered. Afterwards Duoderm is applied to areas where FAST method was performed or where deep boxcar scar was treated. The patient should be informed that 3 days of oozing is possible and that if there is too much oozing then the Duoderm should be changed. But after 3–4 days there will be less oozing, and the Duoderm should be kept in place for 7 days.

In the case of hypertrophic scars, the aim is to reduce the volume of the scar, so the energy should be increased. One pass with treatment density of 1 mm spacing at 40 mJ can be used without risk of pigmentation, but for safety reasons, one pass at 1.2 mm intervals at 30 mJ and one pass at 1.2 mm intervals at 20 mJ are used. (Published with kind permission of © Haewon Jung MD. 2021. All rights reserved).

For seborrheic keratosis (SK), I irradiate it evenly without omission with surgical CO_2 laser handpiece and then peel off the epidermis by gently pushing it with cotton or gauze soaked with boric or normal saline (dermoepidermal sliding effect) [14]. But when the SK is large, thick, and many, it can be treated with a CO_2 fractional laser. The treatment density can be increased to 0.2 mm spacing and the energy lowered to 5 mJ and then the dermoepidermal sliding effect can be used. The remaining part is removed with a surgical handpiece. Scanning size and laser shape should be adjusted to the shape and size of the lesion.

A CO_2 fractional laser can be used to infiltrating the skin booster. Since deep penetration is not required to penetrate the skin booster, the energy is lowered to 5 mJ, the treatment density is increased to 0.7–0.8 mm, irradiated, and the skin booster is applied to the skin. Because the pain is not severe, topical anesthesia is rarely needed. (Published with kind permission of © Yongho Hwang MD. 2021. All rights reserved).

References

1. Yang YJ, Lee GY. Treatment of striae distensae with nonablative fractional laser versus ablative CO(2) fractional laser: a randomized controlled trial. Ann Dermatol. 2011;23(4):481–9.
2. Helou J, Maatouk I, Obeid G, Moutran R, Stephan F, Tomb R. Fractional laser for vitiligo treated by 10,600 nm ablative fractional carbon dioxide laser followed by sun exposure. Lasers Surg Med. 2014;46(6):443–8.
3. Scrimali L, Lomeo G, Nolfo C, Pompili G, Tamburino S, Catalani A, et al. Treatment of hypertrophic scars and keloids with a fractional CO2 laser: a personal experience. J Cosmet Laser Ther. 2010;12(5):218–21.
4. Weiss ET, Geronemus RG. Combining fractional resurfacing and Q-switched ruby laser for tattoo removal. Dermatol Surg. 2011;37(1):97–9.
5. Allemann IB, Goldberg DJ. Basics in dermatological laser applications. Karger Medical and Scientific Publishers; 2011.
6. Fabbrocini G, Annunziata MC, D'Arco V, De Vita V, Lodi G, Mauriello MC, et al. Acne scars: pathogenesis, classification and treatment. Dermatol Res Pract. 2010;2010:893080.
7. Goldsmith LA, Katz SI, Gilchrest BA, Paller AS, Leffell DJ, Wolff K, et al. Fitzpatrick's dermatology in general medicine. New York: McGraw-Hill Professional; 2012.
8. Ogawa R. Total Scar Management. Springer Singapore; 2020.
9. Bogdan Allemann I, Kaufman J. Fractional photothermolysis—an update. Lasers Med Sci. 2010;25(1):137–44.
10. Hruza GJ, Tanzi EL. Lasers and lights. Edinburgh: Elsevier; 2018.
11. Goldman MP. Lasers and energy devices for the skin. [S.I.]: Taylor & Francis; 2013.
12. Schweiger ES, Sundick L. Focal acne scar treatment (FAST), a new approach to atrophic acne scars: a case series. J Drugs Dermatol. 2013;12(10):1163–7.
13. Goldman MP. Cutaneous and cosmetic laser surgery. Philadelphia: Mosby Elsevier; 2006.
14. Lee JD, Lee JK, Oh MJM. Principles and choice of laser treatment in dermatology. Singapore: Springer; 2020.

Part IV

Energy-based Devices and Parameters

13 Fractional Microneedle Radiofrequency and Conductivity

13.1 Overview of Needle RFs

Fractional microneedle radiofrequency (which we will describe in this book as needle RF for) is a device that inserts needles into a skin (minimally invasive) and allows a bipolar radiofrequency (RF) current to flow through to achieve collagen remodeling. RF has a frequency set for each device, and I use the needle RF with 2MHz (Table 13.1). Intensity can be adjusted from level 0 to 100 (%). A repetition refers to the time between pulse durations, which corresponds to frequency (Hz) in lasers. For example, repetition 0.2 s corresponds to 5 Hz. Repetition refers to the time it takes to move the handpiece from one point to another rather than affecting the treatment results, and I usually use 0.5–0.8 s. The needle is a non-insulated needle that is 0.3 mm thick and there are 2 pins; 25 pins with 25 needles arranged 5 × 5 and 16 pins with 16 needles arranged 4 × 4. I mainly use the 25 pin. The biggest advantage of needle RF is that the needle depth can be adjusted, from 0.5 to 3.5 mm. The pulse duration can be adjusted from 50 to 590 ms, but there is no repeat mode by which the current flows or stops repeatedly like the macropulse of the pulsed dye laser (PDL). Recently, there is also a needle RF that can calibrate impedance or temperature correction. The equipment I use cannot calibrate impedance or temperature.

Table 13.1 Specifications of needle RF (Secret[RF], ILOODA, Suwon, Korea)

Max. power	20 W ± 20%
RF frequency	2 MHz ± 20%
Intensity	0–100 level (10 step)
Repetition	0.2/0.5/1/2 s/single
Needle thickness	0.3 mm
Needle figure	25 electrode needle (5 × 5), 7.8 mm × 7.8 mm/pitch 1.95 mm (standard) 16 electrode needle (4 × 4), 7.8 mm × 7.8 mm/pitch 2.6 mm (optional)
Treatment area	1 cm × 1 cm
Adjustable depth	0.5–3.5 mm (0.1 step)
Treatment duration (RF emission)	50 ms–950 ms

13.2 Indications

Needle RF is one of the instruments used for nonablative rejuvenation and has all the indications corresponding to nonablative rejuvenation (Table 13.2). Nonablative rejuvenation has an effect on pores, wrinkles, and skin tightening. Needle RF is effective for scars, as well as pores, wrinkles, and skin tightening, but it's less effec-

J. D. Lee, M. J. M. Oh, *Lasers in Dermatology: Parameters and Choice*,
https://doi.org/10.1007/978-981-19-7568-4_13

Table 13.2 Indications for needle RF

Skin rejuvenation	Diseases
Skin tightening	Acne
Wrinkle	Melasma
Pore	
Acne scar	
Stretch marks	

tive than ablative rejuvenation, so I do not use the needle RF for scar treatment. It is also effective in acne and melasma, but since acne and melasma occur in areas where the depth is shallow, so the needle depth must be adjusted superficially.

13.3 Series Circuit and Parallel Circuit

Because RF is current, it must have a circuit [1]. The circuit can be divided into a series circuit and a parallel circuit depending on the position of resistance. In series and parallel circuits, if there is low resistance and high resistance, what kind of resistance will cause more current to flow and higher electrical energy to produce more temperature?

First, assuming that the voltage is 100 V, and the resistance is 7 Ω and 3 Ω, respectively, for a series circuit, let's calculate power and energy (Fig. 13.1). In a series circuit, the unchanging value is current. Since resistance is 7 + 3 = 10 Ω, current is 10 A. If you look at the resistance of 7 Ω, the voltage is 70 V because current is 10 A and resistance is 7 Ω (V = IR). Since power is 700 W with P = I × V, energy (E = P × t) is 700 J assuming the time is 1 second. For a series circuit, the formula $E = I^2 \times R \times t$ allows for faster calculations (Joule's law). Calculated in the same way, the power and energy generated by the resistance of 3 Ω are 300 W and 300 J, respectively. Therefore, in a series circuit, there is a lot of heat where the resistance is high [2]. For example, in monopolar RF, heat occurs in active electrodes with a narrower area than on ground pads with a wider area because heat occurs where resistance is high in the series circuit (formula below [3]). In addition, if one of the two electrodes during the bipolar RF procedure is not fully in contact with the skin, and only a part of it is contacted, the area is narrowed, and the resistance is increased, a lot of heat may occur on the side that is not fully in contact with the skin, which can cause burns [2]. As such, since the electrode is a series circuit, the current is constant, resulting in heat ($E = I^2 \times R \times t$) in electrodes with high resistance.

$$R = \frac{L}{\sigma A}, R = \rho \frac{L}{A} \left(\because \rho = \frac{1}{\sigma} \right)$$

R: resistance

σ (sigma): conductivity

ρ (rho): resistivity, resistance of a conductor with an area of 1 m^2 and length of 1 m

A: cross-section of tissue experiencing RF current

L: distance between electrodes

Next, for a parallel circuit, assuming the voltage is 100 V, and the resistance is 100 Ω and 10 Ω, respectively, let's calculate power and energy (Fig. 13.2). In a parallel circuit, the unchanging value is voltage. If you look at 100 Ω resistance, current is 1 A because the voltage is 100 V and the resistance is 100 Ω (I = V/R). Since power is P = I X V, power is 100 W, energy (E = P × t) is 100 J assuming the time is 1 second. In parallel circuits, the formula $E = V^2 / R \times t$ allows for faster calculations. Calculated in the same way, the power and energy generated by the resistance of 10 Ω are 1000 W and 1000 J, respectively. Therefore, in parallel circuits, there is more heat on the lower side of resistance. To put it simply, in a parallel circuit, the side with higher resistance has relatively less current, resulting in less heat, and a lot of current flowing on the side with less resistance, resulting in more heat [2]. For example, tissues with greater resistance are fat layers, and tissues with less resistance are skins. When RF treatment is performed, the current flows mainly through the skin, not the fat layer, so that there is not much heat in the fat layer, and heat occurs mainly only in the skin. As such,

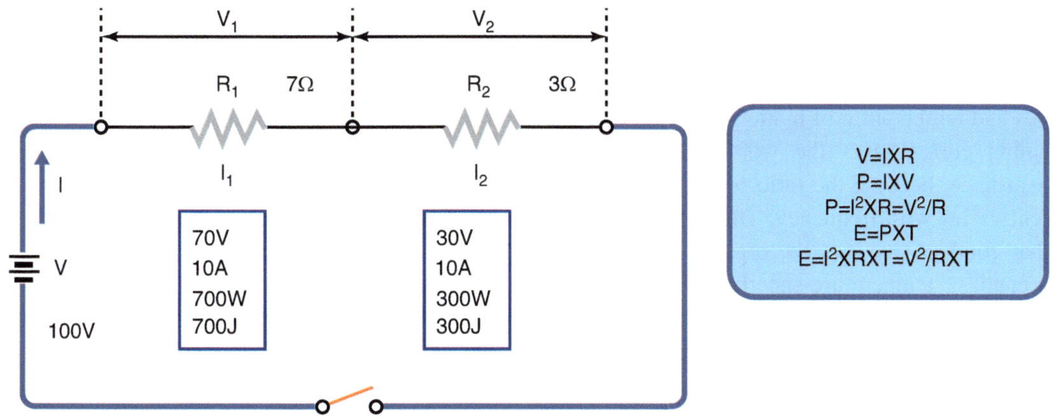

Fig. 13.1 Series circuit. Power (P) and energy (E) when voltage is 100 V and resistance is 7 Ω and 3 Ω, respectively. V: volatage, I: current, R: resistance, P: power, E: energy, T: time

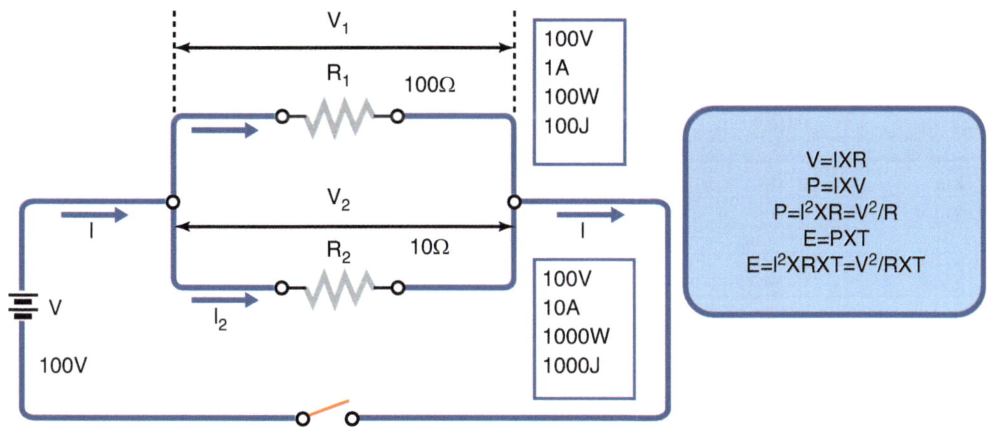

Fig. 13.2 Parallel circuit. Power (P) and energy (E) when the voltage is 100 V and the resistance is 100 Ω and 10 Ω, respectively. V: volatage, I: current, R: resistance, P: power, E: energy, T: time

Table 13.3 Differences in the occurrence of heat in series circuits and parallel circuits

	Circuit	Location of heat
Electrode end	Series circuit	High resistance
Between electrodes	Parallel circuit	Low resistance

since the human tissue is a parallel circuit and the voltage is constant in a parallel circuit, heat ($E = V^2/R \times t$) occurs on the side with less resistance.

In conclusion, the principle of a series circuit applies at the end of an electrode, and the principle of a parallel circuit applies in human tissue between electrodes (Table 13.3).

13.4 Conductivity

As explained earlier, human tissue is a parallel circuit, which causes more heat on the side with less resistance. Conductivity is, by definition, inversely proportional to resistivity ($\rho = \frac{1}{\sigma}$, ρ: resistivity, σ : conductivity) [3]. Thus, human tissue can be said to have more heat on the higher side of conductivity. When RF is used in human tissue, resistance and heat generation are opposites, so the word conductivity is used more often than resistivity to prevent confusion. Also, it is less confusing when we remember that in human tissue, the higher the conductivity, the more heat is generated.

Resistivity is the inherent resistance value of matter that is not related to the length and area of matter, and resistivity only changes in the properties and temperature of matter. In addition, alternating current uses the word impedance, not resistance, because the ratio of voltage and current varies with frequency. Thus, it can be seen that conductivity is, first, organization-specific, second, temperature-specific, and third, frequency-specific. Let's take a closer look.

First, conductivity has different values depending on the human tissue. Looking at Table 13.4, conductivity is the highest in blood, then skin, and the tissues with the lowest conductivity are dry skins and fats. Therefore, when RF therapy is applied to the human body, the current flows into the blood or skin, and the heat is well developed in the blood and skin. In dry skins and fats, the current does not flow well, so there is less heat generation. Basically, the tissue with higher water and blood content shows high conductivity [3]. Therefore, injecting tumescent anesthesia into tissues results in higher conductivity. Also, energy should be lowered in skin with erythema because it has a high conductivity.

Table 13.4 Conductivity of different types of biological tissue at 1 MHz. Reproduced from [3]

Tissue	Conductivity (Sm^{-1})
Blood	0.7
Bone	0.02
Fat	0.03
Dry skin	0.03
Wet skin	0.25

Second, conductivity varies with frequency. From 100 kHz to 1 MHz, conductivity increases with frequency. Beyond that, however, there is no significant change in conductivity in frequency (Fig. 13.3). On the other hand, the conductivity of fat is relatively constant regardless of frequency [3]. So, while using RF with a high frequency may work to raise a high temperature, there is not much difference if it goes beyond 3 MHz. It makes no sense to use RF with a high frequency, especially for lipolysis.

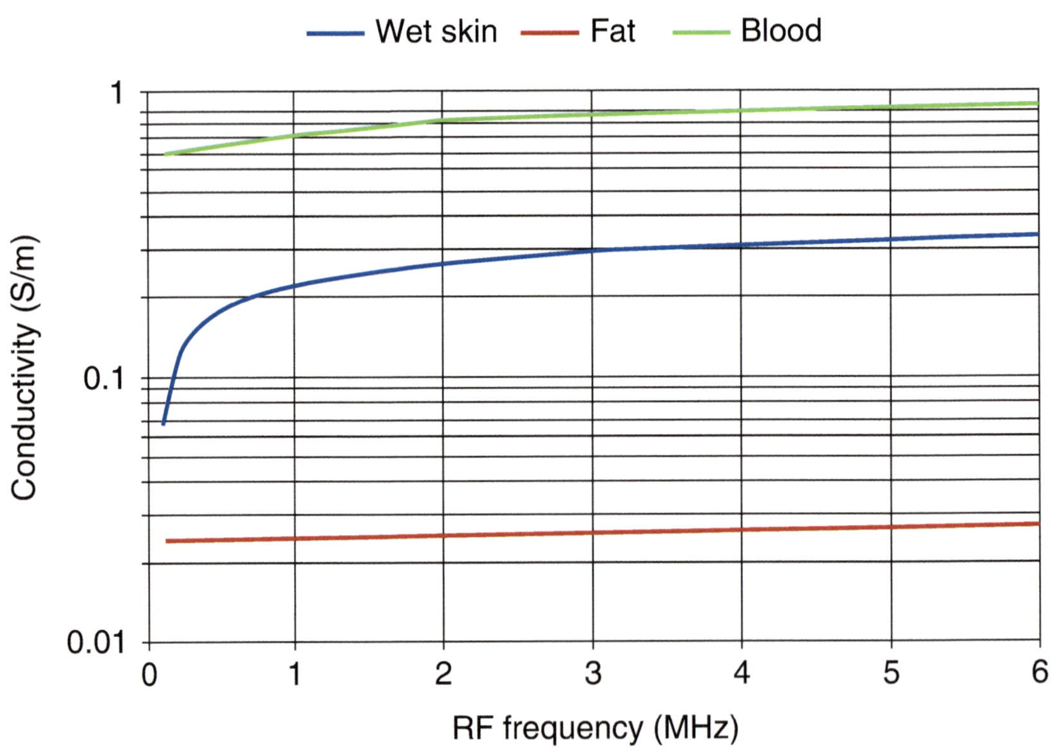

Fig. 13.3 Variation of conductivity of skin components with RF operating frequency. Reproduced from [4]

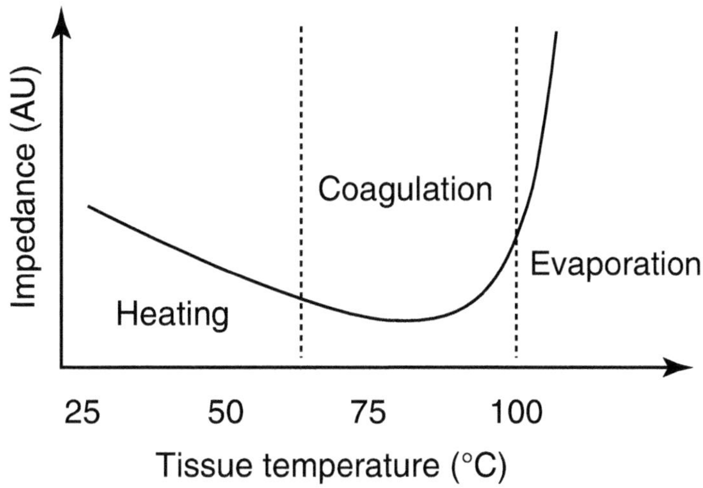

Fig. 13.4 Variation of tissue impedance with temperature. Reproduced from [4]

Third, the conductivity of the tissue varies depending on the temperature. As the temperature of the tissue increases, conductivity increases. For each increase in 1 °C, the impedance decreases by 1.5–2%. In other words, conductivity is increased. It is known that the reason for this increase in conductivity is that viscosity decreases as the temperature of the tissue increases. However, when the temperature goes higher and coagulation occurs, a chemical change occurs in the tissue, which leads to a change in conductivity. In addition, at 90–100 °C, conductivity decreases as vaporization occurs (Fig. 13.4).

Thus, conductivity varies with tissue, frequency, and temperature. Therefore, when performing an RF procedure, even if the procedure is performed on the same area with the same energy on the same patient, sometimes it will not work and sometimes it may have side effects. In particular, if the temperature rises during the procedure, the conductivity goes up and the temperature goes up higher, which increases the likelihood of side effects. Therefore, a device that automatically compensates for impedance (resistance) is needed. In other words, during an RF procedure, the impedance between two electrodes should be measured and applied to the following equation to increase the voltage if the impedance is high, and lower the voltage if the impedance is low, to make the electrical energy constant [2]. In other words, when buying RF equipment, it would be better to buy RF with an automatic impedance compensator.

$$E = \frac{V^2}{R} t$$

E: energy, V: volatage, R: resistance, *t*: time

13.5 Meaning of Parameters in Needle RF

Zheng et al. experimented with adjusting three parameters using needle RF insulated in vivo minipig [5]. The 3 parameters are the penetration depth of the needle, the pulse duration (RF conduction time), and the energy level. The penetration depth was adjusted to 0.5, 1.0, 1.5, 2.0, 2.5, and 3.5 mm, the pulse duration was adjusted to 20, 50, 100, and 1000 ms, and the energy was adjusted to 5.0, 10.0, 20.0, 25.0, 37.5, and 50.0 V. Tissue biopsy was performed immediately after the procedure, 4 days later, and 2 weeks later, respectively.

The results show, first, a cocoon-shaped coagulation column was observed in the dermis layer (Fig. 13.5). Second, on the 4th day after the procedure, reepithelialization occurred, resulting in the formation of mixed cellular infiltration, neovascularization, and granulation tissue. Third, the

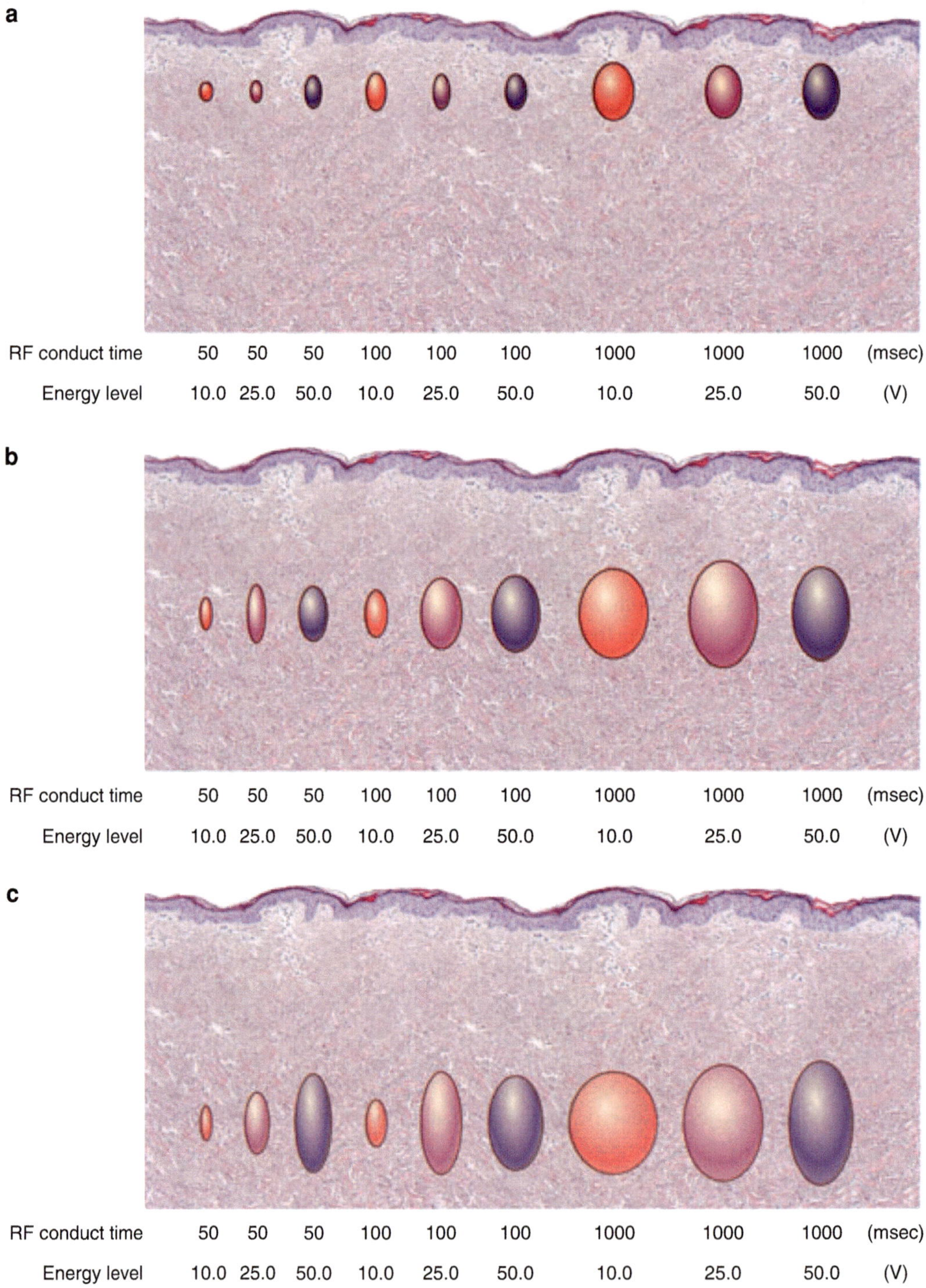

Fig. 13.5 Illustration of biopsy results of needle RF by various parameters. (**a**) Penetration depth 1.5 mm, (**b**), penetration depth 2.5 mm, (**c**), penetration depth 3.5 mm. Reproduced from [5]

Table 13.5 Parameters and meanings of needle RF

Parameters in needle RF	Meanings
Microneedle depth	Location and height & volume of coagulated column
Conduction time	Height & width & volume of coagulated column
Energy level	Intensity of thermal injury

needle penetration depth and pulse duration (RF conduction time) were proportional to the coagulation volume, but the energy level was not related to the coagulation volume. Fourth, energy levels were associated with an intensity of thermal injury rather than the coagulation volume. Fifth, the skin appendages and adipose tissues such as blood vessels, sweat glands, sebaceous glands, and hair follicles were unchanged. However, the coagulation of periadnexal collagen and interstitial collagen has been observed.

Based on the results of Zheng et al., the meaning of parameters in needle RF can be summarized as shown in Table 13.5. Therefore, in order to raise and widen the coagulation column in the dermis, the penetration depth of the needle must be deepened, and the pulse duration must be increased. On the other hand, to induce high tissue denaturation, you need to increase the energy level. In the parameter of needle RF the something to consider is the fact that widening the coagulation column is not unconditionally good, and severe tissue degeneration does not guarantee good results. In addition, taking into account the parameters of fractional photothermolysis, the penetration depth of the needle should be adjusted according to the treatment goals (refer to Sect. 12.7 in Chap. 12). When considering the Arrhenius equation, tissue degeneration must be adjusted by taking into account not only the energy level but also the pulse duration (refer to Sect. 7.3 in Chap. 7).

13.6 Parameters

The parameters of needle RF can be quite complicated because in addition to the energy and pulse duration, the needle depth (penetration depth) varies from site to site, but the principle is not that difficult (Table 13.6).

First of all, if you look at the needle depth, you have to vary the needle depth because the skin thickness is different for each part of the face [6]. And in the thinner the skin (including fat tissue), the energy should be lowered because the current passes through the thin skin, so the current density increases. For example, since the skin around the forehead and eyes is the thinnest, the needle depth should also be lowered, and the energy should also be lowered. On the other hand, because the cheek has no support, so the skin is pushed to the needle, thus the needle depth should be deeper. And the needle depth should be different depending on the treatment goal [7]. For skin tightening, acne, and melasma the needle depth should be shallow, while for pores, scars, and wrinkles the needle depth should be deeper. So, I divide the dermis into papillary dermis and reticular dermis and treat them separately. Because first, aging in the dermis layer occurs first in the papillary dermis and later in the reticular dermis. Second, pigments, face tone, skin texture, etc. are problems of shallow skin, and wrinkles and acne scars are problems of deep skin. Therefore, I first treat the entire face with a needle depth of 0.8 mm with the goal of papillary dermis, and only the parts with deep wrinkles, pores, acne scars, etc. are treated with a deeper needle depth with the goal of reticular dermis. An additional reason for this 2-pass procedure is to reduce the patient's pain.

Lengthening the pulse duration makes the coagulation column longer and wider, so the pulse duration varies depending on the indication. For example, to induce tissue degeneration over a wide range, such as acne, the pulse duration is lengthened. In this case, according to the Arrhenius equation, the energy must also be lowered (AUTO3). Conversely, wrinkles and scars must reduce the pulse duration to induce a narrow range of tissue degeneration, and the energy must also be increased according to the Arrhenius equation (AUTO1).

The parameters need to be adjusted according to the patient. In patients with erythema, the energy should be lowered because of the

Table 13.6 Parameters of needle RF. 25 pin (Secret[RF], ILOODA, Suwon, Korea)

	AUTO1 (skin rejuvenation)			AUTO3 (Active acne, erythema)		
Procedure site	Intensity (%)	RF (ms)	Depth (mm)	Intensity (%)	RF (ms)	Depth (mm)
Forehead	40–50	50–70	0.5–0.8	40–50	50–70	0.5–0.8
Periorbital	40–50	50–70	1.0–1.2	40–50	50–70	1.0–1.2
Cheek	50–60	50–70	1.2–1.5	20–30	150–200	1.5–2.0
Nose	50–60	50–70	1.2–1.5	20–30	150–200	1.2–1.5
Chin	40–50	50–70	1.2–1.5	20–30	150–200	1.2–1.5
Nasolabial fold	50–60	50–70	1.2–2.0	20–30	150–200	1.5–2.5
Neck	40–60	50–70	1.5			
Melasma	20	50	0.8			

increased conductivity caused by the blood, and in patients with thin skin, the needle depth and energy should be lowered. If the patient complains of pain, think of it as a warning end point to lower their energy or lower the needle depth.

Treatment density should be increased for quick effects in the case of papillary dermis. However, in the case of needle RF, the treatment density cannot be adjusted on the machine itself because the needle spacing is fixed. Therefore, treatment density must be adjusted through overlap of stamp. There are two ways to overlap: First, the treatment density can be adjusted by staking or adjusting the overlap when performing the procedure after one shot. Second, the number of passes can be increased (e.g., 2 pass refers to irradiating the entire face, returning to the area where it was first irradiated, and then irradiating the entire face again). However, the method of increasing the pass count is problematic in needle RF procedures. Needle RF causes heat in the dermis, and over time, the blood vessels dilate to cause erythema, at which point when needle RF is irradiated, conductivity increases due to blood vessels, which can cause a sharp rise in temperature. Therefore, I control the treatment density by stacking or adjusting the overlap rather than the method of increasing the number of passes, and only perform 1 pass. When reticular dermis is subsequently treated after treatment with papillary dermis, the procedure should be performed with lower energy than when treating reticular dermis alone because there is already erythema.

The needle RF procedure is painful, so an anesthetic cream is applied, and the occlusion with a plastic wrap is carried out for a long time. I prefer more than 40 min of occlusion with a plastic wrap. I educate my patients to use clobetasol propionate ointment (0.05%), a group 1 steroid to reduce erythema and swelling after the procedure and to prevent acneiform eruption, etc. for 3 times a day for a total of 6 times in 2 days. The interval of the procedure should be spaced out for at least 8–12 weeks, in principle, taking into account the skin regeneration of the dermis, but it is carried out at intervals of 3–4 weeks, since it does not involve strong energy such as CO_2 fractional laser, and the treatment is fractional such as fractional photothermolysis. For quick effect, such as acne, the procedure can be performed every 2 weeks. However, if the erythema is severe, such as rosacea, the erythema will get worse after the needle RF procedure, and because it can last longer, the procedure should be postponed until erythema subsides. Often there are patients with persistent erythema after the procedure. Since there is no way to treat erythema quickly, I explain to all patients before the procedure the possibility that erythema can last a long time and reassure them not to worry because although it lasts longer, it can be sufficiently covered with makeup, and will eventually subside.

References

1. Massarweh NN, Cosgriff N, Slakey DP. Electrosurgery: history, principles, and current and future uses. J Am Coll Surg. 2006;202(3):520–30.
2. Park SH, Yeo WC, Koh WS, Park JW, Noh NK, Yoon CS. Laser Dermatology plastic surgery 2nd ed (Korean). Seoul: Koonja; 2014.
3. Lapidoth M. Radiofrequency in cosmetic dermatology. [S.I.]: Karger; 2014.
4. Issa MCA, Tamura B. Lasers, lights and other technologies. Springer; 2018.
5. Zheng Z, Goo B, Kim DY, Kang JS, Cho SB. Histometric analysis of skin-radiofrequency interaction using a fractionated microneedle delivery system. Dermatol Surg. 2014;40(2):134–41.
6. Alster TS, Graham PM. Microneedling: a review and practical guide. Dermatol Surg. 2018;44(3):397–404.
7. Goldman MP. Lasers and energy devices for the skin. [S.I.]: Taylor & Francis; 2013.

14 Light-Emitting Diode (LED) and Arndt–Schultz Curve

14.1 Overview of LEDs

LEDs have a small semiconductor chip in the center that generates light when current flows [1] (Table 14.1). Thus, LEDs are light, not lasers. There are several advantages of LEDs. First, very little current is needed to produce light. Second, since LEDs are solid semiconductors, there is no need for flash lamps such as filaments or fluorescent lamps, i.e., there is no need for consumables. This is why signs and indoor lamps are changed to LEDs these days. Third, due to quasimonochromaticity (light with a wavelength range of several nanometers) LEDs have target specificity, like a laser. Fourth, hands-free operation is possible because the LEDs can be closely arranged in a large area so that the entire face can be irradiated at once. Fifth, the biggest advantage is the low price. Another advantage is that there are no pain and side effects, and it can be used at any age from infants to the elderly, which is not necessarily an advantage of LEDs, but the advantage of low level light therapy (LLLT, photomodulation).

Table 14.1 Specifications of LEDs (HEALITE II, Lutronic Co. Ltd. Goyang, Korea)

Light source	LEDs (Light Emitting Diodes)		
HEALITE II			
Wavelengths (nm)	800(w/590)	633	415
Intensity (mW/cm^2)—Planar	40–100	30–65	10–30
Intensity (mW/cm^2)—Focused	60–150	45–105	15–30
HEALITE II Combo			
Wavelengths (nm)	830(w/590) + 633	633 + 415	415 + 830 (w/590)
Intensity (mW/cm^2)—Planar	830(w/590): 35–80 633: 20–50	633: 20–50 415: 10–30	415: 10–30 830(w/590): 35–80
Intensity (mW/cm^2)—Focused	830(w/590): 60–150 633: 35–80	633: 35–80 415: 15–50	415: 15–50 830(w/590): 60–150

J. D. Lee, M. J. M. Oh, *Lasers in Dermatology: Parameters and Choice*,
https://doi.org/10.1007/978-981-19-7568-4_14

14.2 Karu's Photo-Biomodulation Band

Photomodulation, one of the photochemical effects must also determine the three parameters of the laser (wavelength, pulse duration, fluence). Wavelength is the most important parameter in photomodulation because without absorption no reaction is possible [2]. Then what wavelength is the most effective wavelength for photomodulation for skin rejuvenation?

Tiina Karu, a well-known Russian photobiologist, stated that photo-biomodulation band suitable for photomodulation is from visible red (around 620 nm) to near infrared (around 1000 nm) [1].

The better the wavelength is absorbed, the shallower the depth of penetration. Conversely, the poorer the absorption, the deeper the penetration depth. In the Fig. 14.1, the y-axis is the optical density (OD), indicating the absorption of the entire skin according to the wavelength regardless of the chromophore. The lower the absorption rate, the deeper the depth of penetration, so as it goes downward on the z-axis, the penetration depth deepens. The green and yellow wavelengths (500–600 nm wavelengths) absorb blood and melanin, making them difficult to penetrate in living tissue. Therefore, green and yellow wavelengths are not suitable for deep penetration. Photomodulation for skin rejuvenation requires a wavelength that can penetrate into the dermis for wound healing and rejuvenation. In Fig. 14.1, we can see that wavelength from 620 nm to 1000 nm is a suitable photo-biomodulation band.

While 633 nm is a slightly longer wavelength than 590 nm by 43 nm, the optical density decreases by 3 OD, from 8 OD to 5 OD. Even though only 3 OD has decreased, the y-axis is reduced by 1000 times because it is expressed in logarithmic units. Also, 830 nm is 5 OD difference than 590 nm, and can penetrate the deepest. LEDs used for skin rejuvenation mainly use 630 nm and 830 nm wavelengths, which is under Karu's photo-biomodulation band [1].

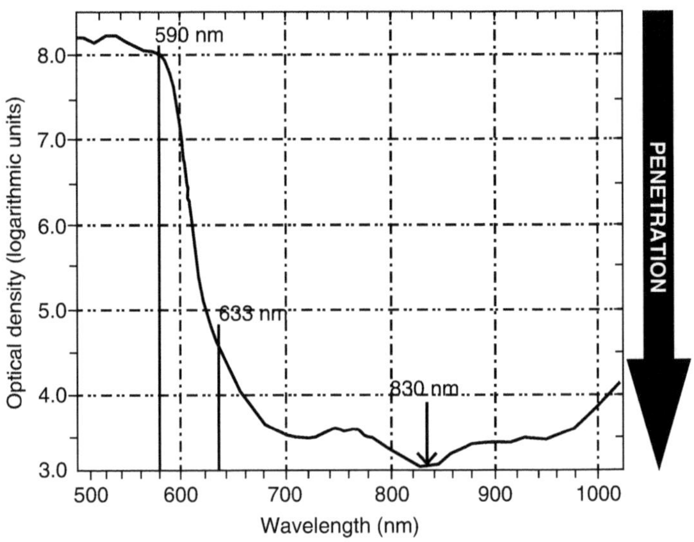

Fig. 14.1 Penetration of broad waveband light through a human hand in vivo. Reproduced from [1]

14.3 Indications

The indications for the LED are as follows [3]. First, blue and red light are used for phototherapy and photodynamic therapy (PDT) to treat acne, second, 620 nm to 1000 nm for LLLT (photomodulation) purposes for wound healing and rejuvenation, and third, there are also 590 nm LEDs (Gentlewave LED, Light BioScience) that have recently been developed for rejuvenation of the epidermis and papillary dermis using yellow light.

14.4 Arndt–Schultz Curve

We will first discuss the Arndt–Schultz law, which is considered as the basic principle of photomodulation. The Arndt–Schultz law is the theory that all drugs and toxic substances stimulate vital activity at low doses but inhibit and destroy vital activity at moderate doses. Substances that cause irritation below harmful levels include antibiotics, snake venom, heat, radiation, and magnetic fields. Figure 14.2 makes this easier to understand. There is no change in cells from A to B, but when more than a certain amount of stimulation is applied, cellular activity increases (B-C). Then cell activity plateaus (C-D) and falls (D-E), and finally cell activity falls below normal level and cause cell damage (E-F) and cell death (F-G). The interval corresponding to LLLT (photomodulation) is the interval from B-E [1].

In other words, photomodulation is a therapeutic method that stimulate cells using photons to increase cell activity rather than causing cell damage or cell death.

Photomodulation is thought to have three effects at the cellular level [1]. First, if photoactivated cells are damaged and inhibited, photomodulation treats these cells. Second, photomodulation makes the cell activity better and faster. For example, it promotes collagen

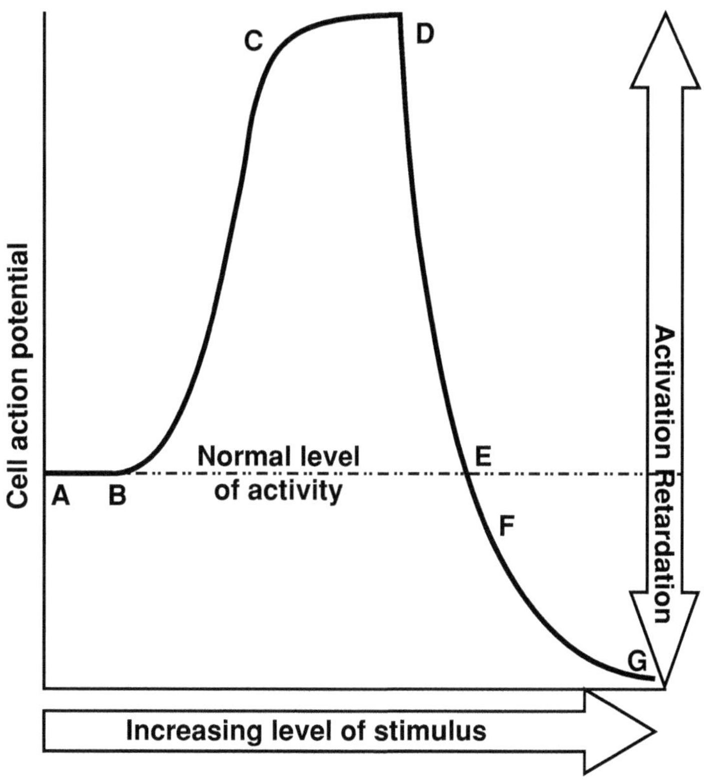

Fig. 14.2 Arndt–Schultz curve by Oshiro and Calderhead. Reproduced from [1]

synthesis of fibroblasts. Third, if there are not enough cells, photomodulation recruits the cells elsewhere and promotes existing cells to proliferate.

14.5 Mechanism of Low-Level Light Therapy (LLLT) by LED

The mechanism of photomodulation can be divided into (a) visible light including 630 nm, under Karu's photo-biomodulation band and (b) near-infrared including 830 nm (Fig. 14.3). Visible light targets the cytochrome C oxidase (CCO) of the mitochondria, and near-infrared light targets the cell membrane. Cytochrome C oxidase or complex IV (CCO) is an end-terminal enzyme of the mitochondria and is involved in the synthesis of adenosine triphosphate (ATP). ATP is used as a fuel for cells and whole organisms [2].

First, visible light is absorbed by the CCO to produce ATP by photochemical cascade and to promote cell wall transport mechanisms such as sodium-potassium pump (Na1/K1-ATPase). Then intracellular/extracellular exchanges between cells and extracellular matrixes increase calcium ions (Ca^{++}) and hydrogen ions (H^{+}), both potent cell-cell signaling compounds. Eventually, the DNA and RNA of the nucleus are made, leading to cell proliferation.

Second, near-infrared rays are absorbed by the cell walls and change the electronic state of the cell wall molecules through photo-physical responses such as rotational and vibrational exchange. It then promotes cell transport mechanisms, allowing calcium ions (Ca^{++}) to increase hydrogen ions (H^{+}) and produce more ATP in the mitochondria. Near-infrared light, unlike visible light, causes an indirect photo-physical response rather than a photochemical cascade. Eventually it induces photomodulation such as cell proliferation.

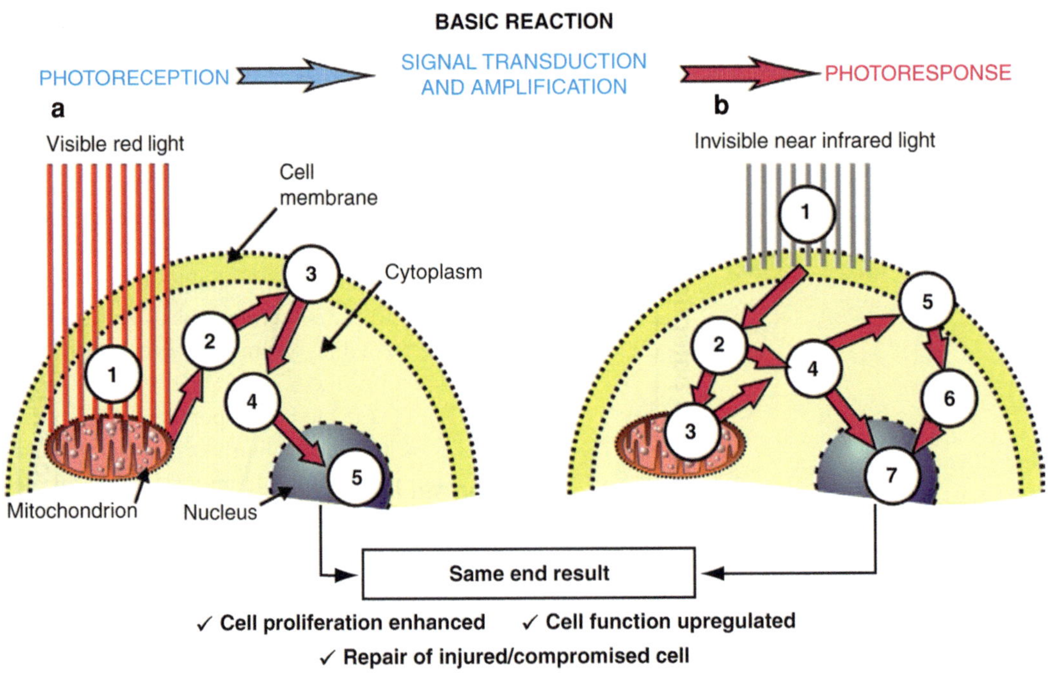

Fig. 14.3 Mechanism of photomodulation. Photomodulations in the case of (**a**) visible red light and (**b**) near infrared light. Reproduced from [4]

14.6 Consensus on LED Effect

Despite these studies, we rarely find clinically noticeable effects of LED. Does LED really work?

In the past, many doubted photomodulation (LLLT) including LED. There were many doubts regarding its clinical efficacy because most studies on photomodulation used cell culture models, and only a few were clinical studies [5]. But recently, there are many clinical studies regarding photomodulation of LED. However, there is no consensus by objective research.

Jagdeo et al. analyzed the effects of LEDs in 31 randomized controlled trials (RCTs) [6]: acne vulgaris (8 trials), herpes simplex and zoster (HSV, HZV) (3 trials), skin rejuvenation (6 trials), acute wound healing (5 trials), psoriasis (3 trials), atopic dermatitis (1 trial), chronic wound healing (2 trials), oral mucositis (1 trial), radiation dermatitis (1 trial), and thigh cellulite reduction (1 trial). Grades of recommendation were assigned based on the Oxford Centre for Evidence-based Medicine-Levels of Evidence. Recommended grades are A, B, C, and D, with A being the highest. The results showed that acne vulgaris, herpes simplex and zoster, and acute wound healing were grade B, and the rest were C or D.

This paper analyzed only the RCTs, which is an objective research method, but the number of papers is too small to make a clear conclusion about the effect of all LEDs. However, we can say LEDs are relatively effective against acne vulgaris, herpes simplex and zoster, and acute wound healing compared to other diseases. But our main interest—skin rejuvenation and thigh cellulite reduction—are grade C and D, respectively, i.e., we cannot yet say that LED is effective for these indications.

For skin rejuvenation, daily use of near infrared LED and red light LED for 8–10 weeks was most effective in improving wrinkles. The parameters vary from paper to paper, making it difficult to present a protocol. There are several papers that state that yellow light LEDs are effective for skin rejuvenation, but no RCTs were found.

Jagdeo et al. recommended LED use despite the fact that there are only three diseases with Recommendation Grade B, because LEDs have few side effects, are affordable and more and more encouraging clinical results are continuously coming out.

14.7 Personal Comments on Photomodulation

Many recent studies on photomodulation have revealed many facts regarding photomodulation effects and its mechanism. However, the exact mechanism is still unknown, and there are many debates about parameters such as energy, distance, and treatment intervals. The main problem is its efficacy. In my personal experience, I have not seen any photomodulation effect through monotherapy with LEDs, and thus use it as an adjuvant therapy. As with the paper mentioned above [6], I believe that LED is effective for acne, herpes simplex and herpes zoster and acute wound healing. Therefore, I use LED for acute wound healing after ablative procedure such as CO_2 fractional laser or severe erythema after laser treatment, and for PDT treatment for acne.

14.8 Parameters

Jagdeo et al. proposed a protocol for each disease based on the analysis results [6].

First, acne. Blue and red light LEDs are recommended for 20 min with the energy of 6–40 mW/cm^2 and 8–100 mW/cm^2, respectively. Treatment period should be 4–8 weeks twice a week.

Second, herpes simplex and herpes zoster. Near infrared LEDs are recommended. Recovery time can be reduced by at least 2 days when LED is used. In addition to oral antiviral drugs, three time a day for 3 days at-home LED is recommended. The parameter should be 33 J/cm^2 for 10 min at 55 mW/cm^2 at 830 nm.

Third, acute wounds. Treatment with yellow light (590 nm) or near infrared LEDs every day until the wound is healed can reduce the duration and erythema of the acute wound, regardless of the cause. Yellow light LEDs are recommended 5 mW/cm^2 for 1–2 min and near-infrared LEDs 5–40 J/cm^2 for 20 min at 50 mW/cm^2 [6].

References

1. Calderhead RG, Vasily DB. Low level light therapy with light-emitting diodes for the aging face. Clin Plast Surg. 2016;43(3):541–50.
2. Calderhead RG. The photobiological basics behind light-emitting diode (LED) phototherapy. Laser Therapy. 2007;16(2):97–108.
3. Opel DR, Hagstrom E, Pace AK, Sisto K, Hirano-Ali SA, Desai S, et al. Light-emitting diodes: a brief review and clinical experience. J Clin Aesthet Dermatol. 2015;8(6):36–44.
4. Nouri K. Lasers in dermatology and medicine: dermatologic applications. Springer International Publishing; 2018.
5. Goldman MP. Cutaneous and cosmetic laser surgery. Philadelphia: Mosby Elsevier; 2006.
6. Jagdeo J, Austin E, Mamalis A, Wong C, Ho D, Siegel DM. Light-emitting diodes in dermatology: a systematic review of randomized controlled trials. Lasers Surg Med. 2018;

15 Skin Care Equipment and Calcium Gradient

15.1 Overview of Skin Care Equipment

Skin care equipment usually refers to equipment that has a skin scrubber and an apparatus capable of performing ultrasound, iontophoresis all in one machine (Table 15.1). Skin care equipment is able to perform very superficial peeling (scaling) using a skin scrubber, and sonophoresis and iontophoresis can be used to penetrate the skin (drug delivery). It is a device used by aestheticians for skin care, which can be mistaken for being insignificant or ineffective because it is not used by doctors, but it is an indispensable piece of equipment for skin care.

Recently, skin care equipment with various features has been launched. There are devices that can cool the skin for soothing after a laser or other procedure, or, conversely, increase the skin temperature to help with blood circulation, and there is also equipment that can perform Ionzyme procedures (Table 15.2). There is also equipment capable of electrophoresis.

Table 15.1 Specifications of skin care equipment (Venus-S, Beautech, Seoul, Korea)

Frequency	1 MHz, 28 kHz
Applicator type	Scrubber/Ultrasound/Iontophoresis

Table 15.2 Specifications of skin care equipment with various features added (CryoDerm, Beautech, Seoul, Korea)

Current type	Galvanic
Cryo	−15 °C ~ +45 °C
Application type	Cryo & Hot handpiece/iontophoresis, Ionzyme

15.2 Functions of Skin and Keratinocyte

The skin has a variety of functions: permeability barrier, protection from pathogens, thermoregulation, sensation, ultraviolet protection, wound repair/regeneration, physical appearance [1]. However, I think there are two main functions of skin. First, the most important function of the skin is the "skin barrier function" that protects the

J. D. Lee, M. J. M. Oh, *Lasers in Dermatology: Parameters and Choice*,
https://doi.org/10.1007/978-981-19-7568-4_15

human body by forming a barrier between the external environment and our body. In other words, it has the function of preventing the leakage of moisture from the outside of our body, preventing the invasion of external pathogens, having the sensory function of detecting and avoiding external stimuli, protecting against ultraviolet rays, recovering quickly when a wound occurs, and eventually protecting our body. Second, it has thermoregulation. Since thermoregulation is not of great concern from the standpoint of laser surgery, I will omit the explanation in this book.

In terms of the skin barrier function, the most important layer of skin is stratum corneum, and the most important cell is keratinocyte, which makes stratum corneum. Keratinocyte finally creates stratum corneum through keratinization. While the human body sustains life, some of the keratinocytes have cells that divide throughout their lives to divide new keratinocytes. These are called stem cells. When stem cells divide, one cell continues to be a stem cell (10%, stem cell), and the other cell is converted into a transient amplifying cell that divides several times over a period of time in the basal layer to supply new cells (50%, amplifying cell). Some of the cells exit the dividing cycle and enter the differentiation process by leaving the basal layer (40%, postmitotic cell) [2]. The keratinocyte that leaves the basal layer changes shape through a differentiation process and moves to the skin surface. Upon reaching the stratum corneum, keratinocyte turns into a nucleus-free corneocyte and then desquamates out of the skin. Thus, keratinocyte functions to protect the skin by constantly differentiating to create new corneocyte, eliminating corneocyte to which external pathogens, stimulants, and antigens are attached.

According to the morphological change of keratinocyte by differentiation, the epidermis is divided into four layers. The basal layer has only one layer and is composed of the only cells that can undergo cell division, and stem cells are also present here. Stratum spinosum consists of 4–8 cell layers and develops an organelle called lamellar granule. The stratum granulosum consists of 1–3 cell layers, while stratum corneum consists of the largest number of layers with 15 layers [2]. The reason why stratum corneum is the thickest of the epidermis layers, at 15 layers, also suggests that stratum corneum plays the most important role as a skin barrier function.

15.3 Calcium Gradient

What factors are involved in regulating the proliferation and differentiation of keratinocyte? Many factors exist, but calcium ions are known to be the most important factor for the proliferation and differentiation of keratinocyte. It was found that when keratinocyte is cultivated, cells proliferate at low concentrations of calcium ions of 0.1 μM or less, but when calcium ions change to high concentrations, cell proliferation is inhibited, and cell differentiation is promoted. The concentration of calcium ions in the lower part of the actual basal layer and stratum spinosum is low, and the concentration of calcium ions increases as the upper layer progresses, resulting in the highest concentration in the upper stratum granulosum (Fig. 15.1). There is also a lamellar body inside the keratinocyte of stratum spinosum

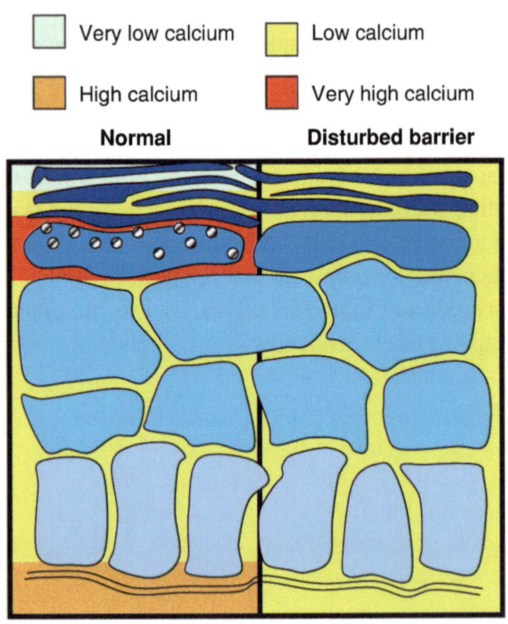

Fig. 15.1 Calcium gradient of the epidermis, the left side is in a normal state, the right side is in a state of impaired barrier function. Reproduced from [3]

and stratum granulosum, which moves to the top of the stratum granulosum cell and attaches itself to the cell membrane and secretes its contents between the cells as exocytosis, creating an extracellular lipid. It is known that the increase in the concentration of calcium ions plays an important role in this process [2].

As such, the difference in concentration of calcium ions in the upper and lower parts of the epidermis is called a calcium gradient. When the epidermis is damaged, the calcium gradient is destroyed, and the skin creates a new epidermis through keratinocyte proliferation, promoting epidermal lipid synthesis, increasing lamellar body secretion, and promoting cytokine synthesis and secretion to restore skin barrier function. A procedure using this principle is iontophoresis. The implementation of iontophoresis on an intact skin artificially destroys the calcium gradient, which has the effect of further strengthening the skin barrier function [4]. In addition, sonophoresis of 1.5–3 MHz also causes changes in calcium gradient, affecting the production of hyaluronic acid and CD44 in the epithelium, affecting epidermal differentiation and lipid synthesis.

15.4 Iontophoresis

Iontophoresis uses galvanic current as a method of penetrating ionized drugs into the skin (ion + introduction). Galvanic current means a very low voltage of direct current. Iontophoresis requires that the molecular weight of the drug to penetrate be small, and because it uses a direct current the drug to penetrate must be ionized. However, nonionized materials can also be transported into the skin under the influence of the movement of water or the movement of other ionized substances (electroosmosis, iontohydrokinesis) [4]. And iontophoresis can reverse epidermal calcium gradient without skin barrier damage, as previously discussed. That is, it is possible to strengthen the skin barrier function without damaging the skin barrier. Representative equipment includes Vitaliont and Ionzyme [2].

The advantages of iontophoresis are that it has an immediate effect, and because only the local area maintains a high concentration of the drug, there are no dangerous side effects compared to other treatment methods, there is no pain such as injection, the drug is easy to control, and the drug can be administered to areas where there are no blood vessels. Iontophoresis is contraindicated in patients using pacemakers, in patients with arrhythmias, and in pregnant women. As a side effect, there is the discomfort of the stinging skin. If lowering the current eliminates this discomfort, the drug penetration effect is reduced, so the physician must use an electric current that patient can tolerate. In addition, an allergic reaction or rash to the drug may occur. And the electrode should be in good contact because blisters or burns may occur due to poor contact of the electrode.

15.5 Vitamin C

A representative drug that penetrates into iontophoresis is vitamin C. The effect of vitamin C is, first, it inhibits melanin synthesis by interfering with tyrosinase. Second, it promotes collagen synthesis and can improve post-inflammatory hyperpigmentation of acne and wrinkles by increasing skin elasticity. Third, it also has antioxidant properties [4]. However, vitamin C has a short duration, so it needs to be repeated. Because ascorbic acid is unstable and oxidizes rapidly in the solution state, stable vitamin C derivatives should be used. Vitamin C can be divided into glucoside type and phosphate type with phosphate group. Among them, the phosphate type is a stable hydrophilic vitamin C derivative. Therefore, when performing iontophoresis, phosphate-type vitamin C derivatives should be used. A representative phosphate-type vitamin C derivative is magnesium L-ascorbyl-2-phosphate (MAP). 4% MAP is used because MAP over 5% is known to have bottleneck effects resulting in reduced effectiveness. The MAP has a low solubility, so it must be mixed into distilled water and wait about 10 min, and a current of 0.3–0.5 mA must be used. The iontophoresis procedure of more than 20 min in 1 procedure is known to be less effective due to the increased fatigue of the gate, so the procedure is performed for 20 min or less. The duration lasts about 72 hours, so the procedure should be performed once every 3–4 days to maintain the effect [4].

15.6 Sonophoresis

Ultrasound refers to sound waves above about 20,000 Hz, a frequency that cannot be detected by the human ear [2]. Ultrasound therapy uses sound waves of 0.5–5 MHz, mainly around 1 MHz. The effect of ultrasound therapy can be broadly divided into thermal effect and non-thermal effect. The thermal effect is caused by the ultrasonic energy being absorbed into the tissue and the temperature of the tissue rising. The thermal effect causes increased blood flow, inducing an inflammatory response, increasing biomembrane permeability, increasing metabolism, increasing collagen tension (during HIFU procedures), increasing pain thresholds, relieving muscle spasticity, changing the rate of nerve conduction, increasing enzyme activity, and changing the contractility of skeletal muscle. The non-thermal effect causes microscopic massage action, which improves the permeability of the cell membrane, enhances protein synthesis, promotes wound healing, makes cavitation, promotes microcirculation, and destroys tissue. In particular, due to cavitation formation, the substance is moved through the skin (transdermal drug delivery).

The effect of the ultrasound therapy machine is mainly the cleaning and peeling effect (skin scrubber), the sonophoresis effect, and the skin barrier strengthening effect. First, purified water can be applied on the skin using a skin cotton pad, and then the cleaning and peeling effect can be achieved using the skin scrubber of the skin care equipment (Fig. 15.2). Second, the sonophoresis effect is a method of transporting drugs into the body through the skin by the vibration of ultrasound. The thermal effect increases the fluidity of the extracellular lipid of stratum corneum and the gap between cells is extended by cavitation formation, forming a temporary pathway to stratum corneum. Third, it is known that skin barrier recovery reactions such as the loss of calcium gradient, the secretion of lamellar body, and the secretion of cytokines occur as ultrasound without the destruction of the barrier and the loss of percutaneous moisture.

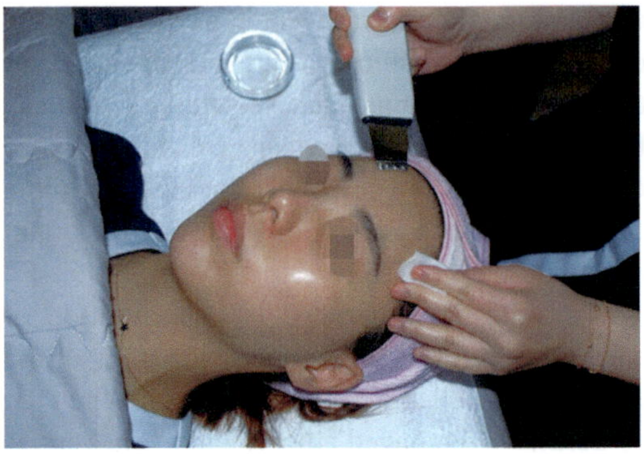

Fig. 15.2 Skin scrub procedure

15.7 Treatment Method

First, the skin must be thoroughly cleaned before iontophoresis is performed. Since iontophoresis uses a direct current, there is an earth handle with a (+) pole and an active electrode with a (−) pole. There are various types of active electrodes depending on their shape, such as a chupa chups-shaped spherical active electrode and a probe-shaped active electrode such as a wire. The procedure involves first moistening the appropriate amount of water in a gauze and wrapping the grounding rod so that the patient can comfortably hold it in their hand. The treatment solution with viscosity is applied evenly to the skin to be treated, and an electric current is flowed and then rubbed evenly into the skin with a spherical active electrode. In the low-viscosity solution, a square cotton pad is inserted into the electrode in the form of a probe so that the solution penetrates the cotton well, and then the active electrode is rubbed evenly into the skin. The intensity of the current starts at a low intensity at first and is gradually increased. It is fixed at the maximum current intensity where the patient does not experience any discomfort. The duration of the procedure is usually 5–10 min.

Sonophoresis usually penetrates the drug using a handpiece with a wide, round ground. If the treatment solution has viscosity, the appropriate amount is evenly spread on the skin to be treated, and the handpiece is attached to the skin, rubbing the entire skin evenly at a speed that is not too hot. If the therapeutic solution has a low viscosity, it is mixed with a transparent ultrasound gel. Sonophoresis can have a peeling effect with scrubber probe. First, cotton that is soaked in clean purified water is applied on the skin. When the end line of the scrubber probe touches the skin and rubs it as if sliding the skin, vibration peels off the aging keratin.

References

1. Goldsmith LA, Katz SI, Gilchrest BA, Paller AS, Leffell DJ, Wolff K, et al. Fitzpatrick's dermatology in general medicine. New York: McGraw-Hill Professional; 2012.
2. Textbook compilation committee in Korean Dermatological Association. Text book of dermatology 6th edition (Korean). Seoul: Daehanuihak; 2014.
3. Proksch E, Brandner JM, Jensen JM. The skin: an indispensable barrier. Exp Dermatol. 2008;17(12):1063–72.
4. Jeong JY. Clinical skin care (Korean). Seoul: MDworld; 2010.

Part V

Treatment of Acne, Scar and Melasma

16 1450 nm Diode Laser and Consensus of Acne Treatment

16.1 Overview and Indications of 1450 nm Diode Lasers

The 1450 nm diode laser is a mid-infrared laser that can be used for nonablative rejuvenation. However, because it is more effective against acne than other mid-infrared lasers, it is more commonly used in the treatment of acne than for nonablative rejuvenation purposes (Table 16.1). Nonablative rejuvenation targets pores, scars, wrinkles, and skin tightening. Because the 1450 nm diode laser has a shallow optical penetration depth compared to other mid-infrared lasers, it is less effective for scarring and wrinkles, and is primarily used for skin texture, pores, and tightening. Other indications are treatment of sebaceous hyperplasia [1] and xanthelasma palpebrarum [2].

The Neobeam laser (Union Medical Co. Ltd. Uijeongbu, Korea) is equipped with a dynamic cooling device (DCD) that can perform epidermal cooling with cryogen spray (A mode). Also, DCD can be turned off for irradiating several passes (T mode), such as the genesis technique. Neobeam lasers have the advantage of being able to use spot sizes up to 10 mm with high outputs, allowing for faster procedures in "T mode" and deeper penetration depth (Fig. 16.1).

The pulse duration can be adjusted from 10 to 200 ms, which can irradiate multiple pulses in a shot, just like the macropulse of a pulsed-dye laser (PDL). DCDs can also be irradiated between pulses. For example, if the pulse duration is set to 125 ms, and 2 pulses are irradiated, and the DCD is set to 20 ms, it is irradiated in the order of 20 ms (DCD), 125 ms (pulse), 20 ms (DCD), 125 ms (pulse), and 20 ms (DCD), so that the total time of one shot is 310 ms.

Table 16.1 Specifications of a 1450 nm diode laser (Neobeam, UnionMedical Co. Ltd. Uijeongbu, Korea)

Laser type	1450 nm diode laser
Spot sizes	6, 8, 10 mm
Mode	A (with cryo), T (toning)
Max. power	25 W
Fluence	Max. 79.6 J/cm^2
Repetition rate	1–10 Hz (step: 1 Hz)
Pulse duration	10–200 ms (step: 1 ms)
Cooling	DCD (dynamic cooling device)

J. D. Lee, M. J. M. Oh, *Lasers in Dermatology: Parameters and Choice*,
https://doi.org/10.1007/978-981-19-7568-4_16

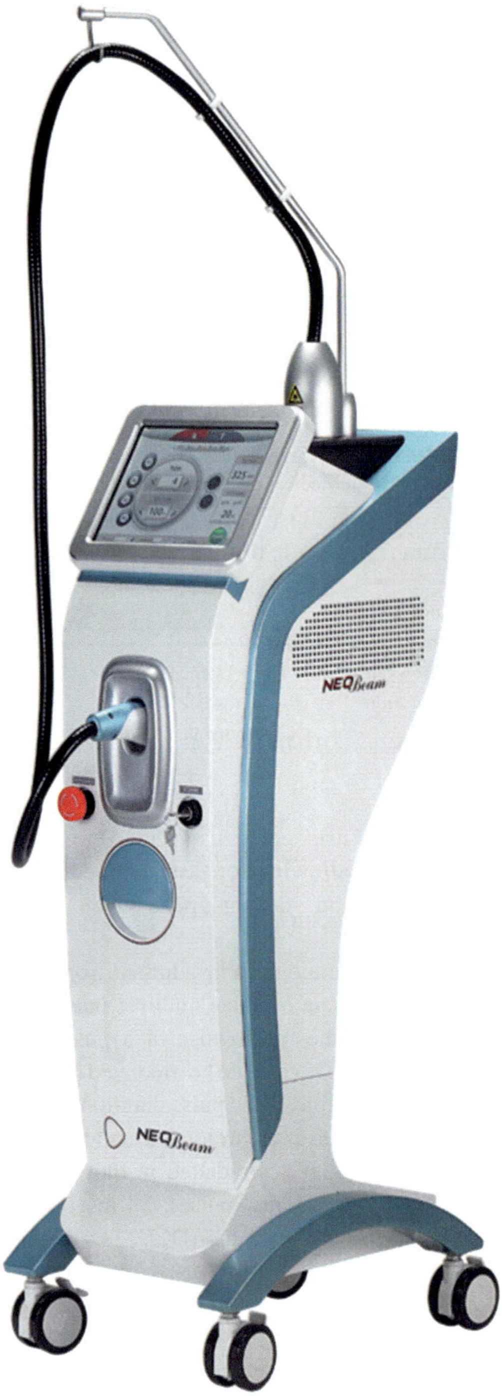

Fig. 16.1 Neobeam laser (UnionMedical Co. Ltd. Uijeongbu, Korea) can increase the spot size to 10 mm, allowing for faster procedures and deeper penetration depth

16.2 Selective Photothermolysis to Target Sebaceous Glands

Sakamoto et al. measured the absorption curve of artificial sebum in the laboratory and observed that the wavelength of the absorption peak was relatively consistent with the absorption curve of fat at 1210, 1390, 1414, 1728, 1760, 2306, and 2346 nm (Fig. 16.2) [3]. In Fig. 16.2, the wavelengths with a higher absorption curve than water are only 1726, 2306, and 2346 nm. Of these, 2306 and 2346 nm cannot be used for the treatment of sebaceous glands because the penetration depth is shallow, and it is difficult to reach the sebaceous glands. Therefore, wavelength near 1726 nm is the most useful wavelength for the treatment of sebaceous glands. However, even at a wavelength of 1726 nm, the absorption coefficient is only 1.2 times higher than that of water. Richard R. Anderson, in his paper "Selective Photothermolysis," stated that in order to be worthy of selective photothermolysis, the absorption coefficient of the target and surrounding tissues must be 10 times different and at least twice as different [4]. Therefore, the 1726 nm wavelength is not a wavelength suitable for acne treatment when the absorption coefficient is considered.

The laser eventually turns the light energy into thermal energy, and our purpose is to damage the target tissue while protecting the surrounding tissue. Therefore, the implication that the absorption coefficient of the target tissue and the surrounding tissue should be at least 2 times should be interpreted to mean that the temperature change of the target tissue should be at least 2 times that of the temperature change of the surrounding tissue. However, temperature changes are affected not only by the absorption coefficient, but also by the specific heat and density (formula below [5]). Given that the product of specific heat and density is 4.2 J/Kcm^3 in dermis and 2.12 J/Kcm^3 in fat, and sebaceous glands are 30% lipid, the product of the specific heat and density of sebaceous glands is 3.62 J/Kcm^3 (Table 16.2) [3, 6]. The actual dermis and fat dif-

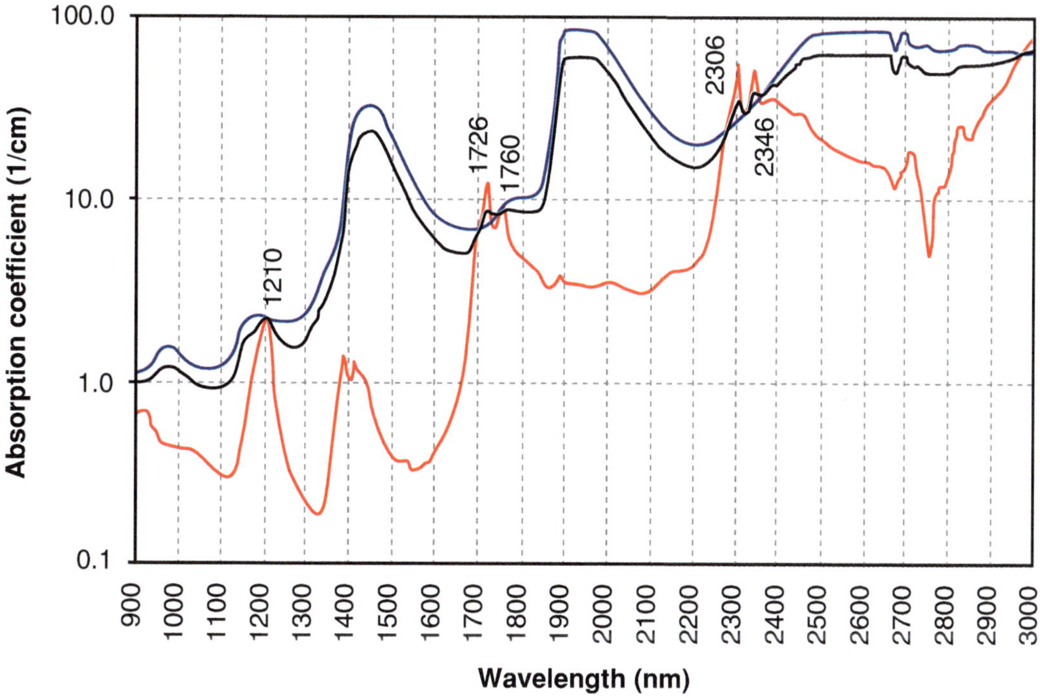

Fig. 16.2 Absorption curve of artificial sebum and water. Reproduced from [3]

Table 16.2 Thermal constants for different biological tissues and materials. Reproduced from [6]

Material	Density ρ (g/cm^3)	Water content (%)	C_w (J/gK)	A (W/mK)
Water	1000	100	4.83	0.58
Blood	900	55	3.22	0.62
Fat	900	–	1.93	0.3
Cartilage	1225	60–70	3.06	0.36
Liver	1220	80	3.42	0.44
Aorta	1000	80	3.76	0.48
Copper	8933	–	0.83	384
Diamond	3510	–	0.502	33,000

fer by 2 times the temperature change, and cryolipolysis using it is effectively used in clinical practice. However, the product of the specific heat and density of the dermis and sebaceous glands does not differ much. In fact, experiments at 1720 nm showed that the temperature change in artificial sebum was only about 1.6 times higher than that of aqueous gel. Therefore, the 1726 nm wavelength is not a suitable wavelength for acne treatment, considering specific heat and density. Nor is a laser with a wavelength of 1726 nm released that we could use it for acne.

On the other hand, a diode laser of 1450 nm is currently available and is known to be effective in acne as well. How is a 1450 nm diode laser effective for acne treatment?

$$\Delta T = \frac{F_z \mu_a}{\rho c}\left(\frac{\tau_r}{\tau_r + \tau_p}\right)^{g/2}$$

ΔT: temperature increase of a desired target
μ_a: absorption coefficient
F_z: local subsurface fluence
ρ: density

c: specific heat

g: geometric factor (1 for planes, 2 for cylinders, and 3 for spheres)

τ_p: laser pulse duration

τ_r: thermal relaxation time of the target (TRT)

16.3 Pulse Duration of 1450 nm Diode Lasers

Next, we'll look at the 1450 nm diode laser. First, let's calculate the pulse duration of a 1450 nm diode laser. Paithnkar et al. reported that because sebaceous glands are at a depth of 200–1000 μm below the stratum corneum, the depth to damage the dermis (where sebaceous glands, including infundibulum, are located) while protecting the epidermis is 400 μm [7]. The penetration depth calculated through the Monte Carlo simulation of a wavelength of 1450 nm was 435 μm, which was consistent.

Let's calculate TRT from the bottom of the stratum corneum to 435 μm, which is our target tissue.

$$\mathrm{TRT} = d^2 / gk$$

d: thickness or diameter of the target, *g*: geometric factor, *k*: thermal diffusivity.

g is a planar because it is the epidermis and the upper part of the dermis under the stratum corneum, ($g = 8$). k has slightly different numbers for each paper. In the paper "extended theory of selective photothermolysis," $k \fallingdotseq 0.1$ mm²/s was seen [8]. *d* is 435 μm, and when calculated by substitution, the TRT is about 236 ms. That is, when selective photothermolysis is applied, the pulse duration can be irradiated to 236 ms or less.

Paithnkar et al. used a laser with a wavelength of 1450 nm (thought to be an early test model for SmoothBeam) with 4 mm spot size, fluence 16 J/cm² and calculated temperature changes over time and depth in in vivo rabbit ear and ex vivo human skin by observing biopsy after irradiation [7]. Based on the above calculations, the total pulse duration was 210 ms, and the total pulse duration was equally divided into four equal parts, and cryogen spray was used between them. Cryogen spray was used in 15 ms before the procedure, 15 ms 3 times between procedures, and 20 ms after the procedure (Fig. 16.3). In addition, 27 patients who developed acne in their backs in a clinical study were treated 4 times every 3 weeks.

Calculations of Monte Carlo simulations and heat transfers showed the highest temperatures at a depth of 150 μm to 88.8 °C, resulting in the highest damage to the upper dermis where the sebaceous gland is located and the epidermis being preserved (Fig. 16.4).

Clinical studies have shown that skin treated with a laser of 1450 nm wavelength has a statistically significant reduction in the number of acne lesions compared to untreated skin ($p < 0.01$). And in 14 of the 15 patients who followed up to 24 weeks, only the skin that irradiated the laser was observed to have no acne lesions. In addition, as a result of the tissue examination of the rabbit ear, damage to the dermis and thermal alteration of sebaceous glands were observed without damage to the epidermis on days 1 and 3 of the procedure. On day 7 of the procedure, the intactness of the sebaceous glands was observed, appearing to have recovered from the initial damage. Therefore, the acne treatment mechanism of the mid-infrared laser is not to completely damage the sebaceous glands with the laser, but to partially damage the sebaceous glands. It is thought that the function of the sebaceous glands,

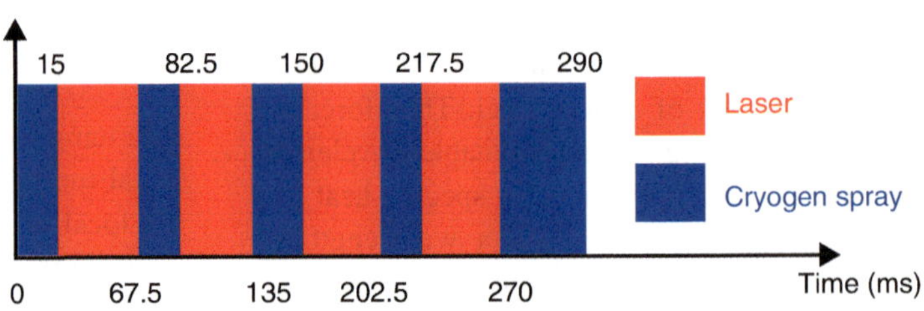

Fig. 16.3 Timing diagram showing alternate cryogen spray and laser pulses used per treatment shot. Reproduced from [7]

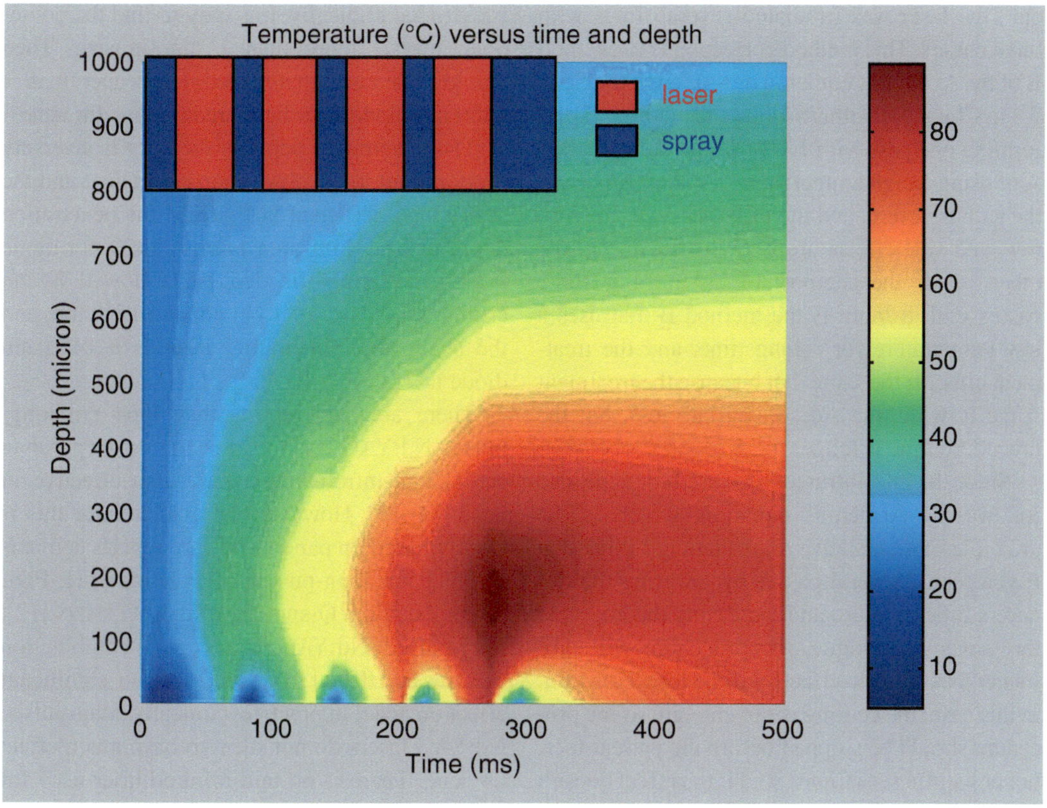

Fig. 16.4 A color plot of calculated temperature versus time and depth. Five cryogen pulses result in epidermal cooling. Thermal heating of the upper dermis is achieved. Reproduced from [7]

which were later recovered, decreased for a considerable period of time, resulting in an improvement in acne.

On the other hand, clinical studies have shown no specific side effects other than erythema and edema. Post-inflammatory hyperpigmentation (PIH) was found in 3 of the 27 patients. One developed severe PIH and the other two developed mild PIH.

16.4 New Parameters

As such, several papers have demonstrated that mid-infrared, especially 1450 nm diode lasers, are effective against acne. However, there are pain during the procedure and side effects (7–39%) that cause PIH to occur frequently in people of color [9], so various parameters have been studied to overcome this.

Yeung et al. applied a 1450 nm diode laser with a new parameter to 26 Chinese patients with facial acne [9]. The spot size is the same as 6 mm, and 3 passes with 8 J/cm^2 were performed so that they did not overlap. Cryogen spray was used briefly for 25 ms to reduce PIH due to cooling. Procedure was performed a total of 4 times at intervals of 3–4 weeks and followed up to 6 months after the final treatment. The result is that after 4 weeks and 6 months of final treatment the average acne lesions are decreased 29% ($p < 0.01$), and 40% ($p < 0.3$), respectively. PIH occurred four times (3.8%) in two patients among the 104 procedures in total. The pain during the procedure was a VAS score of 3.4 to 4.5 out of 10, which was tolerable for most patients.

The authors of this paper consider high fluence of 10 to 14 J/cm^2 to be the cause of pain and PIH when using a 1450 nm diode laser in the past. So instead of lowering the fluence to 8 J/

cm^2, the laser was irradiated several times with three passes. This method corresponds to Method B of the Arrhenius equation described in the Sect. 7.3 in Chap. 7. In other words, the method of performing one pass with 10–14 J/cm^2 is the method A of using a high temperature in a short time, and the pain is severe, and the treatment range is narrow, and side effects are likely to occur. On the other hand, the method of performing three passes with 8 J/cm^2 is the method B that uses a low temperature for a long time, and the treatment effect is the same, but because the treatment range is wide, the side effects are less, but the procedure time is longer.

Since the mid-infrared laser used for acne also follows the Arrhenius equation, which is the principle of nonablative rejuvenation, I think that if you repeat several passes by lowering the fluence a little bit more and increasing the Hz, as in the genesis technique, the procedure will take longer, but the side effects will be less. However, in this case, the cooling is not enough, so the procedure should be stopped before the patient feels hot or painful sensations. And if the effect doesn't seem to be enough, it might be helpful to irradiate the acne lesion with high fluence while cryogen spraying, as with one shot toning of melasma.

16.5 Mechanism of Acne Treatment Using 1450 nm Diode Lasers

The depth of the sebaceous glands is 435 μm below the stratum corneum, and the TRT and pulse duration were determined based on this. However, sebaceous glands in adolescent and young adults are known to be 2 times larger than sebaceous glands in older patients [3], and in acne patients, sebaceous glands are thought to be larger than normal. In addition, if the comedone is extruded clinically, it is easy to find the comedone that is more than 1 mm in size. Then wouldn't a laser that penetrates deeper than a 1450 nm diode laser be more effective for acne?

The penetration depth of the laser is inversely proportional to the absorption coefficient and the scattering coefficient [10]. Thus, the penetration depth of a mid-infrared laser is 1320 nm diode laser penetrating the deepest, followed by an erbium glass laser of 1540 nm and 1550 nm, and the shallowest penetrating laser is a 1450 nm diode laser (Table 16.3).

There are also reports that 1064 nm long-pulsed Nd:YAG lasers that penetrate deeper than actual mid-infrared lasers are also effective in acne [11–13]. However, the evidence for this is mostly based on papers and case reports comparing 532 nm long-pulsed KTP lasers [11], PDL lasers, 1064 nm Q-switched Nd:YAG lasers [12], long-pulsed Nd:YAG lasers with combination therapy and IPL [13] which has no significant effect on acne. In practice, clinically, long-pulsed Nd:YAG lasers do not seem to have much effect on acne. There is no mid-infrared laser used for acne other than a 1450 nm diode laser in private practice.

Why aren't deep-penetrating mid-infrared lasers or long-pulsed Nd:YAG lasers more effective at acne than 1450 nm diode lasers? There's no research on this yet, but I think that first, the 1450 nm diode laser acts on microcomedone, the onset of acne, or sebaceous glands, which are the beginning of acne, rather than the large sebaceous glands seen in inflammatory acne, reducing sebaceous secretion and eventually preventing the development of new acne, which may be the main mechanism of acne treatment. For this reason, I wonder if this mechanism is why the 1450 nm diode laser treatment needs to be repeated not once, but several times, and that acne improves over time after the laser procedure

Table 16.3 Absorption coefficient, effective scattering coefficient, and penetration depth of mid-infrared lasers [10]

	1320 nm	1450 nm	1540 nm
Absorption coefficient	~3 cm^{-1}	20 cm^{-1}	8 cm^{-1}
Effective scattering coefficient	14 cm^{-1}	12 cm^{-1}	11 cm^{-1}
Penetration depth	~1500 μm	300 μm	700 μm

is over. Second, the target tissue is different from the first theory. It may be that the effect of 1450 nm diode laser on acne may be due to the action on the infundibulum, the upper part of the sebaceous glands, rather than the sebaceous glands themselves, to prevent follicular epidermal hyperkeratinization, which is one of the four major causes of acne. Third, the use of a deep-penetrating laser requires high energy because the temperature must be raised to a deeper layer, which can cause severe pain, and if side effects occur, serious side effects such as scarring can occur. For this reason, the mid-infrared laser is not used any more in private practice regardless of the acne therapeutic effect. Currently, only the acne-effective 1450 nm diode laser and the low-cost 1064 nm long-pulsed Nd:YAG laser are in use at private practice.

16.6 Consensus on Acne Treatment

Medication for acne has problems such as incomplete responses, slow onset of action, poor patient compliance, benign intracranial hypertension and lupus-like syndromes (tetracyclines), and potential teratogenicity (systemic isotretinoin). On the other hand, energy-based equipment has advantages such as more rapid onset of action, better patient compliance, fewer adverse events, etc. [6].

However, energy-based devices (LEDs, mid-infrared lasers, PDTs, needle RF, etc.) have the disadvantage of requiring multiple treatments because the effects are temporary, and there is not yet a matched consensus on the appropriate parameters and treatment methods. In particular, there is no consensus that states that it is more effective than medication. The authors of "Fitzpatrick's dermatology in general medicine," a dermatology textbook, believe that energy-based devices are less effective than traditional medications [14]. In addition, the results of a recent Cochrane systemic review conclude that there is still no high-quality evidence of light or laser therapies in acne treatment [15]. Therefore, energy-based device in acne treatment is thought to be the second treatment (medication is the first treatment).

The Global Alliance to improve outcomes in Acne Group recommends LEDs (blue and red light, 415, 635 nm) as the primary treatment among energy-based devices. This is because LEDs have a long treatment period, but they are easy to use and have fewer side effects. In addition, three treatment methods that are known to be the most effective for acne and have a long-lasting effect have been proposed. First, it is a mid-infrared laser, such as a 1450 nm diode laser. Second, photodynamic therapy (PDT) has the best supporting evidence. Third, it is a method of topical drug therapy and combination therapy [16].

Based on the above, I first start treatment with medication for acne. For energy-based devices, PDTs and 1450 nm diode lasers are recommended. However, I also recommend that medications, including oral isotretinoin, should be combined with treatment.

16.7 Parameters

Indications for the 1450 nm diode laser are sebaceous hyperactivity, acne (Fig. 16.5), sebaceous hyperplasia, xanthelasma palpebrarum, and nonablative rejuvenation such as pores and tightening (Table 16.4).

Most of the procedures are performed by first performing the T mode and then applying the A mode to the individual lesions. The T mode is the method B of the Arrhenius equation, such as the genesis technique. The DCD is turned off and the procedure is performed with 10 Hz and 10 mm (largest spot size) for a quick procedure. Multiple shots are irradiated by focusing on areas with a lot of sebaceous secretion, areas with a lot of acne, or areas that need pore treatment and tightening. Fluence is usually used as 12 J/cm^2. Like other nonablative lasers, there is no clinical end point, but if the patient is feeling hot or in pain, this is thought of as a warning end point and the corresponding area is avoided or the fluence is lowered. Since the patient's pain is an important warning end point, anesthetic cream is not

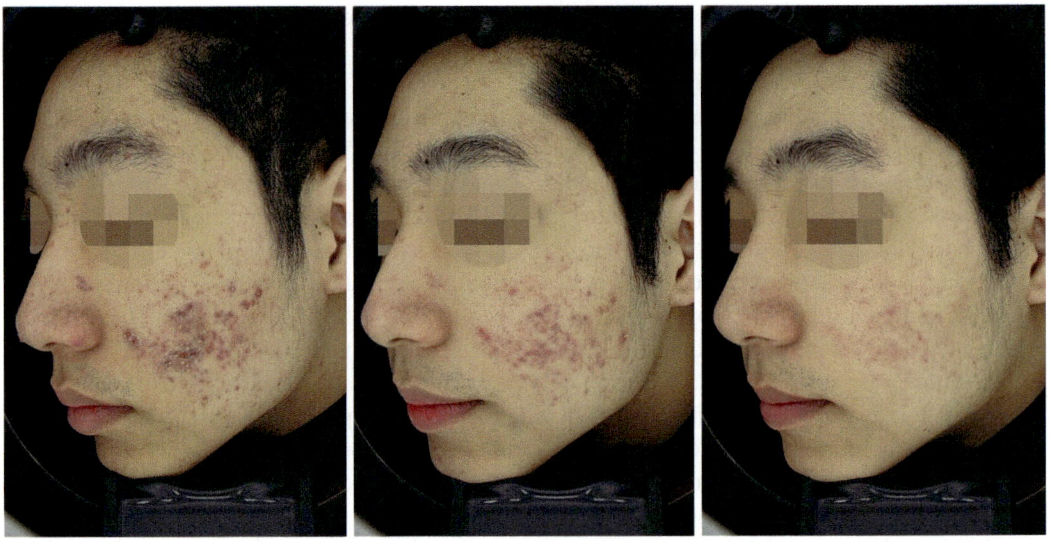

Fig. 16.5 Before and after 1450 nm diode laser procedure. Photo on the left: Before the procedure, Center photo: 3 months after the procedure, Photo at right: 6 months after the procedure (Photos Courtesy of Minho Lee, MD, Bestop clinic, Suwon, Korea. System used: Neobeam, UnionMedical Co. Ltd. Uijeongbu, Korea)

Table 16.4 Parameters of the 1450 nm diode laser (Neobeam, UnionMedical Co. Ltd. Uijeongbu, Korea)

Indications	Spot (mm)	On-time (ms)	Fluence (J/cm^2)	Pulse	DCD (ms)	Pass	Interval (week)	Session
T mode	6		13–15	10 Hz	Off		1–2	3–10
	10		10–15	10 Hz	Off		1–2	3–10
Acne, sebaceous hyperplasia, xanthelasma (A mode)	6	125	7–8	2	20	2–3	1–2	3–10
		200	4–6	2	20	2–3	1–2	3–10
	10	125	4–5	2	20	2–3	1–2	3–10
Pores, tightening (A mode)	6	125	7–8	2	20	3–5	2–3	10–12

applied before the procedure. One thousand shots on half of the face and more than 2000 shots are irradiated on both sides, and with only 4–6 procedures every 2 weeks clinical improvement can be seen. For inflammatory acne or sebaceous hyperplasia, puncture with a needle or CO_2 laser prior to the procedure is recommended. For individual acne or sebaceous hyperplasia, A mode is applied, with a spot size of 10 mm with DCD and multipulse 4–5 J/cm^2 twice at 125 ms (method A of the Arrhenius equation). Patients who are sensitive to pain use 4.1 J/cm^2, while patients who can tolerate pain use 5.1 J/cm^2 for a faster effect. In the case of acne, 2–3 passes are irradiated repeatedly before the patient complains of pain. Note that 2 pass does not mean irradiating a lesion twice, but rather irradiating all lesions throughout the face once and then returning to the primary lesion again and then irradiating the lesion of the entire face again. (Published with kind permission of © Minho Lee MD. 2021. All rights reserved).

In the case of sebaceous hyperplasia or xanthelasma palpebrarum, the slight whitening of the lesion in mode A is seen as a clinical end point and irradiation is repeated [1, 2].

Pores and tightening can be treated with T mode alone, or for further effect A mode with DCD and multipulse twice with 7–8 J/cm^2 at 125 ms, 6 mm spot may be performed. Slight swelling of the target area is seen as the clinical end point, 2–3 passes are performed. The procedure is performed at intervals of at least 10 s and the interval between spots is 5 mm apart to avoid side effects.

References

1. No D, McClaren M, Chotzen V, Kilmer SL. Sebaceous hyperplasia treated with a 1450-nm diode laser. Dermatol Surg. 2004;30(3):382–4.
2. Park EJ, Youn SH, Cho EB, Lee GS, Hann SK, Kim KH, et al. Xanthelasma palpebrarum treatment with a 1,450-nm-diode laser. Dermatol Surg. 2011;37(6):791–6.
3. Sakamoto FH, Doukas AG, Farinelli WA, Tannous Z, Shinn M, Benson S, et al. Selective photothermolysis to target sebaceous glands: theoretical estimation of parameters and preliminary results using a free electron laser. Lasers Surg Med. 2012;44(2):175–83.
4. Anderson RR, Parrish JA. Selective photothermolysis: precise microsurgery by selective absorption of pulsed radiation. Science. 1983;220(4596):524–7.
5. Keyvan N. Lasers in dermatology and medicine. London: Springer-Verlag; 2012.
6. Raulin C, Karsai S. Laser and IPL technology in dermatology and aesthetic medicine. Heidelberg: New York; 2011.
7. Paithankar DY, Ross EV, Saleh BA, Blair MA, Graham BS. Acne treatment with a 1,450 nm wavelength laser and cryogen spray cooling. Lasers Surg Med. 2002;31(2):106–14.
8. Altshuler GB, Anderson RR, Manstein D, Zenzie HH, Smirnov MZ. Extended theory of selective photothermolysis. Lasers Surg Med. 2001;29(5):416–32.
9. Yeung CK, Shek SY, Yu CS, Kono T, Chan HH. Treatment of inflammatory facial acne with 1,450-nm diode laser in type IV to V Asian skin using an optimal combination of laser parameters. Dermatol Surg. 2009;35(4):593–600.
10. Goldman MP. Cutaneous and cosmetic laser surgery. Philadelphia: Mosby Elsevier; 2006.
11. Jeon HC, Cho SY, Lee JH. Does long-pulsed neodymium:yttrium-aluminum-garnet work on acne lesions?: management of acne in Asian patients with a combinational laser treatment. J Dermatol. 2011;38(8):802–5.
12. Bakus AD, Yaghmai D, Massa MC, Garden BC, Garden JM. Sustained benefit after treatment of acne vulgaris using only a novel combination of long-pulsed and Q-switched 1064-nm Nd: YAG lasers. Dermatol Surg. 2018;44(11):1402–10.
13. Mohamed EE, Tawfik K, Elsaie M. Intense pulsed light versus 1,064 long-pulsed neodymium: yttrium-Aluminum- garnet laser in the treatment of facial acne vulgaris. J Clin Diagn Res. 2016;10(7):Wc01-3.
14. Kang S, Fitzpatrick TB. Fitzpatrick's dermatology. New York: McGraw-Hill Education; 2019.
15. Thiboutot DM, Dréno B, Abanmi A, Alexis AF, Araviiskaia E, Barona Cabal MI, et al. Practical management of acne for clinicians: an international consensus from the global Alliance to improve outcomes in acne. J Am Acad Dermatol. 2018;78(2 Suppl 1):S1–S23.e1
16. Allemann IB, Goldberg DJ. Basics in dermatological laser applications. Karger Medical and Scientific Publishers; 2011.

Atrophic Acne Scar and Histology 17

17.1 Subtypes of Atrophic Acne Scars

Jacob et al. divided atrophic acne scars into three types according to their size, depth, and three-dimensional structure [1] (Fig. 17.1). First, an icepick scar is a narrow, deep scar of less than 2 mm in diameter, just like an icepick. The opening in the surface is wider, taking the form of a funnel shaped V. Icepick scars are so deep that they are difficult to treat with laser resurfacing. Second, rolling scars are caused by dermal tethers that connect the dermis to the subcutaneous layer. They have an undulating form with shallow, rounded bases and take the form of an M. The diameter is 4–5 mm. Treatment is done by the removal of the dermal tether. Third, boxcar scars are wider than icepick scars. The base is wide and takes the form of a U, like a boxcar that is upside down. Boxcar scars can be divided into shallow boxcar scars, which can benefit from laser resurfacing, and deep boxcar scars, where the bottom

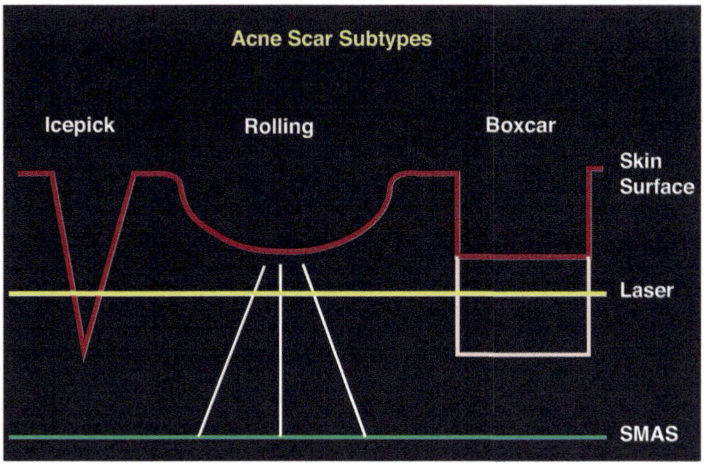

Fig. 17.1 Novel classification system of three basic scar types: icepick, rolling, and boxcar (superficial and deep). *Yellow reference line* denotes the depth of ablation and resurfacing capability of the carbon-dioxide laser. *Green line* represents the superficial musculoaponeurotic system (SMAS) to which fibrous bands adhere, creating rolling scars. Reproduced from [1]

J. D. Lee, M. J. M. Oh, *Lasers in Dermatology: Parameters and Choice*,
https://doi.org/10.1007/978-981-19-7568-4_17

is so deep that laser resurfacing is ineffective. However, all atrophic acne scars cannot be classified into these three types of scars, because they may have more than one characteristic. Thus, the classification of atrophic acne scars by Jacob et al. should be understood as a rough classification concept for approaching treatment.

In real practice, we usually see all of the three atrophic acne scars in a single patient [1]. Most patients have more than one type of atrophic acne scar. I have never seen any patient with only rolling scars or only boxcar scars. Different types of atrophic acne scars coexist in a single patient, with a difference in proportions. Why is this so? I think this because acne itself has various acne symptoms caused by various inflammations. Acne is divided into comedonal lesions such as closed comedone (white head) and open comedone (black head), and inflammatory lesions such as papules, pustules, nodules, and cysts. Comedonal lesions and inflammatory lesions are not different disease entities but are descriptive definitions that describe the various skin changes observed in the progress of disease from closed comedones to inflammatory lesions. Inflammatory lesions, especially papules, pustules, nodules, and cysts, are the same lesions that appear different depending on the severity of inflammation. As a result, all these lesions are found in single patient (pleomorphism). This is why atrophic acne scars caused by inflammation also show various types of scars. Therefore, in the treatment of acne scars, a combination therapy using an effective treatment method for each atrophic acne scar is needed.

17.2 Histology of Atrophic Acne Scars

Lee et al. observed biopsies of 31 atrophic acne scars in 5 patients and described the histological findings of atrophic acne scars [2]. The results showed that keratin plugging was observed in 32% of the hair follicle openings in the epidermis, and a number of multi-channelled tracts were observed. In the dermis, the dermal thickness was reduced and the loss of pilosebaceous units was observed. In addition, inflammatory cell infiltrates were observed in 77%, and in 29% there was an insufficient dense collagen fiber deposition.

Let's consider the meaning of each histological finding. First, the finding that there is keratin plugging in hair follicle openings can be problematic in the case of chemical reconstruction of skin scars method (CROSS). Before performing the CROSS method, keratin plugging should be eliminated through superficial peeling or scaling, so that the CROSS method is more effective. Second, the findings that multi-channelled tracts are observed on the epidermis can also cause problems during the CROSS method. Although it may look like a small sized scar to the naked eye, if TCA flows into multi-channelled tracts during the procedure and a wide area is coagulated, the wound will not heal and may result in a wide scar. Third, the findings of a decrease in dermis thickness are thought to be caused by a decrease in the production of dermis collagen. Fourth, the loss of the pilosebaceous unit, the epidermal appendage, implies that it is vulnerable to reepithelialization due to wounds. Fifth, the infiltration of inflammatory cells is observed. The fact that there is an infiltration of inflammatory cells means that although on the surface it may seem like all the acne is gone, histologically there is still inflammation in the dermis. This means that it is necessary to treat atrophic acne scar with sufficient time after acne treatment, or to combine inflammation treatment when treating scar. Sixth, the observation of the deposition of collagen fibers densely concentrated in the dermis implies that hard and dense collagen fibers (fibrosis) are thought to be made in the dermis to maintain the skin tension weakened by collagen loss. I believe that the fact that this dense fibrous tissue is interfering with collagen reformation is a problem in atrophic acne scar treatment (Fig. 17.2).

Therefore, scar therapy must first re-establish normal collagen tissue. A procedure that makes as much collagen as possible would be advantageous. Second, scar tissue is vulnerable to reepithelialization due to wounds, so procedures that are problematic for regeneration should be avoided. That is, the procedure should not be per-

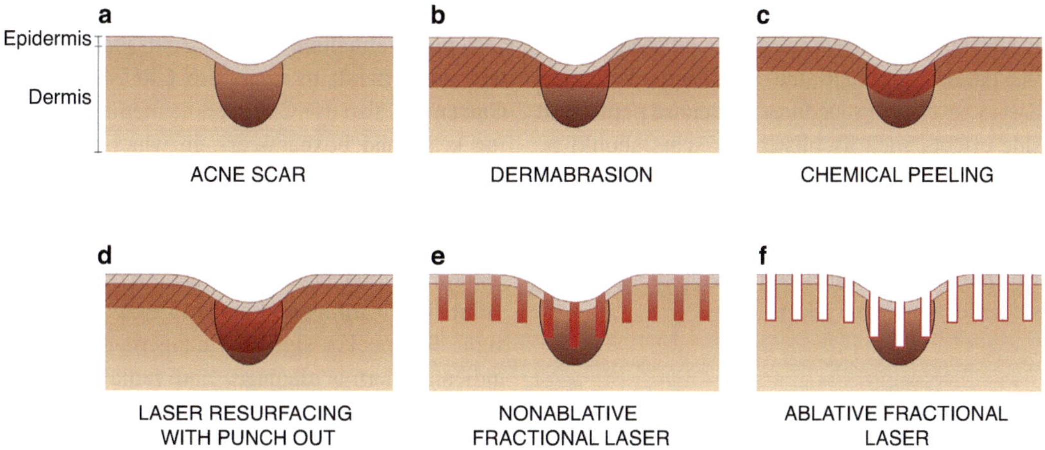

Fig. 17.2 Schematic pictures of atrophic acne scars showing the effectiveness of each scar treatment method. Atrophic acne scars with (**a**) no treatment, treated by (**b**), dermabrasion, (**c**) chemical peeling, (**d**) laser resurfacing with punch-out, (**e**) nonablative fractional laser, and (**f**) ablative fractional laser. Reproduced from [3]

formed too wide or too deeply, and conversely, a narrow and deep procedure (e.g., a pinhole method or fractional laser) is safer. Additionally, a narrow and deep procedure may remove the fibrous tissue in the deeper layers. You also need to have knowledge of wet dressings that help with re-epithelialization. Third, the fibrous tissue that hinders collagen reformation must be eliminated. However, if all the fibrous tissue is removed, the same fibrous tissue occurs again to fill the void. That's why it should be removed little by little.

17.3 Treatment of Atrophic Acne Scars

There are many ways to treat atrophic acne scars. As shown in Table 17.1, it can be classified into five treatment methods according to mechanism [4]. It can also be classified into two types: surgical methods and nonsurgical methods. But I think that the classification of atrophic acne scar treatment is less important, and it is more important to select the treatment method that is suitable for physician by checking the principles and pros and cons of each treatment method.

There is one thing to note here. Scars are not easily treated, and there is no 100% in scar treatment [5]. Patients also understand this, so if having to choose between "efficacy" and "safety," efficacy should come before safety. For example, temporary scabs, bruises, swellings, etc. that occur immediately after the procedure, and erythema or post-inflammatory hyperpigmentation (PIH) that occur after the procedure are visually undesirable side effects but are not permanent, which makes energy levels or procedures that

Table 17.1 Treatments for atrophic acne scars by mechanism [4]

Mechanisms	Modalities
Surgery/movement-related modalities	Punch techniques (punch elevation, punch excision), elliptical excision Botulinum toxin Facelift
Lift-related modalities	Subcision
Volume-related modalities	Soft tissue augmentation, dermal grafting, fat transplant, platelet-rich plasma
Resurfacing modalities	Microdermabrasion, dermabrasion, chemical peeling Chemical reconstruction of skin scars (CROSS) Skin needling (percutaneous collagen induction therapy) Laser resurfacing
Skin-tightening modalities	Lasers (fractional lasers, nonfractional, nonablative lasers, picosecond 755-nm alexandrite laser) Fractional radiofrequency

induce these side effects acceptable in scar treatments, but informed consent will be needed from the patients prior to the procedure. However, energy levels or procedures that cause permanent side effects such as blisters or scars should be avoided. Therefore, it is important to know what scar treatments are effective and in what order they are effective. It is also important to know which treatments are effective without significant side effects in ethnic skin.

17.4 CO_2 Pinhole Method

Ahmed et al. assigned 28 patients with icepick scars to two groups: 14 patients received CO_2 laser irradiation technique (CO_2 pinhole method), and the other 14 patients received TCA CROSS method by 100% TCA [6]. The parameters of the CO_2 laser were 0.12 mm spot size, 1.0 ms pulse duration, 0.9 W, and focused at 99 Hz. There were four sessions at 3-week intervals, and 3 months of follow-up.

There was statistically significant difference in acne scar severity index (patients with 51–70% improvement was 36% in CO_2 pinhole method vs 21% in CROSS method) and qualitative scarring grading system (CO_2 pinhole method > CROSS method) in the improvement results between the two groups. Complications included transient pigmentation and inflammation, which resulted less in CO_2 pinhole method than in CROSS method.

This paper describes that CO_2 pinhole method is more effective than CROSS method in icepick scars. CO_2 pinhole method, like CROSS method, does not require anesthesia, and is more convenient than CROSS therapy, which requires first taking the TCA solution and then administering it. However, the effects on scars other than icepick scars are not shown in this paper. The authors believe that CO_2 pinhole method is more effective than CROSS method because CO_2 pinhole method induces neocollagenesis by thermal damage, which is not present in CROSS method. A technique tip for CO_2 pinhole method is that the skin be pulled back to irradiate the scar base with the tip.

After reviewing this paper, I have attempted CO_2 pinhole method on very small icepick scars that are difficult to treat with CROSS method. Currently I also use CO_2 pinhole method for rolling scars and boxcar scars, in which only 1–2 procedures are necessary for a noticeable improvement in the scar.

There is no exact clinical end point of the CO_2 pinhole method, but I think there is a warning end point. The warning end point I think is a pucker sign. The pucker sign is a dangerous sign that indicates dermis damage, and radial wrinkles form around the irradiated area, as if the skin had risen and wrinkled in all directions just like a grandmother pursing her lips [7]. This is why I stop stacking before the pucker sign appears. When I perform the CO_2 pinhole method on a rolling scar and a boxcar scar, I irradiate it at intervals of 1–3 mm along the border between normal skin and scar, and I also perform 1 or 2 pinhole method in the center of the scar to remove the fibrous tissue of the scar.

17.5 Combination Therapy

Kang et al. used a combination of dot peeling, subcision, and nonablative fractional laser treatment for atrophic acne scars [8]. Dot peeling was done by 100% TCA, and subcision by 29G needle. The nonablative fractional laser was a 1550 nm Er:glass laser, and the parameters were 4 passes using 350–800 spots/cm^2 and 25 mJ per MTZ. Fractional laser was performed 3–4 times in 3–4 week intervals. Dot peeling and subcision were performed at the same time 2 weeks after the fractional laser, for a total of 2 times in 2–3 month intervals. The results showed that the acne scar severity score improved by 55.3%, and 80% of the patients had a "significant" or "marked improvement."

This paper used a combination of three treatments for acne scars. The reason for the combination therapy is described in the paper as follows. Dot peeling is effective on individual atrophic acne scars but is limited to improving overall skin texture. Fractional lasers are effective on improving overall skin texture and on shallow and small atrophic scars, but the effect is limited on icepick scars and boxcar scars. Subcision is also effective for wide boxcar scars and rolling scars. Therefore, it is described that the effects and limitations of these three treatment methods can be complemented to each other by combination therapy, and the overall scar treatment effect can be enhanced.

Combination therapy is known to be more effective than single therapy in acne scars due to the complementary and synergetic effects described above. Acne scar treatment can be divided into first, energy-based methods such as laser and radiofrequency, and second, energy-free procedures such as CROSS, subcision, filler, microneedle therapy system (MTS), and punch techniques. What is important in combination therapy is that treatments with different mechanisms are needed to reduce side effects. For example, laser and radiofrequency may be used in combination, but both procedures are "energy-based" methods and should be avoided. It would be better to combine treatments with different mechanisms, such as laser + subcision or laser + subcision + punch technique. Also, lasers are most effective for scars and should be included in combination therapy as the primary treatment for scars. Subcision is usually the first procedure of the combination therapy [4].

17.6 Order of Combination Therapies

Let's think about the order of combination therapies. When several procedures are performed simultaneously on the same day, what is the principle in choosing the order of combination therapies? I believe that a deep procedure or laser with deep optical penetration detph (OPD) should be performed first, followed by a shallow procedure or laser with shallow OPD. For example, in tattoo removals, CO_2 pinhole method first and 1064 nm Q-switched Nd:YAG lasers later (Kono technique, window technique [9]) may be more effective but may be more dangerous, considering the side effects. In other words, we must put safety first, so "deep procedure → shallow procedure" should be one principle to follow when choosing the order of combination.

I perform the following procedures when treating scars: First, subcision is performed, followed by CO_2 pinhole method, CO_2 fractional laser, and MTS. Subcision is performed on the hypodermis, i.e., just below or to the dermis, CO_2 pinhole method aims to ablate the entire dermis, and CO_2 fractional laser penetrates the epidermis and part of the dermis. But what about MTS? The clinical end point of the MTS is bleeding, which means that it is performed deep in the dermis, which is the same or deeper than the layer that CO_2 fractional laser targets. Then why is MTS performed last? Due to the bleeding of MTS, CO_2 pinhole method and CO_2 fractional laser may not be effective if they are performed after MTS. Thus, according to the principle of order of combination therapies, MTS should be done first, but because of the reasons mentioned above I do it last. Although there are principles, the order of combination therapies may vary depending on the nature or characteristics of the laser or procedure.

17.7 Conclusion

When treating atrophic acne scars, the following principles should be considered. First, a treatment that is more effective must be selected, unless it has a risk of permanent side effects. Second, because of various acne symptoms, various types of scars are present on the face at the same time. Therefore, only one procedure does not yield satisfactory results. Third, combination therapy has a synergic effect. Fourth, each treatment method has a different therapeutic effect for each type of scar. The first three criteria were reviewed above. Here, we will review the last principle.

Bhargava et al. reviewed 89 review articles on the treatment of acne scars [4]. According to the quality of evidence, they were classified as level I–IV. The smaller the number, the higher the evidence. The result was as follows: First, there was no paper showing high evidence in the treatment of acne scars. Second, fractional lasers and radiofrequency waves were highly effective with most atrophic acne scars without serious side effects. Third, combination therapy is more effective than monotherapy.

Table 17.2 important to note in this paper. This table shows the effect of each scar type according to various treatment methods. The effects vary depending on the type of treatment and the type of scar.

According to the four principles, the procedure should be selected as follows: First, the darkest blue that corresponds to "effective" must be selected. Second, because various types of acne scars are present on the face at the same time, four separate treatments for four types of scars must be selected for effective treatment. Third, because combination treatment is more effective, effective treatment for the four types of scars should be combined.

I use the Table 17.2 as follows:

1. Ice pick scars

   The most effective methods for icepick scars are the CROSS method and punch excision. But I choose CROSS method because patients are reluctant to have surgery, and after punch excision scars do not disappear, but somewhat recur after punch excision. However, considering the histological findings of atrophic acne scars and the comparative papers of CO_2 pinhole method, I mainly use CO_2 pinhole method instead of CROSS method.
2. Rolling scars and boxcar scars

   Subcision, MTS, fractional lasers, and needle RF are effective in rolling scars and boxcar scars. I used to perform subcision, MTS, and fractional lasers, but these days I only use subcision and fractional lasers due to its convenience.
3. Deep boxcar scars

   Ablative lasers, punch elevation, and punch excision are effective in deep boxcar scars. But since punch elevation and punch excision are both surgical procedures, ablative lasers are preferred. However, ablative lasers have the possibility of serious side effects, so I use the FAST method by CO_2 fractional laser (refer to Sect. 12.8 in Chap. 12). In addition, CO_2 pinhole method is performed to the borders of the deep boxcar scars.

When combination therapies are performed on the same day, I perform in this order: subcision for rolling scars, CO_2 pinhole method for ice pick scars and deep box car scars, and FAST method with fractional laser for rolling scars, shallow boxcar scars and deep boxcar scars. And Finally, PDRN is applied to the skin to facilitate wound healing. Where only some areas underwent the CO_2 pinhole method, no dressing is necessary. In large areas where FAST method has been performed, Duoderm dressing is recommended. The patient is advised to replace the Duoderm if there is too much discharge during 3–4 days, otherwise it should be maintained for 10 days.

Table 17.2 Effectiveness of treatment methods according to the type of atrophic acne scar. Reproduced from [4]

Type of Treatment	Modality[a]	Icepick Scars	Rolling Scars	Shallow Boxcar Scars	Deep Boxcar Scars
Resurfacing	Microdermabrasion	Less effective	Ineffective	Less effective	Ineffective
	Dermabrasion	Less effective	Ineffective	Less effective	Less effective
	Peels	Less effective	Ineffective	Less effective	Ineffective
	CROSS	Effective	Ineffective	Effective	Ineffective
	Needling	Ineffective	Effective	Effective	Less effective
	Ablative laser	Less effective	Effective	Effective	Effective
Lifting-related	Subcision	Less effective	Effective	Less effective	Less effective
Volume-related	Filler	Ineffective	Effective	Less effective	Less effective
	Platelet rich plasma[b]	Ineffective	Less effective	Less effective	Less effective
Skin Tightening	Fractional/nonablative lasers	Less effective	Effective	Effective	Less effective
	Fractional radiofrequency	Less effective	Effective	Effective	Less effective
Surgery/movement-related	Punch elevation	Ineffective	Ineffective	Effective	Effective
	Punch excision	Effective	Ineffective	Less effective	Effective

Effective Less effective Ineffective

References

1. Thiboutot D, Gollnick H, Bettoli V, Dreno B, Kang S, Leyden JJ, et al. New insights into the management of acne: an update from the global alliance to improve outcomes in Acne group. J Am Acad Dermatol. 2009;60(5 Suppl):S1–50.
2. Lee WJ, Jung HJ, Lim HJ, Jang YH, Lee SJ, Kim DW. Serial sections of atrophic acne scars help in the interpretation of microscopic findings and the selection of good therapeutic modalities. J Eur Acad Dermatol Venereol. 2013;27(5):643–6.
3. You HJ, Kim DW, Yoon ES, Park SH. Comparison of four different lasers for acne scars: resurfacing and fractional lasers. J Plast Reconstr Aesthet Surg. 2016;69(4):e87–95.
4. Bhargava S, Cunha PR, Lee J, Kroumpouzos G. Acne scarring management: systematic review and evaluation of the evidence. Am J Clin Dermatol. 2018;19(4):459–77.
5. Dreno B. Acne: physical treatment. Clin Dermatol. 2004;22(5):429–33.
6. Ahmed R, Mohammed G, Ismail N, Elakhras A. Randomized clinical trial of CO(2) LASER pinpoint irradiation technique versus chemical reconstruction of skin scars (CROSS) in treating ice pick acne scars. J Cosmet Laser Ther. 2014;16(1):8–13.
7. Wanner M, Sakamoto FH, Avram MM, Anderson RR. Immediate skin responses to laser and light treatments: warning endpoints: how to avoid side effects. J Am Acad Dermatol. 2016;74(5):807–19.
8. Kang WH, Kim YJ, Pyo WS, Park SJ, Kim JH. Atrophic acne scar treatment using triple combination therapy: dot peeling, subcision and fractional laser. J Cosmet Laser Ther. 2009;11(4):212–5.
9. Lee JD, Lee JK, Oh MJM. Principles and choice of laser treatment in dermatology. Singapore: Springer; 2020.

18 Melasma and Melanogenesis

"What are the diagnostic criteria for melasma?" "What causes melasma?" "What is the effect of laser toning?" "How should we treat melasma?" This chapter will reflect on these four questions.

18.1 Diagnosis of Melasma

Melasma is a common hypermelanosis that occurs in areas exposed to sunlight, especially the face. It occurs rarely before puberty and is commonly observed in women, especially women of child-bearing age. It is also observed in 10% of men. New melasma often arise, and existing melasma may worsen during pregnancy. Symptoms appear as brown macules with irregular borders and occur symmetrically in the photodistribution of sunlight on the face. They are often fused in a reticular pattern. They are darkened by sunlight, which makes them worse during summer and improve during winter, i.e., there is a seasonal change. Melasma is common among Asian and Hispanic women who live in areas with strong sunlight. Melasma occurs frequently in patients with Fitzpatrick skin types IV, V, and VI [1].

The differential diagnosis for melasma includes nevus of Ota, abnormal bilateral nevus of Ota like macule (ABNOM, Hori's macules), medication-induced hyperpigmentation, erythema dyschromicum perstans (EDP), Lichen planus pigmentosus, abrupt demarcation between sideburn and the lighter skin posteriorly, lichenoid drug eruption, Riel's melanosis, post-inflammatory hyperpigmentation (PIH), maturational dyschromia, periorbital hyperpigmentation, acanthosis nigricans, ephelides, lentigines, exogenous ochronosis, etc. [2].

Rodriques et al. mentioned two features of melasma that are helpful in differentiating from other pigmentation disorders [2]. First, melasma occur in the orbital rim and rarely in the mandible. Second, melasma are neither dark, such as pigmentation by medication-induced hyperpigmentation or erythema dyschromicum perstans (EDP) nor gray like cement. In practice, however, it is often difficult to differently diagnose melasma.

Because melasma has no clear diagnostic criteria, diagnosis by exclusion must be performed. Still, the characteristics of melasma that I think are helpful with diagnosis are: First, melasma is brownish. Melasma is divided into epidermal type, dermal type, and mixed type according to the location of the pigment, but most melasma are either an epidermal type or a mixed type. In mixed type melasma, dermal melanin pigmentations are observed in the dermis close to the surface layer. Therefore, it looks brown, not gray or blue. Second, the border of melasma is blurry rather than irregular. Melasma does not have the same clear boundaries as lentigo, which makes it difficult to divide the boundaries with normal skin. Third, melasma appears symmetrically bilateral and occurs at the site of sunlight exposure. If it occurs unilaterally, or if it occurs in a

J. D. Lee, M. J. M. Oh, *Lasers in Dermatology: Parameters and Choice*,
https://doi.org/10.1007/978-981-19-7568-4_18

non-sunlight exposed area, it is not likely to be melasma. Fourth, melasma is often fused into a reticular pattern. The melasma do not consist of independent brown patches, but are connected to each other, most of which form a single patch.

18.2 Issues of Melasma

Laser treatment of melasma may cause three problems. First, latent melasma may convert to actual melasma. Second, existing melasma may get worse. Third, after laser treatment melasma can occur even in areas not irradiated by laser. We will review these three problems one by one.

First, when intense pulsed lights (IPL) were popular in private practice, post-IPL pigmentations similar to melasma were often found. Negishi et al. studied this phenomenon by comparing normal pictures with pictures taken with ultraviolet (UV) cameras [3]. A survey of 223 Japanese women found that 63 (28.3%) had melasma that could not be seen under normal light but could be seen with UV light. That is, latent melasma was observed. In addition, clinical findings showed that in patients who had latent melasma by UV light, new melasma occurred in the clinically same area after IPL. During laser treatment, it is important to keep in mind that even though we cannot see melasma when we examine the patient's face with our bare eyes, there is always a possibility of latent melasma.

Second, when treating melasma with laser parameters known to be effective in other pigmentation disorders, melasma may seem to disappear at first, but becomes darker with time, and then with another laser treatment it may seem to disappear again, only to become darker again [4, 5]. Thus, the vicious cycle. If melasma is not diagnosed accurately, and treated like another pigmentation disorder, melasma can get worse. Therefore, accurate diagnosis is important in melasma.

Third, after laser treatment melasma can occur even in areas not irradiated by laser. Lee et al. treated a 37-year-old female patient with ABNOM with 1064 nm Q-switched Nd:YAG laser five times at four-week intervals. A month later melasma was observed around the ABNOM [6]. Melasma occurred in areas not irradiated by laser.

The three problems reviewed above—latent melasma converting to actual melasma, existing melasma getting worse, new found melasma after treating other pigmentation disorders such as ABNOM—may happen during laser treatment in private practice. These situations gave both the doctor and the patients a hard time. So in the past, lasers were contraindicated in treating melasma.

18.3 Activated Melanocyte

Why do these happen? The pathogenesis of melasma is not well known, but biologically active melanocytes, genetic causes, hormonal effects, and UV light are known to be important [7]. Other causes may include birth control pills, estrogen replacement therapy, mild ovarian or thyroid dysfunction, ovarian tumors, cosmetics, nutrition, phototoxicity, photoallergic drugs, and epilepsy drugs [7]. I especially believe that activated melanocytes are the fundamental issue [8]. That is, melasma can be considered to be a state in which melanin synthesis is active.

Kang et al. compared histological examination of melasma skin and surrounding normal skin in 56 Korean melasma patients [9]. The results showed that melanin was significantly increased in the epidermis, especially in the basal layer. In addition, a statistically significant increase in solar elastosis was observed in melasma skin compared to normal skin. Electron microscopic findings revealed that melanocytes in melasma skin had more mitochondria, Golgi apparatus, rough endoplasmic reticulum, and ribosomes than normal melanocytes (Fig. 18.1). In other words, melanocytes in the melasma skin are "activated melanocytes" which are more activated than normal to make melanin, and actually made more melanosomes.

So even though we do not know the exact cause of melasma, wouldn't inhibiting melanogenesis improve melasma?

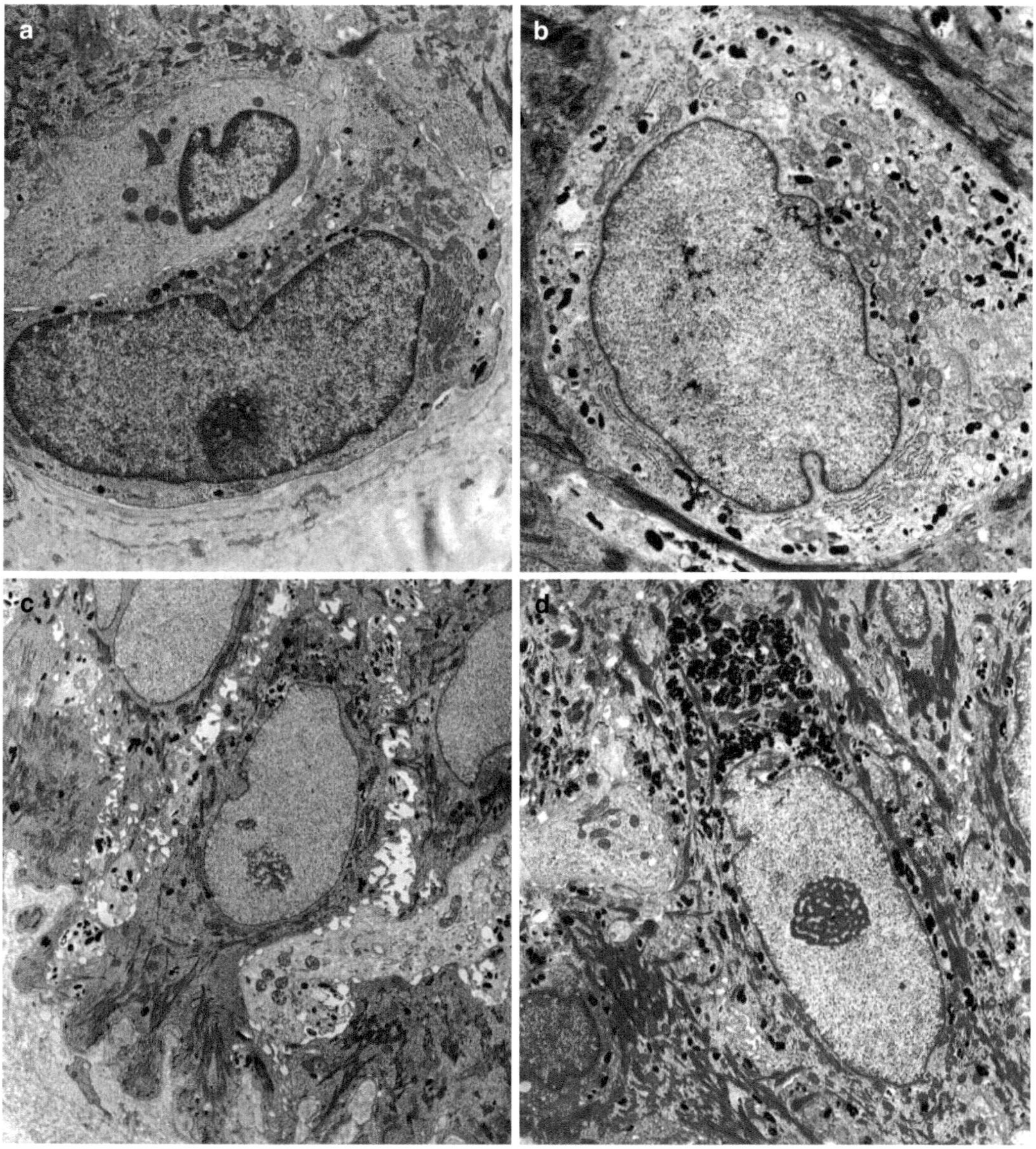

Fig. 18.1 Electron microscopy of perilesional skin and melasma skin. Melanocytes in (**a**) perilesional skin and (**b**) melasma skin. Lesional melanocytes were filled with more mitochondria, Golgi apparatus, rough endoplasmic reticulum, and ribosomes in the perikaryon than were normal skin melanocytes. Keratinocytes in (**c**) perilesional skin and (**d**) melasma skin. Reproduced from [9]

18.4 Melanogenesis

The biosynthesis process of melanin shows that the amino acid tyrosine is converted into DOPA, DOPAquinone by the enzyme tyrosinase, and then through various processes, finally eumelanin called DHI and DHICA are made, and pheomelanin is finally made by glutathione or cysteine in DOPAquinone. The transformation of tyrosine into DOPA by tyrosinase during this process is an important rate limiting step in determining the rate of melanogenesis [1]. That's why hydroquinone, a tyrosinase inhibitor, is known to be the most powerful depigmenting agent. Thus, melanin is the final product produced by the oxidation of the amino acid tyrosine by the enzyme tyrosinase. Therefore, antioxidants that prevent oxidation will also help in whitening.

The organelle that synthesizes melanin is the melanosome within melanocyte. The melanosome is formed in the Golgi body and has an elongated oval shape. Melanosome matures through the biosynthesis process of melanin. According to the degree of maturity, melanosome is divided into four stages. The melanosome in stages 1 and 2 are "the stage where there is no melanin yet" and "the stage with pheomelanin only," respectively, and the skin with melanosome in stages 1 and 2 looks brighter. The melanosome in stages 3 and 4 is made of eumelanin and the skin with melanosome in stages 3 and 4 appears dark [10].

The number and density of melanocytes are constant regardless of race and skin color [11]. So the reason for the difference in skin color is not because of the number of melanocyte. The difference in skin color is determined, first, by the activity of melanogenesis in the melanocyte, second, by the proportion of mature melanosome described above, and third, by the migration and distribution of melanosome to keratinocyte.

When the melanosome is full of melanin, the melanosome moves to the dendrite for delivery to keratinocyte. The melanosome travels to the dendrite through the microtubule, a cytoskeleton protein involved in substance transfer, in which proteins such as kinesin and dynein are involved [1]. Niacinamide is a drug that inhibits the delivery process of this melanosome and is used as a raw material for whitening cosmetics that reduce pigmentation [12].

The melanosomes, located above the nucleus of keratinocyte, are thought to decompose during keratinization. This is because even in dark skin types, the structure of melanosome is not observed in the corneocyte of the stratum corneum, the outermost layer of the skin. Several recent studies have shown that melanosome breaks down through autophagy, and melanosome slowly breaks down as autophagy action is impaired in dark skin [7].

18.5 Signaling Pathway

What are the signaling pathways that regulate melanogenesis? Not all of the signaling pathways of melanogenesis are yet known. Let's take a look at just a few known facts.

First, a key regulator of melanogenesis is known to be the Microphthalmia-associated Transcription Factor (MITF) in the nucleus of melanocyte. The determining enzymes of melanogenesis are tyrosinase, TRP-1 and TRP-2, both of which are transcription products of MITF.

The most commonly known signaling pathway today is the cAMP/PKA pathway (Fig. 18.2). By ultraviolet light, proopiomelanocortin (POMC) is expressed in keratinocyte through a p53 tumor suppressor, and β-endorphin and α-MSH are produced. α-MSH secreted outside the cell increases cAMP (cyclic AMP) and PKA (Protein Kinase A) in melanocyte through MC1R of the surrounding melanocytic membranes, activating cAMP Response Element-Binding protein (CREB), and finally making melanin through MITF [14].

Except for the cAMP/PKA pathway, there are Wnt pathway (Wnt/β-catenin pathway) and MAPK pathway (MAP Kinase pathway). Kondo et al. have recently reported DKK1 (Dickkopf-related protein 1) and NRG1 (Neuregulin-1) as paracrine factors secreted from fibroblasts [14]. DKK1 is a factor secreted by fibroblasts in the dermis of the palms and soles and inhibits the Wnt pathway (Wnt/β-catenin pathway). NRG1 is highly expressed in fibroblasts in dark-skinned patients and regulates the MAPK pathway (MAP Kinase pathway) through ErbB3 or ErbB4 receptors. It can be seen that fibroblasts are also involved in melanogenesis.

Much is not yet known about the signaling pathway that regulates melanogenesis. The more information is revealed about the signaling pathway, the newer depigmenting agents will be able to be developed. But the first thing we note in the signaling pathway at this point in time is the fact that melanogenesis begins through ultraviolet light and keratinocyte. This suggests that a lifestyle that reduces ultraviolet rays and a healthy keratinocyte are important. Second, not only the

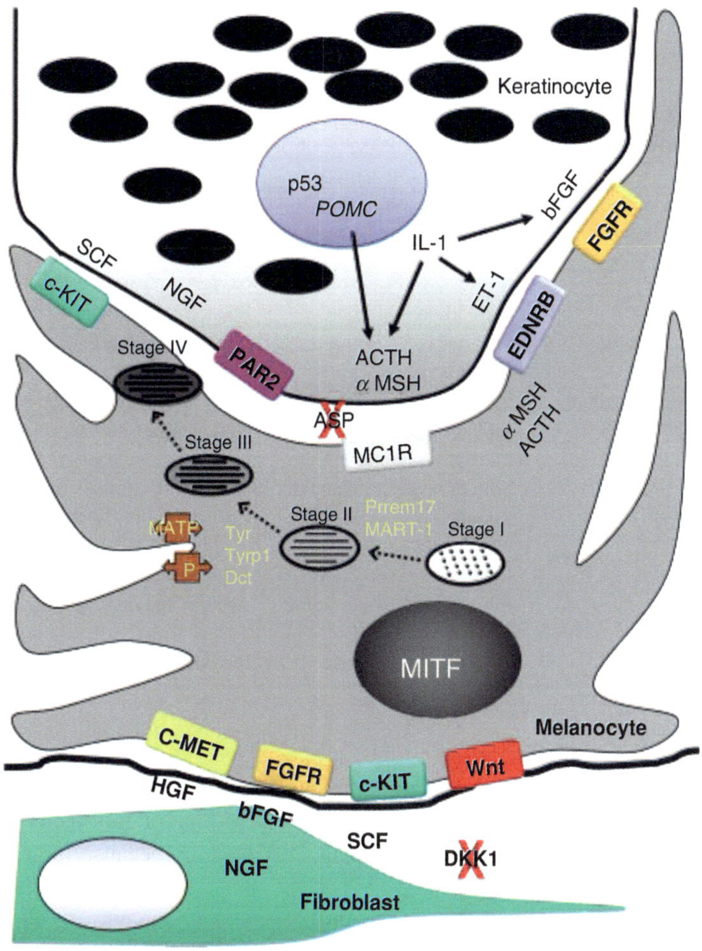

Fig. 18.2 Various factors that regulate the function of melanocyte and signaling pathways. Reproduced from [13]

epidermis, but also the fibroblasts of the dermis are involved in the signaling pathway. Therefore, the procedure to make the dermis healthy will also help in brightening. Third, as recent studies on the causes of melasma have been conducted, it has been known that melanocyte, keratinocyte, fibroblasts, as well as vascular endothelial cells and sebaceous cells, are also involved in hyperpigmentation [15]. Therefore, brightening treatment does not end with simply removing pigments or applying sunscreen well, but also suggests that it is important to make the entire skin healthy.

18.6 Depigmenting Agents and Melanogenesis

Depending on melanin biosynthesis and signaling pathway, depigmenting agents can be classified into 3 main categories (Table 18.1). These are depigmenting agents before melanogenesis, depigmenting agents during melanogenesis and depigmenting agents after melanogenesis [12]. A representative drug for depigmenting agents before melanogenesis is tranexamic acid. Representative drugs of depigmenting agents during melanogenesis are hydroquinone and

Table 18.1 Classification of depigmenting agents according to melanogenesis. Reproduced from [12]

Stage of melanin synthesis	Deposition	Active molecules
Before melanin synthesis	Tyrosinase transcription	Tretinoin, c-2 ceramide
	Tyrosinase glycosylation	$PaSSO_3Ca$
	Inhibition of plasmin	Tranexamic acid
During melanin synthesis	Tyrosinase inhibition	Hydroquinone, mequinol, azelaic acid, kojic acid, arbutin, deoxyarbutin, licorice extract, rucinol, 2,5-dimethyl-4-hydroxy-3(2H)-furanone, N-acetyl glucosamine, resveratrol, oxyresveratrol, ellagic acid, methyl gentisate, 4-hydroxyanisole
	Peroxidase inhibition	Phenolic compounds
	Reactive oxygen species scavengers	Ascorbic acid, ascorbic acid palmitate, thioctic acid, hydrocumarins
After melanin synthesis	Tyrosinase degradation	Linoleic acid, α-linoleic acid
	Inhibition of melanosome transfer	Niacinamide, serine protease inhibitors, retinoids, lecithins, neoglycoproteins, soybean trypsin inhibitor
	Skin turnover acceleration	Lactic acid, glycolic acid, linoleic acid, retinoic acid
	Regulation of melanocyte environment	Corticosteroids, glabridin
	Interaction with copper	Kojic acid, ascorbic acid
	Inhibition of melanosome maturation	Arbutin and deoxyarbutin
	Inhibition of protease activated receptor 2	Soybean trypsin inhibitor

ascorbic acid, and for depigmenting agents after melanogenesis, niacinamide and glycolic acid.

So at what stage does laser toning work?

18.7 Effects of Laser Toning

Next, we will look at two papers that studied the effects of laser toning.

Mun et al. performed laser toning by 1064 nm Q-switched Nd:YAG laser in 16 patients and observed the melasma lesion by electron microscopy and reconstructed it into 3D images [16]. The results were as follows. First, the volume of the melanocytes was reduced and the number of melanosomes was reduced. Second, the "dendrectomy" phenomenon, in which the melanocyte dendrite was reduced, was observed (Fig. 18.3). Third, mature melanosomes of stage IV decreased, and fourth, degraded melanosomes and traces were observed. Fifth, immature melanosomes in stages I and II were unchanged (Fig. 18.4).

What is interesting about this paper is the "dendrectomy" phenomenon, which is the reduction of the dendrites of melanocytes. The authors of this paper assume that the reason for this is because stage IV melanosomes are located more on the dendrite than any other parts of the melanocyte, so due to the thermolytic effect of laser the dendrite disappears [16]. I regard this phenomenon as "inactivation of melanocyte." The most important role of melanocytes is to make melanosomes and deliver them to keratinocytes. Thus, the reduced dendrites imply that the role of melanocytes has ceased. I think that laser toning induces melanocyte inactivation. In addition, after laser toning, melanosomes in the melanocytes disappear, the volume of melanocytes become smaller, and nuclear fission is reduced, which I believe are all signs of melanocyte inactivation.

I also believe that the mechanism of brightening of melasma by laser toning is due to dendrectomy rather than by breaking the melanosome. In the subcellular selective photothermolysis paper, the melanosomes of the zebrafish were broken by laser toning (Fig. 5.4). But if the melanosome breaks inside the cell, does this result in making the overall melasma tone brighter? Melanosomes

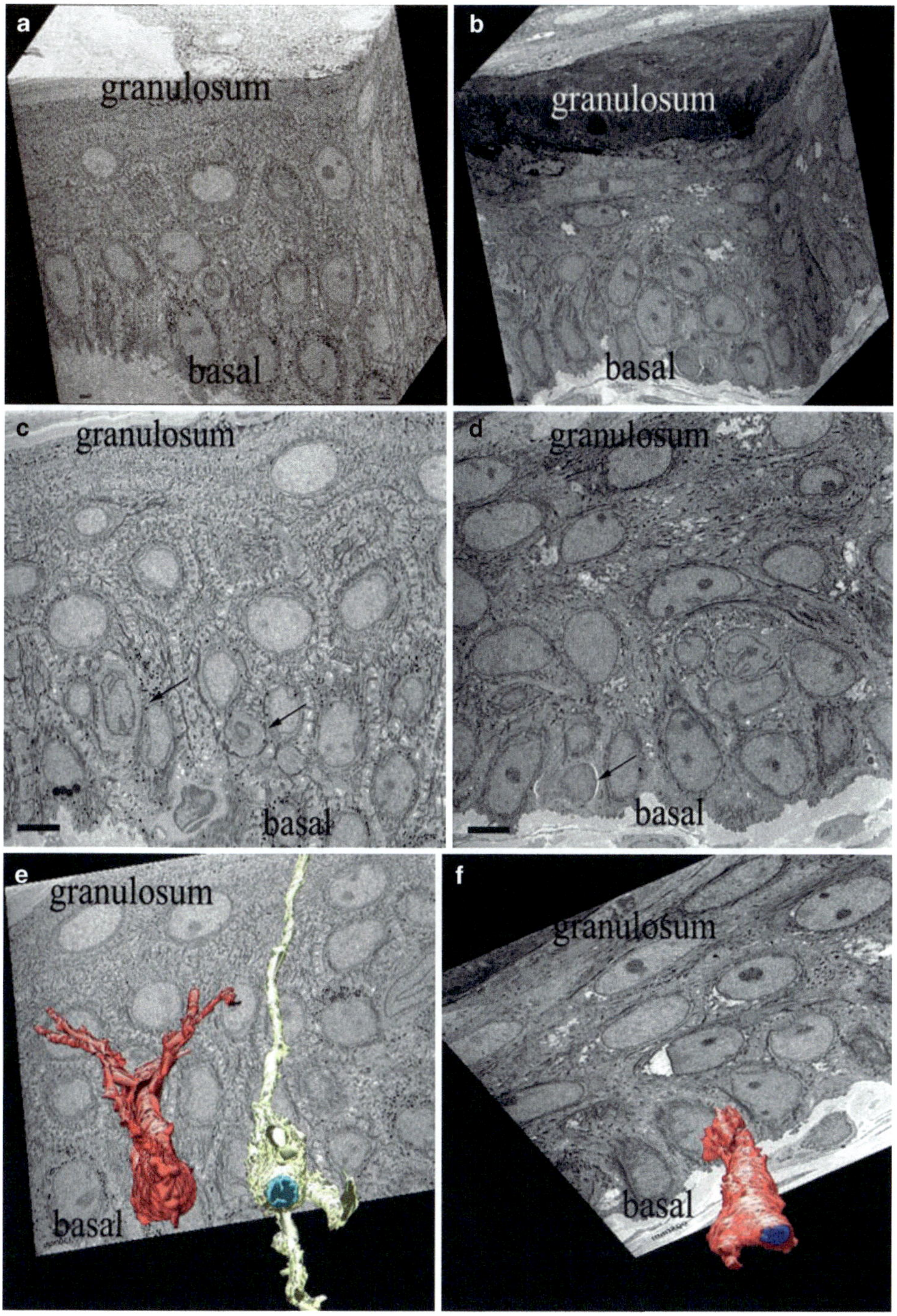

Fig. 18.3 3D structures of melanocytes in the epidermis layer of melasma patients. (**a**), (**c**), and (**e**) Images of prelaser treatment and (**b**), (**d**), and (**f**) images of post-laser treatment. 3D volume of over 500 serial images using 3VIEW was showed by IMOD (**a** and **b**). (**c**) and (**d**) One of the serial images for 3D reconstruction of (**e**) and (**f**). Arrows of (**c**) and (**d**) show the reconstructed melanocytes in (**e**) and (**f**). The size bar of (**c**) and (**d**) is 5 μm. The images (**e**) and (**f**) show the surface model of melanocytes showing cell body and their dendrites. Each nucleus was assigned a separate color (**e**, cyan blue; **f**, blue). Melanocytes in melasma patient have many dendrites and stretch from basal layer to granulosum layer (**e**). After laser toning treatment, the 3D structure of melanocytes contained fewer dendrites (**f**). Reproduced from [16]

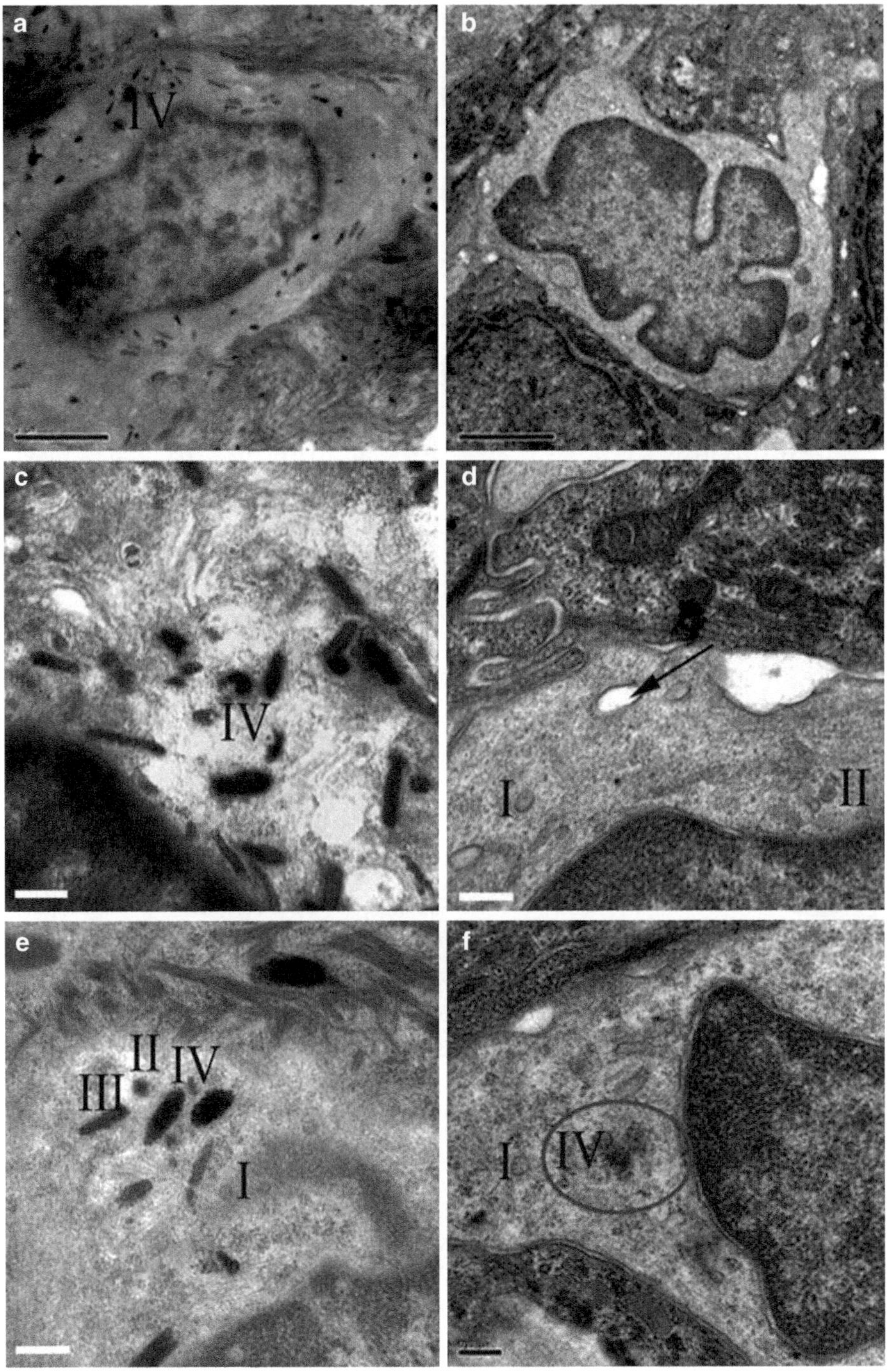

Fig. 18.4 Transmission electron microscopy images of melanosomes in melanocytes of melasma patient. The image of melanocyte from a melasma patient (**a**, **c**, **e**) and that after post-laser treatment (**b**, **d**, **f**) were compared for investigation of the ultrastructural change of melanosome after laser treatment. Melanocytes in melasma patients without laser treatment have many melanosomes (**a**, **c**, **e**). After laser toning treatment, the melanocytes had far fewer melanosomes (**b**, **d**, **f**) and remnant (**d**) and lysed form (**f**) of Stage IV melanosome in melanocyte was observed. Arrow of (**d**) shows the remnant of Stage IV melanosome. Lysed Stage IV melanosome was represented as circle in (**f**). However, melanosomes in the early stage like Stages I and II were observed without any change (**d**, **f**). The size bar of (**a**) and (**b**) is 2 μm and that of (**c**–**f**) is 0.2 μm. Reproduced from [16]

broken by laser toning do not disappear out of the cell but remain broken inside the keratinocytes or melanocytes. When the melanin breaks up and spreads, it appears bright microscopically, but the overall amount of melanin remains unchanged. In other words, there is no big difference when seen with eyes. This is the reason we cannot clinically observe immediate brightening after laser toning. I think dendrectomy prevents melanocytes from delivering melanosomes to the keratinocytes for at least 2 weeks, so during the epidermal turnover, melanosome-free keratinocytes develop and the face brightens. This is the reason why laser toning doesn't immediately improve melasma, but brightens the face after 4 weeks, after an epidermal turnover.

One more thing to mention is that many think that laser toning only damages melanosomes in melanocytes. However, most melanosomes are in keratinocytes, and melanocytes have mature melanosomes in their dendrites, which disappear after dendrectomy while immature melanosomes (stage I, II) are not affected by laser toning, i.e., the melanocytes do not become brighter or disappear. Therefore, laser toning not only improves the appearance of melasma but also brightens the overall tone of the face.

Kim et al. observed changes before and after laser toning through histopathological examination [17]. Compared with nonlesional skin, samples from melasma lesions showed increased reactivity in melanin and in melanogenesis-associated proteins, including α-melanocyte-stimulating hormone (α-MSH), tyrosinase, tyrosinase-related protein (TRP)-1, TRP-2, nerve growth factor (NGF), and stem cell factor (SCF). After laser treatment, the melasma skin showed a decrease in the number of melanosomes and reduced expression of melanogenesis-associated proteins.

This paper shows that laser toning reduces the proteins involved in melanogenesis. In other words, laser toning does not simply break melanosomes, but inhibits melanin synthesis, which is not permanent, but melanin production temporarily stops, resulting in brightening.

Based on the two papers above, the brightening effect of laser toning is due to first, inhibition of melanin synthesis and second, by blocking the transmission of melanosome.

However, laser toning does not block all stages of melanogenesis and signaling pathways, so laser toning alone does not improve all melasma. Also, if other steps can be blocked in a different way, better results may be achieved (Fig. 18.2). For example, it will be important to apply sunscreen well so that it can block between UV rays and keratinocyte. A tranexamic acid that can block between keratinocyte and melanocyte will also help. Various procedures aimed at dermal fibroblasts to improve the dermis will also be helpful.

18.8 Effective Therapy

After analyzing several histological papers on melasma and the causes of melasma, I think the probable mechanism of melasma is as follows [18].

> In patients with genetically or hormonally sensitive skin, inflammation may be caused by chronic irritation, such as UV rays or cosmetics, this may break the epidermal barrier, resulting in damaged basement membrane and inflammation in the dermis. In order to protect the damaged skin, pigmentations appear on the epidermal layer, thus melasma occurs.

Therefore, I think the following methods may be helpful in treating melasma (Table 18.2):

First, because we do not know 100% of the causes of melasma, we cannot treat melasma 100%. But if the patient takes birth control pills, switching them to low-dose estrogen contraceptives (e.g., Yaz®) may be helpful. Also, causative treatment such as avoiding chronic irritation (e.g., cosmetics) and thorough sun protection is most important for melasma treatment (behavior modification therapy).

Second, the damaged skin needs to be repaired. The epidermal layer will benefit from moisturizers and iontophoresis. The basement membrane will benefit from less irritating peeling such as 50% glycolic acid (GA) and genesis technique. To improve the dermis, nonablative lasers, genesis technique, and intradermal injections of hyaluronic acid, also known as "injectable glow" may be helpful.

Table 18.2 Probable causes and effective therapy of melasma. Reproduced from [18]

Etiologies—genetics, hormone, UV, cosmetics, etc.
1. Epidermal barrier dysfunction—Moisturizer, iontophoresis
2. Basement membrane disruption—Superficial peeling (50% GA), genesis technique
3. Dermal inflammation—Nonablative rejuvenation, genesis technique, "injectable glow"
4. Hyperpigmentation
1. Decrease the activity of melanocyte—Laser toning
2. Inhibit melanosome formation—Tranexamic acid, vit C, glabridin
3. Promote melanosome degradation
I. Epidermal melanin removal—Laser toning, 755-nm long-pulsed laser
II. Dermal melanin removal—1064-nm Q-switched laser

Third, to reduce the activity of melanocytes, laser toning is performed which has an effect of dendrectomy on melanocytes. Topical whitening medications to prevent melanin production may be helpful. Tranexamic acid, ascorbic acid (vitamin C), glabridin, and niacinamide are economical without side effects.

Finally, pigmentation that is already on the skin is regarded as the pigmentation itself and removed with a pigmentation laser. However, because the laser may worsen melasma, an appropriate laser with no side effects should be chosen, and the energy should be weak. I use laser toning and 755 nm long-pulsed alexandrite laser for epidermal melasma (refer to Sect. 2.8 in Chap. 2). Laser toning is performed on the whole face with a PTP mode of 2.1–2.5 J/cm^2, and then one shot toning is performed at 4 J/cm^2 or less (refer to Sect. 5.4 in Chap. 5). The energy used for epidermal pigmentations in long-pulsed alexandrite lasers is usually 16–20 J/cm^2, but I use 8–10 J/cm^2 in the treatment of melasma, and I consider the clinical end point as delayed perilesional erythema which occurs usually when patients are finished with their face pack and ready to go home (refer to Sect. 10.7 in Chap. 10). Pigmentations that still persist even after prolonged epidermal melasma treatment, or pigmentations that are gray or blue are considered dermal melasma and can be treated by 1064 nm Q-switched Nd:YAG laser by increasing the energy, similar to tattoo treatment.

18.9 Advices on Melasma Treatment

I have been treating melasma for over 15 years and learned a lot through trial and error. The following is a list of advices that may be helpful to those who are new to melasma treatment [19].

First, when a melasma patient first visits, you should check what treatment has been attempted before. You should also ask if the treatment was effective or if there were any side effects. If there were no side effects and it was effective, and only the recurrence is the problem then the same procedure may be repeated. But if there were side effects, treatment changes should be considered. For example, if laser toning has been performed in the past and mottled hypopigmentation has occurred, then laser toning should not be attempted again, and it can be expected that it will not easily improve with conventional melasma treatment.

Second, you should not tell patients that melasma can be cured 100%. Despite all the melasma treatments, including behavioral therapy, medication, and laser treatment, melasma cannot be treated 100%. In addition, multiple repeated treatments are required. Recently I think that laser toning should be performed 20–30 times instead of 10 times when treating dermal melasma.

Third, the emphasis should not be on brightening the entire face, but on improving the dark pigmentation to match the overall face tone. This applies to all pigmentation treatments, including melasma. It is not easy to brighten the tone of the whole face. It is easier to make dark lentigines or melasma lighter, and this also has fewer side effects.

Fourth, combination treatments are needed. There are many causes and mechanisms of melasma, and there is no single treatment for melasma. However, as explained above, the underlying mechanism of each treatment should be considered so that the mechanism does not overlap.

Fifth, not everyone responds the same to each treatment. Some patients may develop side effects. Therefore, the patient should be carefully monitored whenever treatment is performed to see if there are any signs of improvement or side effects.

Sixth, melasma recur. Therefore, a maintenance treatment should be prepared in advance. Prevention through behavioral therapy is also necessary, and sufficient consultation with the patient is needed in regard to dermal environment improvement and laser toning repetition.

References

1. Goldsmith LA, Katz SI, Gilchrest BA, Paller AS, Leffell DJ, Wolff K, et al. Fitzpatrick's dermatology in general medicine. New York: McGraw-Hill Professional; 2012.
2. Rodrigues M, Pandya AG. Melasma: clinical diagnosis and management options. Australas J Dermatol. 2015;56(3):151–63.
3. Negishi K, Kushikata N, Tezuka Y, Takeuchi K, Miyamoto E, Wakamatsu S. Study of the incidence and nature of "very subtle epidermal melasma" in relation to intense pulsed light treatment. Dermatol Surg. 2004;30(6):881–6. discussion 6
4. Choi CP, Yim SM, Seo SH, Ahn HH, Kye YC, Choi JE. Retreatment using a dual mode of low-fluence Q-switched and long-pulse Nd:YAG laser in patients with melasma aggravation after previous therapy. J Cosmet Laser Ther. 2015;17(3):129–34.
5. Wattanakrai P, Mornchan R, Eimpunth S. Low-fluence Q-switched neodymium-doped yttrium aluminum garnet (1,064 nm) laser for the treatment of facial melasma in Asians. Dermatol Surg. 2010;36(1):76–87.
6. Lee WJ, Kim YJ, Noh TK, Chang SE. Formation of new melasma lesions in the periorbital area following high-fluence, 1064-nm, Q-switched Nd/YAG laser. J Cosmet Laser Ther. 2013;15(3):163–5.
7. Kang S, Fitzpatrick TB. Fitzpatrick's dermatology. New York: McGraw-Hill Education; 2019.
8. Kang HY, Bahadoran P, Suzuki I, Zugaj D, Khemis A, Passeron T, et al. In vivo reflectance confocal microscopy detects pigmentary changes in melasma at a cellular level resolution. Exp Dermatol. 2010;19(8):e228–33.
9. Kang WH, Yoon KH, Lee ES, Kim J, Lee KB, Yim H, et al. Melasma: histopathological characteristics in 56 Korean patients. Br J Dermatol. 2002;146(2):228–37.
10. Textbook compilation committee in Korean Dermatological Association. Text book of dermatology 6th edition (Korean). Seoul: Daehanuihak; 2014.
11. Bolognia J, Schaffer JV, Cerroni L. Dermatology: Elsevier; 2018.
12. Shankar K, Godse K, Aurangabadkar S, Lahiri K, Mysore V, Ganjoo A, et al. Evidence-based treatment for melasma: expert opinion and a review. Dermatol Ther (Heidelb). 2014;4(2):165–86.
13. Yamaguchi Y, Brenner M, Hearing VJ. The regulation of skin pigmentation. J Biol Chem. 2007;282(38):27557–61.
14. Kondo T, Hearing VJ. Update on the regulation of mammalian melanocyte function and skin pigmentation. Expert Rev Dermatol. 2011;6(1):97–108.
15. Passeron T, Picardo M. Melasma, a photoaging disorder. Pigment Cell Melanoma Res. 2018;31(4):461–5.
16. Mun JY, Jeong SY, Kim JH, Han SS, Kim IH. A low fluence Q-switched Nd:YAG laser modifies the 3D structure of melanocyte and ultrastructure of melanosome by subcellular-selective photothermolysis. J Electron Microsc. 2011;60(1):11–8.
17. Kim JE, Chang SE, Yeo UC, Haw S, Kim IH. Histopathological study of the treatment of melasma lesions using a low-fluence Q-switched 1064-nm neodymium:yttrium-aluminium-garnet laser. Clin Exp Dermatol. 2013;38(2):167–71.
18. Lee JD, Lee JK, Oh MJM. Principles and choice of laser treatment in dermatology. Singapore: Springer; 2020.
19. Trivedi MK, Yang FC, Cho BK. A review of laser and light therapy in melasma. Int J Womens Dermatol. 2017;3(1):11–20.

Part VI

Side Effects and Complications of Lasers

19 Pathogenesis and Treatment of Post-Inflammatory Hyperpigmentation (PIH)

19.1 Overview of PIH

The definition of PIH is "a common condition caused by numerous preceding cutaneous insults" [1]. Causes include drug reactions, phototoxicity reactions, inflammation, physical irritation or damage, allergic reactions, and inflammation diseases. Diagnosis of PIH is made when there is a hyperpigmented patch in the area of inflammation. PIH is prevalent and lasts longer in darker skin types (Fitzpatrick skin types III ~ VI). Wood's lamps can be used to distinguish epidermal and dermal PIH. Biopsy reveals "pigment incontinence" (epidermal pigment falling into the dermis, where they do not belong) and "melanophages" (melanocytes falling into the dermis or macrophages phagocytosing dermal pigments). Melanin is increased in both the epidermis and the dermis. Treatment of PIH is difficult but spontaneous resolution is possible for epidermal PIH.

19.2 Epidemiology and Possible Etiology of PIH

PIH can occur at any age and in any skin types, and there is no difference in the incidence of men and women. However, it occurs more often in Fitzpatrick skin types IV, V, and VI. This may be due to "hyperactive melanocyte," which are found in patients with darker skin types, which cause hypersensitivity to the same inflammation [2].

In summary, PIH occurs frequently in Koreans with Fitzpatrick skin types IV and V. Hyperactive melanocytes which are also the cause of melasma are considered to be a fundamental problem of PIH.

19.3 Predicting PIH Occurrence

Since laser is also one of the underlying causes of PIH, people with a higher likelihood of PIH should be careful when using lasers. Is there a way to predict PIH occurrence in patients before laser treatment?

First, Fitzpatrick skin types IV and V can be distinguished through a questionnaire. For example, if you answer "No" to the question "Does your skin tan in summer?," your skin type is I, II, III. If you answer "Yes" to that question, the next question will be "Does it turn red and then black? (skin type IV), Or does it become black right away? (skin type V)." Second, find out if any PIH has already occurred on the patient's skin. If the patient already has PIH, there is a higher likelihood of PIH after laser treatment [3]. Third, if the skin tone of finger joints is darker than the surrounding skin, the probability of developing PIH is known to be high [3] (Fig. 19.1). Fourth, if the

J. D. Lee, M. J. M. Oh, *Lasers in Dermatology: Parameters and Choice*,
https://doi.org/10.1007/978-981-19-7568-4_19

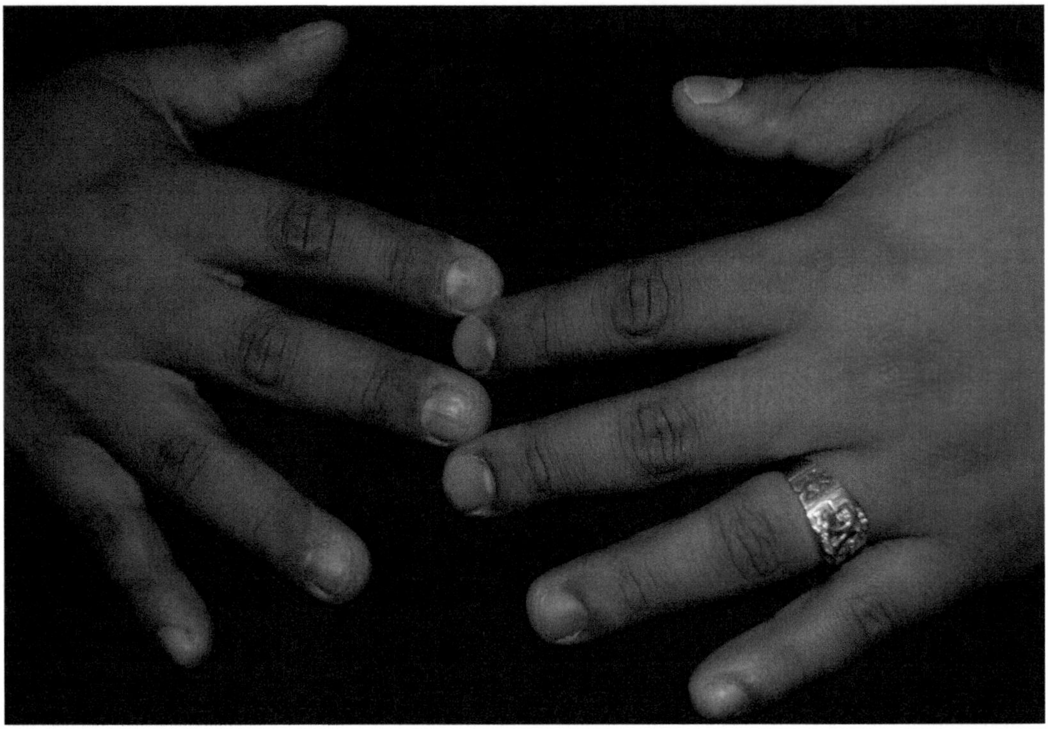

Fig. 19.1 Pigmentation observed in the finger joints of a 24-year-old male patient

patient's skin seems dark to the laser physician, then PIH is more likely [4]. Care should be taken when performing laser procedures on these patients.

Other prognostic factors of PIH are also being discussed. Kang et al. investigated PIH related factors in 516 Korean patients with solar lentigines treated with 532 nm Q-switched Nd:YAG lasers [5]. The overall incidence of PIH was 20.3% (105/516 patients). Patients with erythematous lentigines presented with PIH more frequently compared with those without erythematous lentigines. And facial diffuse dyschromia such as melasma, freckles, photoaging-associated mottled pigmentation was significantly associated with PIH. Furthermore, PIH occurred more frequently in patients with invisible pores and velvety skin (Table 19.1). However, age, sex, and especially Fitzpatrick skin type and season of treatment showed little association with PIH.

Table 19.1 Predisposing factors of occurrence of PIH associated with treatment of solar lentigines using a Q-switched 532-nm Nd:YAG laser [5]

Predisposing factors of occurrence of PIH associated with treatment of 516 patients with solar lentigines using a Q-switched 532-nm Nd:YAG laser
1. Invisible pore (velvety skin)
2. Erythema on lentigo
3. Facial diffuse dyschromia (e.g. melasma)

19.4 Prognostic Factors of PIH and Chromatic Tendency

The degree of PIH is known to vary depending on the color of the skin, degree and depth of inflammation, degree of damage to the dermoepidermal junction, inflammatory state, and the stability of melanocytes. Takiwaki et al. reported that erythema and melanin index are directly proportional. That is, the more severe erythema, the darker the PIH [6].

Ruiz-Maldonado and Orozco-Covarrubias suggested the "individual chromatic tendency" hypothesis [7]. Individuals tend to have different pigmentation tendencies. Depending on the unique characteristics of the individual's melanocytes, after skin inflammation or injury, melanin production could be high, low, or normal. This is genetically determined and is not related to the patient's skin type.

Then how can we reduce PIH? First, inflammation should be prevented during laser procedure, and procedures that do not damage the dermo-epidermal junction should be performed. And if inflammation develops, it should be quickly dealt with. In particular, severe erythema is a red flag of PIH. Therefore, if there is severe erythema after laser treatment, active actions should be taken. Despite these actions, PIH may occur because individuals tend to have different pigmentation development tendencies. Therefore, patients should be informed in advance of the possibility of developing PIH, and PIH should be treated safely for faster resolution.

19.5 Prognosis of PIH

Epidermal PIH disappears after 6–12 months, but it may take several years for dermal PIH resolution. PIH recovery time differs by site, in which the PIH of the face usually disappear after 6 months, while PIH of the body or upper limbs lasts 1–2 years, and the lower limb 3–4 years [3]. However, if the underlying cause is not resolved and inflammation persists, new PIH may occur even if the existing PIH disappears. This is why it is important to find and resolve the underlying cause of inflammation.

19.6 Pathogenesis of PIH

PIH may be seen as the skin's "normal response" to inflammatory stimuli [6]. In other words, it may be thought of as a normal process in which pigmentations are produced to protect the post-inflammatory damaged skin from UV rays. What is the specific pathogenesis of PIH?

The following is the summary of the PIH pathogenesis in various papers, that I summarized. I would like to notify in advance that the mechanism for PIH has not yet been fully understood and there are many controversial issues.

First, due to the inflammatory response of the epidermal layer, arachidonic acid is secreted and oxidized to produce cytokines such as prostaglandin (PG) and leukotriene (LT). In vitro studies have shown that leukotriene C_4, leukotriene D_4, prostaglandin E_2, histamine, and thromboxane B_2 have properties that stimulate melanocytes [7]. These cytokines increase the activity of melanocytes and immune cells, increasing melanin synthesis and increasing melanin delivery to surrounding keratinocytes [9]. Arachidonic acid is present in the cell membrane (Fig. 19.2).

Second, the basement membrane is destroyed due to inflammation. Melanocytes or keratinocytes with melanin in the basal layer drop to the upper dermis [9] and is phagocytosed by macrophages. The phenomenon in which melanin, which should not be present in dermis, is found in dermis, is called "pigment incontinence."

Third, keratinocytes, fibroblasts, endothelial cells, and inflammatory cells crosstalk with each other to regulate pigmentations. In other words, the epidermis and the dermis interact with each other to regulate pigmentations. For example, treatment with a very high-power Q-switched laser in nanoseconds results in photothermal and photomechanical effects on melanin. Undesired effects also take place: superficial vessels are damaged and inflammatory mediators from vascular endothelial cells and inflammatory cells crosstalk to activate melanocytes. An important inflammatory mediator from endothelial cells is nitric oxide (NO). NO is known to induce and enhance melanin formation after UV exposure [3]. In addition, PIH after purpura by vascular lasers, is known to be associated with hemosiderin infiltration.

The three pathophysiology of PIH are summarized below, by location (Table 19.2).

Phenomena that take place during laser treatment occur in the microscopic environment. Then how does PIH occur in this microscopic

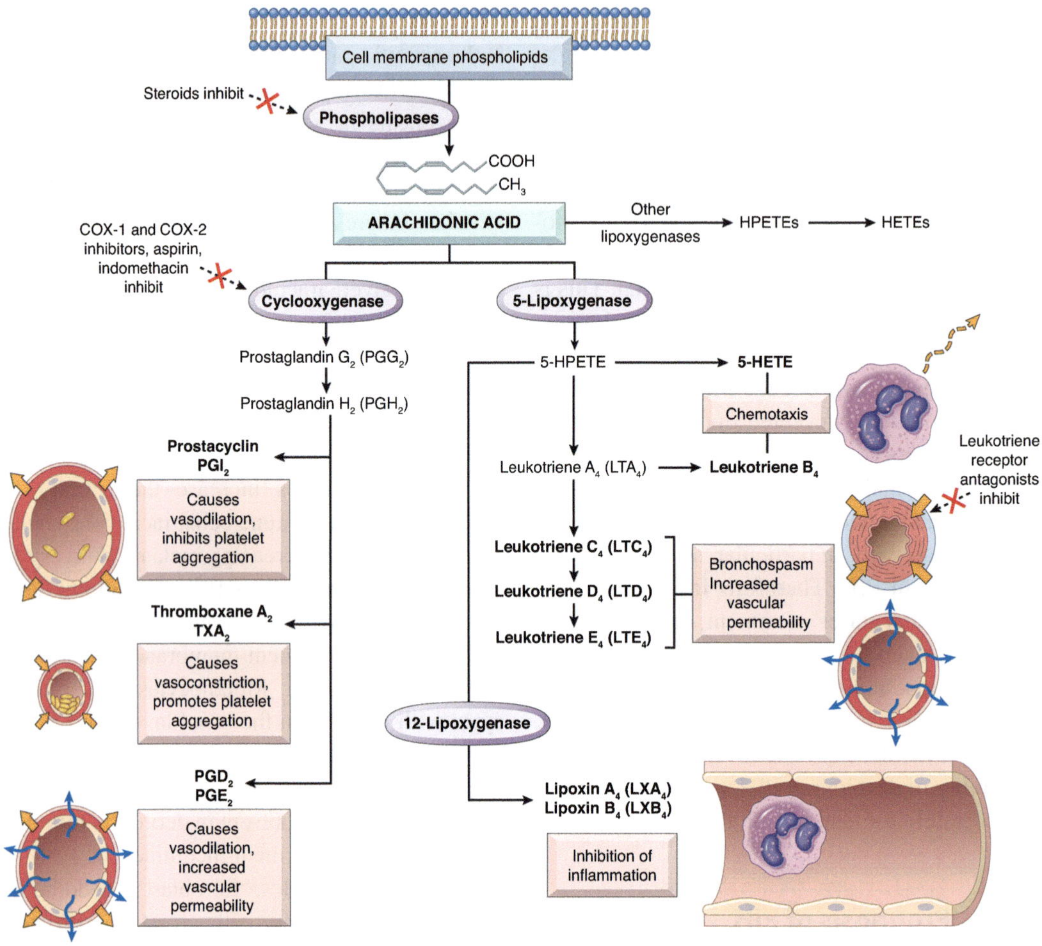

Fig. 19.2 Production of arachidonic acid metabolites and their roles in inflammation. Note the enzymatic activities whose inhibition through pharmacologic intervention blocks major pathways (denoted with a red X). COX-1, COX-2, Cyclooxygenase 1 and 2; HETE, hydroxyeicosatetraenoic acid; HPETE, hydroperoxyeicosatetraenoic acid. Reproduced from [8]

Table 19.2 Pathophysiology of PIH by location. PG: prostaglandin, LT: leutotriene, NO: nitric oxide

Pathophysiology of PIH	Location
1. Release and oxidation of arachidonic acid to PG and LT	Cell membrane
2. Pigment incontinence	Dermoepidermal junction
3. NO from endothelial cells, hemosiderin	Vessels

environment? For example, let's think about pigmentation treatment with a Q-switched laser. When the temperature of melanin rises sharply by a Q-switched laser, an explosion (shock wave) occurs in the melanosomes. The explosion itself and the melanosome fragments broken by the explosion both break the nucleus and the cell membrane (first cause of PIH). If the explosive force is stronger, the dermoepidermal junction below the basal layer is destroyed, resulting in keratinocytes with melanosomes or melanocytes dropping to the dermis (second cause of PIH). If the explosive force is much stronger, this will lead to the destruction of blood vessels in the upper dermis, leading to the release of NO and hemosiderin (third cause of PIH).

So how can we reduce PIH during laser treatment? First, less explosive force should be used to reduce surrounding damage. At first, low energy should be used, and if it isn't effective, it should be raised gradually. Second, long-pulsed lasers are safer than Q-switched lasers. I think if we coagulate the cells (coagulation of photothermal effect) without breaking them (shockwave of photomechanical effect), less arachidonic acid may be released. Third, the basal layer and the dermoepidermal junction should be strengthened. I think the Genesis technique strengthens the basal layer and dermoepidermal junction. The Genesis technique will be discussed in detail in "Chap. 7." Fourth, purpura should be avoided during vascular treatment, and procedures that reduce flushing or telangiectasia should be added. Finally, procedures that may cause skin irritation should be avoided.

Out of these three, what is most common pathogenesis for PIH? I think the first cause of PIH (breaking of cell membranes) is the most common mechanism because it occurs first. Therefore, avoiding high energy or procedures that may break cell membranes are the most important preventive measures in reducing PIH.

19.7 Treatment of Post-Laser PIH

PIH treatment can be divided into three by treatment period. First, prevention. Second, treatment of the underlying inflammatory condition [6]. Third, treatment of PIH itself (Table 19.3).

First, PIH prevention. We will not discuss details here because this has been described above, and all throughout this book I will explain which lasers and which parameters to choose.

Second, treatment of the underlying inflammatory condition is needed. Because there are a number of underlying causes, appropriate treatment according to the underlying cause should be taken [10]. For example, in the case of acne, the treatment of inflammation of acne should first proceed. In particular, the underlying cause of PIH we are interested in is side effects after laser procedure. If PIH developed after the laser procedure, then the same laser procedure should not be repeated. If there is remnant inflammation or a possibility of developing PIH, the inflammation should be reduced as soon as possible.

Table 19.3 Treatment of PIH by time

Treatment of PIH
1. Prevention
2. Treatment of the underlying inflammatory condition
3. Treatment of PIH itself

The best medication for inflammation in the skin is steroids. Steroids are known to help restore and protect epidermal barrier function by minimizing inflammation and protecting the skin in the inflammatory stage of wound healing process. Also, steroids theoretically inhibit the release of prostaglandin (PG) and leukotriene (LT) derived from arachidonic acid. In other words, steroid suppresses the first cause of PIH described above.

Cheyasak et al. treated 40 subjects with atrophic acne scars with an ablative fractional laser on both sides of the face. Post-operatively, clobetasol propionate 0.05% ointment (group 1 steroid) was applied to one randomly selected side of the face for the first 2 days, followed by an application of petrolatum jelly for the rest of the week. Petrolatum was applied to the other side for 7 days [11]. The side of the face treated with petrolatum alone had statistically significantly higher incidence of PIH (75%) after laser irradiation than the side of the face treated with topical corticosteroids and petrolatum (40%). The PIH occurring on the petrolatum-treated sides had significantly higher intensity and was spread over a significantly larger area, compared with the corticosteroid and petrolatum treated sides. In conclusion, a short-term application of topical corticosteroids postoperatively is associated with a decreased risk of PIH after laser procedure.

But there are many concerns about the use of steroids. Cheyasak et al. the author of this paper addresses these concerns as follows. First, there is concern that the anti-proliferative effects of steroids may interfere with fibroblast activity and prevent new collagen formation, thus preventing scar improvement. But after 12 weeks, there was no difference in scar improvement between the two groups. Second, steroids may cause acneiform eruptions, but this is less likely because steroids were used short-term, for only 2 days.

Third, postoperative infection occurred in two patients, but in these cases, the fractional coverage was increased by more than 80%. Higher coverage seems to be the cause rather than steroid use.

Based on this paper, I give a small amount of group 1 steroids to patients with strong or long-lasting erythema after laser treatment and tell them to apply this generously three times a day for 2 days.

Third, treatment of PIH itself. This can be divided into two phases, "inflammatory phase" and "non-inflammatory phase" depending on active inflammation. First, in "inflammatory phase" there is active inflammation. For example, acne is still active and PIH is accompanied by inflammation. In this case, as in the second PIH treatment described above, acne treatment and inflammation treatment should be given priority. And since the primary cause of PIH is hyperactive melanocytes, I think that the rest of PIH treatment is the same as melasma treatment. For example, it is possible to apply the so-called laser toning to reduce the activity of melanocytes and eliminate melanosomes without side effects.

In "non-inflammatory phase" inflammation is completely reduced and there is no erythema. This is a very interesting period. PIH is caused by "temporarily" increased activity of melanocytes due to an underlying cause of inflammation. However, if there is no underlying cause of inflammation and if there is no active inflammation, then the melanocyte activity will be reduced, unlike melasma. I consider PIH in this phase as pigmentations, and pigmentation treatment is possible. Stronger laser toning, long-pulsed alexandrite laser, or even IPL may be used to treat this PIH. Various other whitening agents and chemical peels may be of help.

For reference, Winhoven et al. reported a case in which a 23-year-old woman with acne and severe PIH took isotretinoin which resulted in dramatic improvement of acne and PIH [12]. Although the paper above is just a case report, I too often observe significant improvement in PIH in acne patients taking isotretinoin at low doses (10–20 mg/day).

19.8 Conclusion

PIH after laser treatment is troublesome and difficult for both patients and doctors. PIH prevention should first be taken into account. If post-laser PIH risk seems high, it is most important to get proper treatment as soon as possible. However, once PIH occurs, it does not disappear easily. I also went through many difficult situations due to PIH.

Finally, for physicians in trouble because of PIH, I would like to recommend "time," the most important method. Some say that dermal PIH may not go away, but most PIHs will go away because they are mostly epidermal. This is the biggest difference between melasma and PIH. In addition, in melasma it is hard to know the exact cause, so there is no fundamental treatment. But PIH disappears when the temporary underlying cause (inflammation) disappears. The only question is when it will go away. Therefore, if you persuade your patient and take enough time to treat PIH, PIH will disappear.

Remember, "Time is on our side!"

References

1. Goldsmith LA, Katz SI, Gilchrest BA, Paller AS, Leffell DJ, Wolff K, et al. Fitzpatrick's dermatology in general medicine. New York: McGraw-Hill Professional; 2012.
2. Callender VD, St Surin-Lord S, Davis EC, Maclin M. Postinflammatory hyperpigmentation: etiologic and therapeutic considerations. Am J Clin Dermatol. 2011;12(2):87–99.
3. Committee C, Chun S, Kim IH, Kang JS, Park SH, Chung KY, et al. Laser and light treatment in Asian skin. Paju: Koonja; 2016.
4. Lee JD, Lee JK, Oh MJM. Principles and choice of laser treatment in dermatology. Singapore: Springer; 2020.
5. Kang HJ, Na JI, Lee JH, Roh MR, Ko JY, Chang SE. Postinflammatory hyperpigmentation associated with treatment of solar lentigines using a Q-switched 532-nm Nd: YAG laser: a multicenter survey. J Dermatolog Treat. 2017;28(5):447–51.
6. Eimpunth S, Wanitphadeedecha R, Manuskiatti W. A focused review on acne-induced and aesthetic procedure-related postinflammatory hyperpigmentation in Asians. J Eur Acad Dermatol Venereol. 2013;27(Suppl 1):7–18.

7. Silpa-Archa N, Kohli I, Chaowattanapanit S, Lim HW, Hamzavi I. Postinflammatory hyperpigmentation: a comprehensive overview: epidemiology, pathogenesis, clinical presentation, and noninvasive assessment technique. J Am Acad Dermatol. 2017;77(4):591–605.
8. Kumar V, Abbas AK, Aster JC, Robbins SL, Cotran RS. Robbins and Cotran pathologic basis of disease. Philadelphia, PA: Elsevier; 2014.
9. Lacz NL, Vafaie J, Kihiczak NI, Schwartz RA. Postinflammatory hyperpigmentation: a common but troubling condition. Int J Dermatol. 2004;43(5):362–5.
10. Davis EC, Callender VD. Postinflammatory hyperpigmentation: a review of the epidemiology, clinical features, and treatment options in skin of color. J Clin Aesthet Dermatol. 2010;3(7):20–31.
11. Cheyasak N, Manuskiatti W, Maneeprasopchoke P, Wanitphakdeedecha R. Topical corticosteroids minimise the risk of postinflammatory hyper-pigmentation after ablative fractional CO2 laser resurfacing in Asians. Acta Derm Venereol. 2015;95(2):201–5.
12. Winhoven SM, Ahmed I, Owen CM, Lear JT. Postinflammatory hyperpigmentation in an Asian patient: a dramatic response to oral isotretinoin (13-cis-retinoic acid). Br J Dermatol. 2005;152(2):368–9.

20 Complications and Management of Laser Therapy

20.1 Side Effects and Complications

Before we get into the laser's side effect and complication, let's start with the terminology. A side effect is a phenomenon that is directly related to a particular procedure itself and is expected to occur outside of the main effect. For example, purpura that occurs after a PDL laser and pinpoint bleeding or crusting that occurs after a Q-switched laser [1]. It is usually temporary and self-limited. A complication or adverse event is an undesirable and unexpected phenomenon that occurs after a particular procedure [2]. Complication is important because proper diagnosis and treatment are required [1]. For a practitioner who starts a laser for the first time, it is difficult to differentiate between side effects and complication. That's why when first buying a laser, I recommend that the practitioner himself or his or her family first try the laser and then observe and write down the skin reactions that change over time from day to day.

Complication can be divided into mild, intermediate, and severe depending on the severity (Table 20.1). Minor complications are complications that are relatively easy to treat, such as acne, milia, purpura, and urticaria. Intermediate complications are complications that are not easily treated, such as PIH, hypopigmentation, crusting, blistering, line of demarcation, paradoxical hypertrichosis, prolonged post-laser resurfacing, etc. Major complications are complications that cannot be completely treated, such as scarring, indentation, infection, sensory nerve injury, etc., and should be avoided because of the sequelae.

Table 20.1 Complication of lasers [3, 4]

Minor complications	Intermediate complications	Major complications
Acne/milia Acneiform eruption Purpura Urticaria Recall phenomenon	Hyperpigmentation (PIH) Hypopigmentation Crusting/vesiculation or blistering Line of demarcation Paradoxical hypertrichosis Prolonged post-laser resurfacing erythema Burn Textural imperfection Delayed reepithelialization	Scarring Indentation Infections (bacterial, viral, yeast) Sensory nerve injury Ocular damage

J. D. Lee, M. J. M. Oh, *Lasers in Dermatology: Parameters and Choice*,
https://doi.org/10.1007/978-981-19-7568-4_20

20.2 Side Effects

20.2.1 Erythema

Side effects of laser include erythema, edema, purpura, pain, crusting, and oozing, but in this book, we will only look at erythema.

Erythema is a phenomenon caused by heat scattering and can occur in any laser procedure, and the erythema that occurs after a nonablative laser procedure usually disappears within 24 hours [3]. However, the erythema that occurs after an ablative laser procedure often persists from weeks to months [3]. Erythema frequently occurs especially in periorbital areas. In addition, erythema occurs more in fair skins than in dark skins and occurs more if there is a history of rosacea, plethoric skin, or if the patient has stated that they have sensitive skin [4], or if topical tretinoin is applied prior to the procedure [2].

Perifollicular erythema and edema occur after laser hair removal, which usually disappear within a few hours [3]. If erythema persists for more than 24 hours after epilation, I consider it a warning end point and recommend that the patient visit the hospital immediately.

The treatment of erythema usually does not require any special treatment other than reassurance of the patient [5]. To quickly relieve erythema, icepacks, oral steroids, and topical steroids can help [3]. Topical ascorbic acid can also help reduce the strength and duration of erythema after ablative rejuvenation [2].

The erythema that occurs after a laser procedure usually isn't a big concern, but it should be considered a warning end point after pulse stacking, multiple passes, high energy, or inadequate cooling [2].

20.3 Important Complications

20.3.1 Acneiform Eruption

Acneiform eruption is a complication in which comedones are not observed and inflammatory lesions such as papules and pustules occur, either because of the procedure itself or because of the treatment after the procedure. The incidence varies from procedure to procedure, with an incidence of 3–15% for ablative rejuvenation [6] and 2–10% for fractional laser procedures [7]. This is a mild, self-limited complication. Acneiform eruption is also thought of as simple folliculitis, which appears as a wound healing response [6]. If acneiform eruption is severe, acne medications or methylprednisolone are used [7]. I prescribe doxycycline (50 mg bid) and methylprednisolone (4 mg qd) for 3 days.

20.3.2 Hypopigmentation

Hypopigmentation is a rarer complication than post inflammatory hyperpigmentation (PIH) and while it can be temporary, it can sometimes persist permanently. It is notorious for being hard to treat [3]. Hypopigmentation occurs most often after traditional ablative rejuvenation with CO_2 lasers, chemical peeling with phenol, deep mechanical peeling, and is known to occur well in patients with white porcelain-like appearance [4].

The mechanism is first, the complete destruction of melanocytes in the epidermis and hair follicles due to excessive thermal damage. And second, inflammation caused by laser procedures results in inhibiting melanin synthesis of melanocyte (malfunctioning melanocyte) [3].

Hypopigmentation can be divided into three types depending on the course. First, "relative" hypopigmentation. After treating solar lentigo or epidermal pigmentations with laser, the crusting drops or exfoliates and looks relatively whiter than the surrounding normal skin [3]. A representative example is the tiger print (footprint) that occurs after IPL (Fig. 20.1) [8]. Second, excessive energy or lack of cooling can cause "permanent" hypopigmentation if not only the melanosomes but also the melanocytes are damaged. Third, "delayed" hypopigmentation. This is the case when permanent hypopigmentation occurs 6–12 months after ablative rejuvenation [2]. Some authors believe that after ablative rejuvenation, a new collagen bundle is produced in the dermis, which reflects light, resulting in delayed hypopigmentation [3].

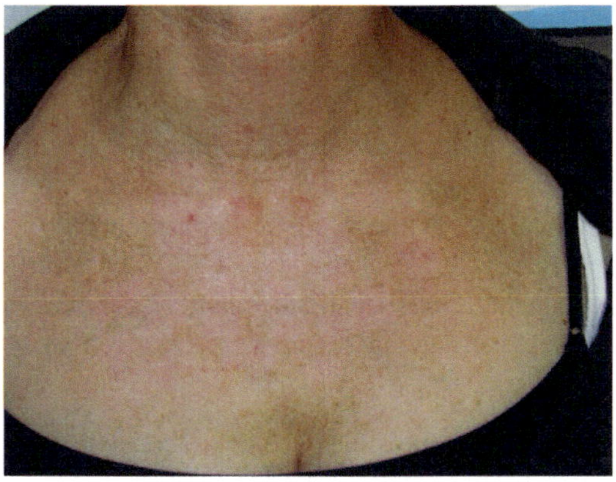

Fig. 20.1 Reticulated hypopigmentation after IPL treatment. This likely resulted from actinic bronzing that caused increased absorption of light. This is transient; with subsequent treatments the dyspigmentation will even out. Reproduced from [2]

The treatment of hypopigmentation includes phototherapy such as narrow-band UVB or excimer lasers, and there are some reports that fractional lasers are helpful [3]. However, because hypopigmentation is not easy to treat, we should not tell the patient that hypopigmentation will fully recover over time. It is psychologically better for the patient to have "the joy of partial improvement of hypopigmentation in an unexpected situation" than the disappointment that "the hypopigmentation is not fully recovered" [4].

20.3.3 Crusting and Vesiculation (Blistering)

Both crusting and blisters mean epidermal damage. Crusting occurs by suprabasal necrosis, and vesiculation or blistering occurs at the cleavage at the dermo-epidermal junction. This is caused by thermal damage and occurs when high fluence is used, when cooling fails, when pulse stacking or high repetition rate is performed, when the procedure is performed on a tanned patient, or when cosmetics are not well removed [3]. There is no specific treatment for crusting and blisters, only supportive therapy. OTC antibiotic ointments such as neomycin or bacitracin are not recommended because they can cause allergic contact dermatitis (ACD) and are less effective for wound healing than petrolatum [2]. For the treatment of crusting, periodic application of ointment based on petrolatum may help, as well as cleansing and not touching the affected area. For small blistering, if it has not already burst, the affected area should not be touched and should be covered with a non-adhesive dressing or drained with a disinfected needle followed by sterile dressing [3].

In the case of large blistering, there is concern that changes in skin color or skin texture during re-epithelialization will occur as the epithelium falls, but most of the time it is treated well without sequelae with only supportive therapy. However, other causes such as inflammation or vesicular diseases should be considered for differential diagnosis [4].

20.3.4 Paradoxical Darkening

Paradoxical darkening refers to the phenomenon in which a tattoo becomes darker after laser tattoo treatment. It is particularly common in white, skin-colored, pink, and red tattoos, and is known to occur in beauty tattoos such as makeup tattoos, which mainly uses these colors. The mechanism is due to the chemical transformation from red-toned ferric oxide (Fe_2O_3) to black ferrous oxide (FeO). In addition, titanium dioxide, which is used for white or bright color tattoos, is also known as the cause [9]. In this case, although laser is used to remove the tattoo, it turns darker, and the number of treatments increases, which puts both the patient and the doctor in a precarious situation. Therefore, before tattoo treatment, the patient should be informed that paradoxical darkening may occur.

Some laser texts recommend a test shot before tattoo treatment to prevent paradoxical darkening [9], but this is difficult to realistically perform in private practice. As a treatment for paradoxical darkening, ablative fractional lasers help. Although paradoxical darkening is generally accepted as a complication of laser treatment, one laser text considers paradoxical darkening as a part of treatment process for tattoos because if you continue laser treatment, the tattoo that turned darker eventually becomes lighter [10].

20.3.5 Paradoxical Hypertrichosis

The most confusing side effect of laser hair removal is paradoxical hypertrichosis (Fig. 20.2). Paradoxical hypertrichosis is the phenomenon in which hair increases after laser hair removal. Paradoxical hypertrichosis is known to occur in about 5% of the Mediterranean and Middle Eastern races and is usually permanent once they occur. This occurs on or near the area where laser removal procedure has been performed [9]. It usually affects the jaw line, cheeks, neck, shoulders, back, and upper arms, and is more likely to be closer to the torso than the treatment region [12]. It is more common in Fitzpatrick skin types III and IV, and in people whose forehead hairline is unclear [9]. Also, it may occur if the procedure interval is more than 8 weeks, pulse duration is short, or the wavelength or fluence is not appropriate (Table 20.2). Therefore, when performing laser hair removal of fine hair in the beard area in female patients, the patients should be informed in advance that paradoxical hypertrichosis is likely to occur and that multiple laser hair removal procedures may be needed [11].

The mechanism is not yet known, but it is suggested that subtherapeutic thermal injury to the follicular vasculature may induce an inflammatory response caused by heat, increasing blood flow, and increasing growth factor, resulting in thicker hair [11]. Low level laser therapy (LLLT) mechanism suggests that weak light rather stimulates hair follicles and leads them to the anagen phase, resulting in thicker hair [12].

Table 20.2 Factors associated with paradoxical hypertrichosis. Reproduced from [11]

Contributing Factors to Paradoxical Hypertrichosis
Thick hair
Dark hair color
Depth of treated hair—Superficial
Presence of underlying untreated hormonal conditions (polycystic ovarian syndrome)
Use of hormone supplements or medications (corticosteroids)
Presence of post-treatment side effects (crusting, erythema, edema, hyperpigmentation)
Suboptimal treatment fluences—Too low, yet enough energy to stimulate hair growth
Anatomic site (face and neck)
Sex (female; possibly because of sampling)
Darker skin types (III–VI)

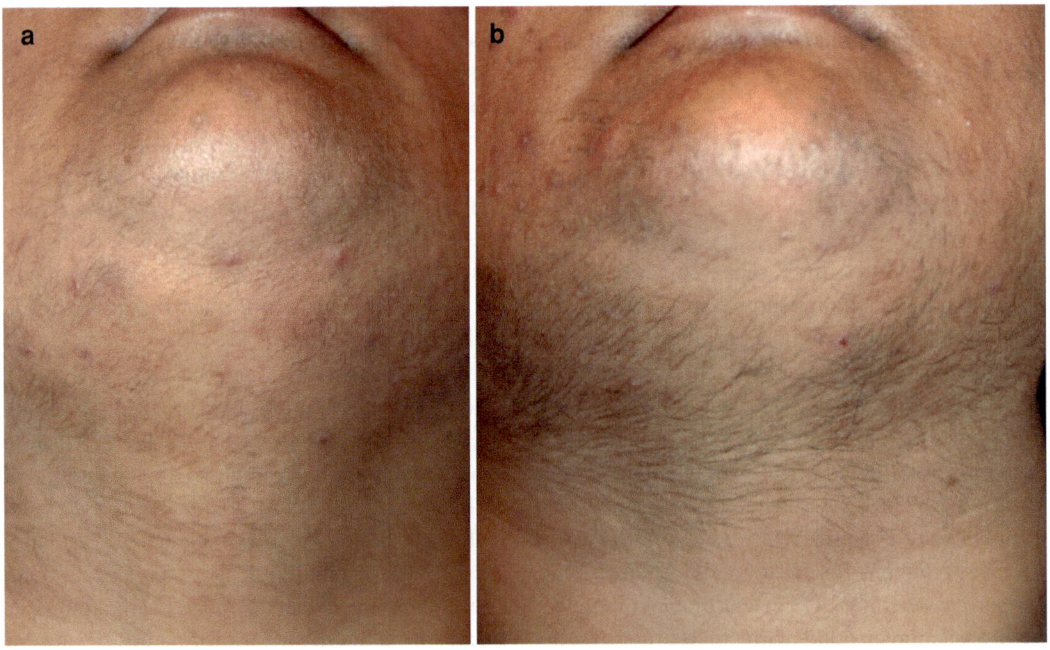

Fig. 20.2 Photographs of a 22-year-old woman (skin type IV) (**a**) before and (**b**) after two treatments with a long-pulse 755-nm alexandrite laser of the chin and beard area with the GentleLASE (Candela Corp, Wayland, MA): 18-mm spot size, energy level of 20 J/cm^2, and 3-ms pulse. Reproduced from [11]

Therefore, in order to reduce paradoxical hypertrichosis, appropriate sufficiently high fluence should be used for laser hair removal. To prevent the effect of LLLT, cold pack should be used to shrink blood vessels and prevent the activation of inflammatory cells.

Recently, several researchers have recommended that laser hair removal be continued to treat paradoxical hypertrichosis, including not only the existing laser hair removal site, but also the site where paradoxical hypertrichosis has occurred. The fluence should be increased, and a filter with a short wavelength should be used in the case of IPL, and the surrounding area should be cooled sufficiently. A method of irradiating 2 passes on the procedure site or irradiating one more pass a week after one pass has been proposed [11].

20.3.6 Prolonged Post-Laser Resurfacing Erythema

The time standard for "prolonged" in prolonged post-laser resurfacing erythema is not clear, but some laser experts have suggested 4 days for nonablative fractional procedures and 4 weeks for ablative procedures. Persistent erythema is important because it can leave sequelae such as scars and PIH. Like erythema, it occurs well in plethoric skin or rosacea. Differential diagnosis is *Candida albicnas* infection, irritant contact dermatitis (ICD), or allergic contact dermatitis (ACD).

Sunscreen and vitamin C serum is helpful for treatment, and avoiding caffeine, excessive exercise, alcohol, spicy foods, etc. is recommended to prevent erythema from getting worse. Short-term topical steroid application may help with pruritus. LEDs and vascular lasers such as IPL or PDL may also be used [3].

20.3.7 Textural Imperfection

Textural imperfection may appear by treating only a portion of the face, but even if the entire face is treated, this may still occur due to different response in a portion of the face. Usually, mild textural imperfection is treated passively (not treated). The textural imperfection caused by edema improves later, and some textural imperfections disappear naturally without special treatment. In addition, most cosmetic procedures involve multiple laser procedures, and textural imperfection caused by the initial procedure may be corrected by subsequent procedures.

If textural imperfection is not corrected after a few months, treatment is needed. Deep and noticeable depressions are corrected with fillers or fat transplantation. Fine textural imperfection is treated with a fractional laser. Sometimes subcision is performed if the depression is severe, or intralesional triamcinolone is performed if a nodule is present [4].

20.3.8 Scarring

Scars are the most serious and most fearful complication that occurs with laser procedures. Scars occur due to irreversible damage to collagen and epidermal appendage, when stem cells fail to replace damaged cells. In particular, care should be taken when using long-pulsed lasers because long-pulsed lasers can cause scarring well with irreversible collagen degeneration. For example, if the tattoo is irradiated during laser hair removal, the long-pulsed laser will heat the tattoo and damage the surrounding dermis, which can cause scarring [3].

This commonly occurs in the mandible, anterior neck, and infraorbital area. Therefore, when performing procedures in this area, the parameters should be lowered [2]. Risk factors include excessive fluence, inadequate cooling, post-procedure infection, pulse stacking or repeated irradiation, crusting and blistering not treated properly [3]. Patient factors include history of isotretinoin, keloid, and radiation therapy [2].

Scars are not just due to parameters, but also caused by a variety of causes, including the patient's individual healing ability and skin type, whether the skin is damaged before the procedure, and skin health and moisture. Therefore, since scarring cannot be predicted with certainty in advance, it is important to inform all patients undergoing ablative procedures of the risk of scarring in advance [4].

An important point in scar treatment is to prevent the occurrence of scars early on. Severe and persistent erythema, which has an initial induration or early textural imperfection, should be detected early and actively treated. For hypertrophic scars, steroid intralesional injection, silicone gel, 5-FU injection, PDL, etc. are used. Atrophic scars can be treated with ablative or nonablative fractional lasers or fillers [3].

20.3.9 Infection

Infection is important because it breaks down the epidermal barrier and increases the risk of developing scarring. Depending on the source of infection, there is bacterial infection, viral infection, and yeast infection [3].

The causative agent of bacterial infection is mainly *Staphylococcus aureus*. There is a high risk of occurrence after an ablative procedure that damages the epidermal barrier, resulting in crusting and oozing. In particular, it is thought to be caused by excessive occlusive dressing, which is performed early after the procedure. The incidence is highest within 4–8 h after the ablative procedure. Pain is an important sign in the diagnosis, and bacterial infection should be suspected if crusting or erosion and erythema occur topically and are accompanied by pain. Bacterial infections that occur after fractional lasers occur partially in deeper depths, so when there is slight erythema and edema, or if wound healing suddenly worsens, bacterial infection must be suspected. Treatment involves first bacterial culture and the use of oral antibiotics and antiseptic agents [3].

Viral infections usually appear when the herpes simplex virus (HSV) is reactivated. In particular, it occurs frequently around the mouth after a laser procedure. Crusting and blistering accompanied by pain occur, and superficial erosion with burning and tingling sensations occurs. Therefore, since differentiation from bacterial infection is very difficult, it is necessary to use antiviral drugs empirically with bacterial culture [3]. In particular, in the case of ablative procedures, antiviral drugs should be used prophylactically before and after the procedure. Recently, however, questions have been raised about the usefulness of prophylactic antiviral drugs. Trelles reported that of patients not given prophylactic antiviral drugs, less than 1% of 600 patients developed reactivation of HSV with ablative rejuvenation. Campbell and Goldman reported that in just 1.1% of the 373 people who received CO_2 fractional laser, herpes simplex developed. Despite the low incidence, the use of prophylactic antiviral drugs is still recommended because disseminated HSV infection leaves very serious scars [5].

Yeast infection is a very rare complication, the main causative agent of which is *Candida albicans*. It occurs mainly after the ablative procedure, and erythema and pruritus are the main symptoms. The timing of occurrence is unusual. It occurs mainly on the 7–14th day after the procedure. Treatment includes oral antifungal and topical antifungal agents [3].

20.3.10 Ocular Damage

Ocular damage is an uncommon complication, but in the event of ocular damage, the cause is mostly laser [4]. Caution should be exercised because ocular damage leaves the patient with irreversible sequelae such as blindness. Before the procedure, the patient should wear an opaque goggle or an eye shield that is inserted inside the eyelids. And the practitioner and everyone in the laser room should wear safety glasses.

The laser has many safeguards to prevent ocular damage. Most lasers are noncollimated and pulsed pulse. This is because first, of the 4 properties of a laser that distinguish it from light, there is collimation, but the laser outside the handpiece is usually divergent. For example, the laser beam of the CO_2 laser is focused on the tip. On the other hand, if the tip is moved away from the skin, it is defocused. Second, a laser can be a continuous pulse, but mechanically it is a pulsed pulse. This is because the laser will not fire unless the button on the foot-pedal or handpiece is pressed continuously or repeatedly.

Ocular damage can be divided into corneal, vitreous, and retinal damage. Almost all lasers can cause superficial corneal damage, but this is a very rare complication unless you shoot directly with the eyes open. Also, minor scratches that occur in cornea are not a problem because they recover quickly. Vitreous damage is also possible, and vitreous damage caused by actual PDL has been reported. Vitreous damage is a problem with the operator rather than the patient. When the procedure is performed with the safety lens incompletely covering the operator's eye, the laser can enter the operator's eye. When laser energy enters the vitreous, it damages the vitreous, causing a threadlike object floating in the visual field. Some lasers such as the 1064 nm Nd:YAG laser can cause retinal damage. Even an experienced operator or an engineer may make the mistake considering the laser turned off or in standby, resulting in retinal damage. When retinal damage occurs, visual field defects or blindness may occur, which may be permanent.

For ocular damage, prevention is of the utmost importance. Before the procedure, appropriate goggles, protective gear, and safety glasses should be worn. In particular, the laser tip should not be directed towards the eye when the power is on and looking inside the handpiece to check the condition of the lens should be avoided [4] (Table 20.3).

Table 20.3 Laser complications per treatment modality. Reproduced from [3]

Laser procedure	Complications	Management
Laser hair removal	Hyperpigmentation	Sun protection Lightening creams
	Hypopigmentation	Narrowband UVB/excimer laser/fractional lasers
	Crusting/blistering	Petrolatum-based ointments Anti-septic treatment Avoidance of "picking" of the crust
	Folliculitis	Antiseptic treatment and in some cases oral antibiotics
	Scarring	Corticosteroid injections and PDL for hypertrophic scars Fractional ablative or non-ablative treatment for atrophic scars
	Paradoxical hypertrichosis	Adequate fluences with cooling. Adequate pre- and post-treatment cooling in particular to the adjacent areas
	Acne	Topical and systemic standard acne therapy
Tattoo removal	Blistering	As above Reduce subsequent fluences with less overlap
	Hyperpigmentation	As above
	Hypopigmentation	As above
	Scarring	As above
	Darkening of cosmetic tattoos	Treatment subsequently with 1064-nm Nd:YAG and/or fractional ablative therapy
	Infections	Prompt systemic antibacterial and antiviral agents Topical antibiotics (care of contact dermatitis particularly following ablative procedures)
	Allergic reactions	Systemic antihistamines and corticosteroids
	Immediate pigment darkening following previous gold therapy treatment (Chrysiasis)	Factional ablative laser tattoo removal Difficult to treat but switch to 1064-nm Nd:YAG Fractional ablative laser pigment removal

(continued)

Table 20.3 (continued)

Laser procedure	Complications	Management
Laser treatment for vascular lesions	Bruising	Longer pulse widths and lower fluence (with PDL) Shor-term use of topical corticosteroids in intense purpura (particularly to avoid PIH in the higher skin types)
	Hyperpigmentation	As above
	Hypopigmentation	As above
	Scarring	As above
	Indentation	Filler injections or autologous fat transfer
Ablative and non-ablative procedures	Infection	As above
	Hyperpigmentation	As above
	Hypopigmentation	As above
	Scarring	As above
	Milia/acne	Switch to light-based topical treatments and standard acne therapy Milia extraction may be performed
	Prolonged erythema	Sun protection Vitamin C serum PDL/IPL
	Contact dermatitis	Limit the use of topical agents to non-irritating Avoidance of "alcohol-containing" products
	Line of demarcation	"Feathering" the edges with lower fluences and density

References

1. Carniol P, Sadick NS. Clinical procedures in laser skin rejuvenation. CRC Press; 2007.
2. Keyvan N. Lasers in dermatology and medicine. London: Springer-Verlag; 2012.
3. Al-Niaimi F. Laser and energy-based devices' complications in dermatology. J Cosmet Laser Ther. 2016;18(1):25–30.
4. Alam M, Warycha M. Complications of lasers and light treatments. Dermatol Ther. 2011;24(6):571–80.
5. Hruza GJ, Tanzi EL. Lasers and lights. Edinburgh: Elsevier; 2018.
6. Hruza GJ, Avram M. Lasers and lights: procedures in cosmetic dermatology series, 3e. London: Saunders; 2013.
7. AlNomair N, Nazarian R, Marmur E. Complications in lasers, lights, and radiofrequency devices. Facial Plast Surg. 2012;28(3):340–6.
8. Goldman MP, Weiss RA, Weiss MA. Intense pulsed light as a nonablative approach to photoaging. Dermatol Surg. 2005;31(9 Pt 2):1179–87. discussion 87.
9. Allemann IB, Goldberg DJ. Basics in dermatological laser applications. Karger Medical and Scientific Publishers; 2011.
10. Serup J, Bäumler W. Diagnosis and therapy of tattoo complications: with atlas of illustrative cases. Karger Medical and Scientific Publishers; 2017.
11. Desai S, Mahmoud BH, Bhatia AC, Hamzavi IH. Paradoxical hypertrichosis after laser therapy: a review. Dermatol Surg. 2010;36(3):291–8.
12. Lee W. Principles of IPL and its uses (Korean). Seoul: MDworld; 2008.

GPSR Compliance

The European Union's (EU) General Product Safety Regulation (GPSR) is a set of rules that requires consumer products to be safe and our obligations to ensure this.

If you have any concerns about our products, you can contact us on ProductSafety@springernature.com

In case Publisher is established outside the EU, the EU authorized representative is:

Springer Nature Customer Service Center GmbH
Europaplatz 3
69115 Heidelberg, Germany

Batch number: 10732801

Printed by Printforce, the Netherlands